TRAINING GUIDE
FOR THE DENTAL TEAM

M000106555

Coding
Companion

CDT®
2021

Includes e-book access

ADA American Dental Association®
America's leading advocate for oral health

Copyright © 2021 by the American Dental Association. All rights reserved. Except as permitted under the Copyright Act of 1976, no part of this publication may be reproduced, stored in a retrieval system, or transmitted, in any form or by any means, electronic, photocopying, recording, or otherwise, without the prior written permission of ADA, 211 East Chicago Avenue, Chicago, Illinois, 60611.

Book ISBN: 978-1-68447-066-2

E-book ISBN: 978-1-68447-067-9

ADA Product No.: J451BT

Acknowledgements

The ADA would like to acknowledge contributions made by the following individuals to this publication, in addition to the chapter authors:

Editorial Panel – Council on Dental Benefit Programs' Coding and Transactions Subcommittee
Dr. Roderick Adams; Dr. Thomas a'Becket; Dr. Rodney Hill; Dr. James Hollingsworth; Dr. Randall Markarian (ex-officio); Dr. Cynthia Olenwine; Dr. King Scott; Dr. Jessica Stilley-Mallah; and Dr. Hope Watson (ex-officio)

ADA Practice Institute – Center for Dental Benefits, Coding and Quality
Dr. Krishna Aravamudhan, Senior Director; Dennis McHugh, Manager; Frank Pokorny, MBA, FACD (hon.), Senior Manager; and Stacy Starnes, Dental Codes Advisor

ADA Department of Product Development and Sales
Kathy Pulkrabek, Manager/Editor, Professional Products and Pamela Woolf, Senior Manager, Product Development

We also want to acknowledge the permissions to reprint:

- Artwork provided by Glidewell Laboratories used in the discussion of Implant procedures, which are captioned: "Image courtesy of Glidewell Laboratories."

- Artwork provided by Zest Dental Solutions used in the discussion of Implant procedures, which are captioned: "Image courtesy of Zest Dental Solutions."

CDT 2021 Coding Companion
Table of Contents

Section 1

The CDT Code: What It Is and How To Use It

A Brief History

The CDT Code was first published in 1969 as the "Uniform Code on Dental Procedures and Nomenclature" in the *Journal of the American Dental Association*. It originally consisted of numbers and a brief name, or nomenclature. Since 1990, the CDT Code has been published in the American Dental Association's dental reference manual titled *Current Dental Terminology (CDT)*. The CDT Code version published in CDT-1 (1990) was marked by the addition of descriptors (a written narrative that provides further definition and the intended use of a dental procedure code) for most of the procedure codes.

The American Dental Association is the copyright owner and publisher of the CDT Code. New versions are published every year and become effective January 1st.

Federal regulations and legislation arising from the Health Insurance Portability and Accountability Act of 1996 (HIPAA) require all payers to accept HIPAA standard electronic dental claim. One data element on the electronic dental claim is the dental procedure code, which must be from the CDT Code – specifically the version that is in effect on the date of service.

Purpose

The CDT Code supports uniform, consistent, and accurate documentation of services delivered. This information is used in several ways:

- To provide for the efficient processing of dental claims
- To populate an electronic health record (EHR)
- To record services to be delivered in a treatment plan

Note: Treatment plans must be developed according to professional standards, not according to provisions of the dental benefit contract. Always keep in mind that the existence of a procedure code does not guarantee that the procedure is a covered service.

Categories of Service

The CDT Code is organized into twelve categories of service, each with its own series of five-digit alphanumeric codes. These categories:

- Exist solely as a means to organize the CDT Code.
- Reflect dental services that are considered similar in purpose.
- Contain CDT codes that are available to document services delivered by anyone acting within the scope of their state law (for example, a dentist in general practice uses D7140 that is found in the oral and maxillofacial surgery category to document an extraction).

#	Name	Code Range	Description in Commonly Used Terms*
I.	Diagnostic	D0100–D0999	Examinations, X-rays, pathology lab procedures
II.	Preventive	D1000–D1999	Cleanings (prophy), fluoride, sealants
III.	Restorative	D2000–D2999	Fillings, crowns and other related procedures
IV.	Endodontics	D3000–D3999	Root canals
V.	Periodontics	D4000–D4999	Surgical and non-surgical treatments of the gums and tooth supporting bone
VI.	Prosthodontics – removable	D5000–D5899	Dentures – partials and "flippers"
VII.	Maxillofacial Prosthetics	D5900–D5999	Facial, ocular and various other prostheses.
VIII.	Implant Services	D6000–D6199	Implants and implant restorations
IX.	Prosthodontics – fixed	D6200–D6999	Cemented bridges
X.	Oral & Maxillofacial Surgery	D7000–D7999	Extractions, surgical procedures, biopsies, treatment of fractures and injuries
XI.	Orthodontics	D8000–D8999	Braces
XII.	Adjunctive General Services	D9000–D9999	Miscellaneous services including anesthesia, professional visits, therapeutic drugs, bleaching, occlusal adjustment

* The language used in the "description" column has been simplified using common non-clinical terms. It is not technical terminology.

 © American Dental Association

Note: Documentation of services provided may necessitate selection of CDT Codes from different categories of service. Two illustrative scenarios follow. Section 4 "Alphabetic Index to the CDT Code" in *CDT 2021: Current Dental Terminology* will also help you locate an applicable procedure code.

Scenario Description	Procedure Delivered	Category of Service
1. Implant Case – Four-unit Fixed Partial Denture	Radiographs	Diagnostic D0100–D0999
	Implant body placement	Implant Services D6000–D6199
	Implant supported retainers	
	Pontics	Prosthodontics, fixed D6200–D6999
2. Orthodontic Case – Treatment Planning	Pre-treatment examination	Orthodontics D8000–D8999
	Radiographs	Diagnostic D0100–D0999
	Diagnostic casts	
	Case presentation	Adjunctive General Services D9000–D9999

The CDT Code: What It Is and How to Use It

Subcategories

All CDT Code categories of service are subdivided into one or more subcategories to aid navigation through the code set. For example, subcategories in the Diagnostic category of service include:

- Clinical Oral Evaluations
- Diagnostic Imaging
- Tests and Examinations

Note: CDT Code entries are *not always* in numerical order within a category of service or subcategory. As the CDT Code grows and evolves, there are times when there is no sequential number available for new entry that is related to an existing code. Such out of sequence listings are in the following Categories of Service (or subcategories therein): Diagnostic; Restorative; Periodontics; Maxillofacial Prosthetics; Implant Services; Oral & Maxillofacial Surgery; Adjunctive General Services.

Components of a CDT Code Entry

Every dental procedure code within a category of service has at least the first two and sometimes all three of the following components:

Procedure Code – A five-character alphanumeric code beginning with the letter "D" that identifies a specific dental procedure. Each procedure code is printed in **boldface** type in the CDT manual and cannot be changed or abbreviated.

> **Dental Procedure Code – five character alphanumeric beginning with "D"**
>
> **(D1351)**   **sealant – per tooth**
> Mechanically and/or chemically prepared enamel surface sealed to prevent decay.

Nomenclature – The written, literal definition of a procedure code. Each code has a nomenclature that is printed in **boldface** type in the CDT manual. Nomenclature may be abbreviated only when printed on claim forms or other documents that are subject to space limitation. Any such abbreviation does not constitute a change to the nomenclature.

> **Nomenclature (name) – written title of the procedure**
>
> **D1351**   **(sealant – per tooth)**
> Mechanically and/or chemically prepared enamel surface sealed to prevent decay.

Descriptor – A written narrative that provides further definition and describes the intended use of a dental procedure code. A descriptor is not provided for every procedure code. Descriptors that apply to a series of procedure codes may precede that series of codes; otherwise a descriptor will follow the applicable procedure code and its nomenclature. When present, descriptors are printed in regular typeface in the CDT manual. Descriptors as published cannot be added, abbreviated or otherwise changed.

D1351   sealant—per tooth
Mechanically and/or chemically prepared enamel surface sealed to prevent decay.

⬆
Descriptor – Narrative providing further definition and describes the intended use of the procedure

Descriptors are a very important component. Understanding the descriptor can help determine whether the procedure code accurately describes the service provided to a patient. This information can also help resolve questions about the accuracy of claim submissions.

Note: Your practice management software may not include entire CDT Code entries as some, due to space limitations, truncate nomenclatures and omit descriptors. With the current CDT Manual at hand you will have the complete entries for all CDT codes, which will help you select the appropriate code to document and report the service delivered.

What If There Is No Code Describing a Procedure?

The complete CDT Code entry, described above, published in *CDT 2021: Current Dental Terminology*, is used to determine the procedure code for documenting and reporting a service provided to a patient. But, what if there is no CDT code that, in the dentist's opinion, is applicable to the service? The available and appropriate option is to use an "unspecified procedure, by report" code, also known as a "999" code. These codes (e.g., **D2999 unspecified restorative procedure, by report**) are in every category of service, and when used must include a supporting narrative that explains the service provided.

A third-party payer may request additional documentation of certain procedures regardless of the presence of the narrative. Note, too, that dental benefit plan coverage limitations and exclusions, and where applicable the provisions of a participating provider agreement, affect third-party payer claim adjudication and reimbursement.

Narratives for "By Report" Codes

There are two types of CDT codes that require an explanatory narrative. The first and most readily known type are the "unspecified...procedure, by report" codes found in every category of service. Second are those codes in several categories that include "by report" in their nomenclatures – as seen in the following two examples:

D5862 precision attachment, by report
Each set of male and female components should be reported as one precision attachment. Describe the type of attachment used.

D6100 implant removal, by report
This procedure involves the surgical removal of an implant. Describe procedure.

When preparing a narrative report, first try and put yourself in the claim examiner's position. Your goal is to describe what you did and why, in a writing style and tone of an explanation to a friendly colleague. A good report is a clear and concise narrative that includes, as needed:

- Clinical condition of the oral cavity
- Description of the procedure performed
- Specific reasons why the procedure was needed, or extra time or material was needed
- How new technology enabled delivery
- Specific information required by a participating provider contract

Both the ADA Dental Claim Form and the HIPAA standard electronic dental claim transaction support transmittal of your narrative. If the "Remarks" field on the paper form does not provide enough space for you to say what you need to say, additional sheets may be included. Check with your practice management system vendor to learn how a narrative is included on your electronic claim submission.

Clarity is crucial. Do not assume that the reader will be familiar with acronyms or abbreviations you use on your patient records. Be sure to proofread the text before inclusion with the claim submission.

What do you think of this "by report" narrative?

> 1/2 carp anestetic 4% w/10.5 epinephrine administered. Explained procedure with patient's mother. Laser gingivectomy #8 and #9 and frenulectomy for max ant. Patient tolerated procedure well. Coagulation observed. Removed 2 mm of hyperplastic gingival #8 and 1.5 mm on #9 in facial and contured interseptal region. Raised max labial attendant 5 mm. Coagulation observed. POIG. Patient given rinse and cold sore meds for topical anesthisia.

It is a real-life example – shown exactly as submitted – that looks more like quickly written notes from the patient's record, with acronyms, misspellings and abbreviations that may confuse the reader. The entire claim was returned unprocessed.

Acronyms, abbreviations, and misspelled words hinder understanding. Narrative templates should be avoided, but if used the dentist remains obligated to review and approve the completed work before submission.

Now let's look at how the returned report narrative might have looked if written clearly.

> Patient age 5 presented with hyperplastic gingival tissue, and short and taut lingual frenum. Parent stated that child suffered from Aichmophobia, which could be diminished by anesthesia and use of laser in lieu of scalpel.
>
> Administered 1/2 carpule 4% Citanest Forte DENTAL with epinephrine. Used laser to: 1) remove 2 mm of hyperplastic gingival tissue from #8 and 1.5 mm on #9; 2) excise lingual frenum; and 3) cauterize wound. Coagulation was observed.
>
> Patient received post-operative instructions, oral antibiotic (amoxicillin) and oral analgesic (benzocaine) before release. Procedures delivered were: D4211 (gingivectomy or gingivoplasty); D7962 (lingual frenectomy [frenulectomy]); D9215 (local anesthesia); D9630 (drugs dispensed for home use).

This is a clear and concise report that answers the "what and why" questions the claims reviewer will be asking. It establishes clinical need and the procedure's positive outcome as expected.

CDT Code Maintenance: Additions, Revisions and Deletions

The ADA's Council on Dental Benefit Programs (CDBP) is responsible for CDT Code maintenance. In 2012, it established its Code Maintenance Committee (CMC), which convenes annually to vote on CDT Code action requests. Accepted requests are incorporated into the next version, which is effective on January 1st yearly.

Features of the maintenance process now in place are:

1. The CMC, a decision-making body comprised of 20 organizations representing diverse sectors of the dental community (such as third-party payers and dental specialties, including public health dentistry), that votes to accept, amend or decline a CDT Code action request.

2. A summary of action requests to be addressed at each CMC meeting is posted for download on *ADA.org/cdt*, including information on how to obtain a copy of the complete request form.

3. During a CMC meeting the chair encourages submitters of action requests and any other interested party to voice their comments on any requests to the committee's members.

4. During a CMC meeting the committee members discuss action requests and cast their votes.

5. The ADA Council on Dental Benefit Programs sends notices of action taken to each person or entity that submitted a CDT Code action request and posts the results on *ADA.org/cdt*.

Please visit the ADA's web page *ADA.org/cdt* for more information.

The CDT Code changes for many reasons, including technology or materials that have led to new procedures not currently in the taxonomy, or the need to improve clarity and accuracy of nomenclature and descriptors. <u>Anyone</u> may submit an action request.

For further assistance please contact the ADA Member Service Center at 312.440.2500.

Dental Procedure Codes (CDT) and Diagnosis Codes (ICD)

Dentists, through education and experience, diagnose a patient's oral health prior to treatment plan preparation and delivery of necessary dental services. However, for diagnoses, codified clinical documentation or reporting on a dental claim is not a routine activity. Change is afoot and your colleagues on the ADA Council on Dental Benefit Programs offer a look ahead to help you prepare for documenting and reporting diagnosis codes if and when required.

Both the ADA Dental Claim Form and the HIPAA standard electronic dental claim transaction are able to report up to four diagnosis codes. This capability was added to the claim forms with the expectation that ICD (International Classification of Diseases) would, at some point, become a required data element for dental claim adjudication.

Why should dentists be concerned with ICD codes when the ADA has developed SNODENT?

SNODENT is a clinical terminology designed for use with electronic health records, and it differs from ICD in three ways:

1. It is an input code set.
2. It has broader scope and specificity.
3. It may be mapped to ICD as needed on a dental claim.

Federal regulations published under the auspices of HIPAA's Administrative Simplification provisions specify only ICD codes as valid on claim submissions.

Most – but not all – diagnoses will be reported using an entry from the "Diseases of Oral Cavity" in ICD-10-CM (K00–K14 series). ICD-10-CM became the HIPAA standard on October 1, 2015. It is a code set maintained by federal government agencies and available online at *www.cms.gov/Medicare/Coding/ICD10*.

Dentists and their staff are urged to familiarize themselves with the particulars of patients' dental benefits plans claim preparation and submission requirements. In addition, pay close attention to communications from dental plans regarding additional benefits for services connected to systemic health or about dental plans' intentions to require diagnostic codes on dental claim submissions.

Note: There is no immediate and universal mandate to include an ICD-10-CM code on all dental claims. We also emphasize that dental benefit plans are unlikely to establish identical diagnostic code reporting requirements in the foreseeable future. You should check with each plan for its requirements.

Section 3 contains the appendix titled "CDT Code to ICD (Diagnosis) Code Cross-Walk," an aid to recordkeeping and claim preparation. Tables in this appendix link frequently reported CDT codes with one or more possible ICD-10-CM diagnostic codes. Please note that these tables are not all inclusive but do serve as a guide for commonly occurring conditions.

Dentists, by virtue of their clinical education, experience, and professional ethics, are the individuals responsible for diagnosis. As such, a dentist is also obligated to select the appropriate diagnosis code for patient records and claim submission. It is quite possible that other diagnoses and their associated codes may be appropriate for a given clinical scenario.

As you study these tables, please note:

1. Some address a single CDT code (e.g., preventive resin restoration), and others include a suite of related procedure codes (e.g., resin-based composite).

2. Likewise, the number of suggested ICD-10-CM diagnosis codes in a table can range from one (e.g., gingival recession for eight graft codes) to more than 10.

3. Several contain suggested diagnosis codes that are not from the "Diseases of the Oral Cavity" section ICD-10-CM; there are circumstances (e.g., vehicle accidents, workers compensation) where other sections of the ICD code set has pertinent entries.

4. Most of the frequently cited ICD codes applicable to dental procedures are found in the Kxx series (Diseases of oral cavity and salivary glands), and to a lesser degree from three other series – Rxx (symptoms, signs and abnormal clinical and laboratory findings); Sxx (injury, poisoning and certain other consequences of external causes); and Zxx (factors influencing health status and contact with health services).

5. Some ICD code terms contain words that are not commonly used in the US. These words, identified by an asterisk (*), are defined in the ADA online glossary: *ADA.org/en/publications/cdt/glossary-of-dental-clinical-and-administrative-ter*

Similar CDT to ICD tables are posted in the ADA's Center for Professional Success (CPS) website at *https://success.ADA.org/en/dental-benefits/icd-and-cdt-codes*.

These online tables may be updated more frequently than those in print as changes to ICD-10-CM occur on a schedule that differs from the CDT Code's timetable.

 © American Dental Association

Dental Procedure Codes vs. Medical Procedure Codes

The CDT Code is the source for procedure codes used when submitting claims to dental benefit plans on either the ADA Dental Claim Form or the HIPAA standard electronic dental claim transaction. There may be times when a dentist's services are submitted to a patient's medical benefit plan. When this happens, not only is there a different claim form, but there are also different procedure codes that must be used. None of these are developed or maintained by the ADA.

Filing claims with a patient's medical benefit plan can be done using the "1500" paper form or HIPAA electronic equivalent. Information on the 1500 Claim Form, including completion instructions, can be found at the American Medical Association's (AMA) National Uniform Claim Committee website *www.nucc.org*.

Medical procedure codes come from two sources, the AMA's Current Procedure Terminology (CPT) code set and the federal government's Healthcare Common Procedure Code Set (HCPCS). All medical diagnosis codes come from the federal government's International Classification of Diseases-10th Revision-Clinical Modification (ICD-10-CM) code set.

Note: When selecting a medical procedure code, the rule of thumb is to first look at the CPT code set to determine if there is an appropriate code to use. If there is none, a HCPCS code may be used.

Sources for medical procedure codes include, but are not limited to:

- American Medical Association
  https://commerce.ama-assn.org/store
  800.621.8335

- Centers for Medicare and Medicaid Services (HCPCS)
  www.cms.hhs.gov/HCPCSReleaseCodeSets

One source of dental to medical procedure cross coding information is:

- ADA Catalog
  Medical-Dental Cross Coding with Confidence by Charles Blair, D.D.S.
  ADAcatalog.org
  800.947.4746

Sources for ICD-10-CM diagnosis codes include, but are not limited to:

- National Center for Health Statistics
  https://www.cdc.gov/nchs/icd/index.htm

- PMIC Coding and Compliance
  http://icd10coding.com

Claim Rejection: Payer Misuse of the CDT Code or Something Else?

Some claims will be rejected by a third-party payer and the reason for denial helps determine what should be done next. "The existence of a dental procedure code does not mean that the procedure is a covered or reimbursed benefit," is a quote from the preface of the first (1990) and every later edition of the CDT manual. This is an important concept as available coverage is determined by dental benefit plan design. Plan limitations and exclusions vary, which means a procedure that is covered by one patient's benefit plan may not be covered by another patient's plan.

In August 2000, HIPAA (Health Insurance Portability and Accountability Act of 1996) Subtitle F (Administrative Simplification) regulations named the Code on Dental Procedures and Nomenclature (CDT Code) as the federal standard for reporting dental procedures on electronic dental claims. Some have interpreted this to mean that since the CDT Code is a national standard, payers must provide reimbursement for any valid procedure code reported on a claim. This is an erroneous interpretation as the HIPAA regulations are limited to four statements:

1. A standard electronic dental claim may only contain procedures found in the CDT Code.

2. A dentist must submit the procedure code that is valid on the date of service.

3. A payer may not refuse to accept for processing a claim with a valid procedure code.

4. A payer's benefit plan design and adjudication policies apply when processing a claim.

In other words, HIPAA establishes a standard for communicating information about services provided to a patient. HIPAA does not influence a payer's claim adjudication process (e.g., application of policies and benefit limitations and exclusions).

An explanation of benefits that shows reimbursement for fewer services or for different procedure codes than reported on the claim raises eyebrows and prompts dentists to call the ADA and ask, "How can this happen? Isn't the third-party payer doing something wrong or illegal? It looks like the CDT Code is being misused." The first step in answering these questions and concerns is to look at what guidance is in place concerning CDT Code use:

- A third-party payer is supposed to use the code number (e.g., D0120), its nomenclature and its descriptor as written.

- The ADA defines procedure code bundling as "the systematic combining of distinct dental procedures by third-party payers that results in a reduced benefit for the patient/beneficiary." Procedure code bundling is frowned upon by the ADA.

  However, dentists who have signed participating provider agreements with third-party payers may be bound to plan provisions that limit or exclude coverage for concurrent procedures.

- HIPAA requires the procedure code reported on a claim be from the CDT Code version that is effective on the date of service. Yet neither HIPAA, ADA policy nor the CDT Code itself require that a third-party payer cover every listed dental procedure.

- Covered dental procedures are identified in the contract between the plan purchaser and the third-party payer.

Many patients do not understand how dental benefit programs work and that coverage limitations and exclusions may limit reimbursement for necessary care. Such a misunderstanding is compounded when EOB language suggests that the dentist is at fault. Ensuring patients understand the limitations of their dental plan prior to treatment may help avoid problems and maintain a strong dentist-patient relationship.

Some dental claim adjudication practices are appropriate when based on plan design and should be clearly explained on the EOB to prevent misunderstandings. Other situations, where the EOB message suggests the dentist is in error, may pose problems. Each of these conditions is illustrated in the following examples:

- **Acceptable EOB explanation**: A claim for a full mouth debridement and a two-surface restoration is adjudicated, and only the D4355 is reimbursed. The EOB message states that the benefit plan has limitations and exclusions, one of which is that the plan does not cover any restorative procedure delivered on the same day as a D4355. In this example, the payer has not paid for the procedure due to benefit plan design limitations – there is no suggestion that the dentist has done anything improper.

- **Unacceptable EOB explanation**: The dentist reports a D1110 on the claim because the patient is 13 years old with predominantly adult dentition, but the EOB lists D1120 with a message that this is the correct code for a patient under the age of 15. In this example, the payer is wrong, as the message implies that the dentist reported the incorrect prophylaxis procedure code. Here the payer ignored the CDT Code's descriptor where dentition, not age, is the criterion for reporting an adult versus child prophylaxis. What the payer should do when the benefit plan specifies an age-based benefit limitation is accept the claim as submitted and note on the EOB that the claim has been adjudicated based on benefit plan design.

The second example illustrates why it is important that the dental office help the patient understand the clinical basis for treatment. In this case, the type of prophylaxis is determined by the state of the patient's dentition, not age, even though the patient's benefit may be determined by age.

Dental benefit plan limitations and exclusions affect how a claim is adjudicated and, as noted above, a payer may reject or not reimburse a claim in accordance with the benefit plan's provisions. Just as benefit plan designs vary, there is variation in participating provider contract provisions, and if you have one (or more) each must be reviewed to see how claim submission and processing may be affected. The ADA Contract Analysis Service, an ADA member benefit, can identify areas of provider contract provisions that may be of concern and be addressed before signing the contract. More information on the Contract Analysis Service is available here: *ADA.org/en/member-center/member-benefits/legal-resources/contract-analysis-service*.

Participating provider contracts are between the dentist and payer. These contracts may include provisions that require you to accept least expensive alternative treatment (LEAT) reimbursement, or agree to reimbursement based on payer guidelines instead of specific procedure codes reported on a claim. A dentist who signs a participating provider contract is generally bound to its legally sound provisions. Likewise, the payer is also bound to the contract provisions and cannot obligate you to do something that is beyond the signed agreement.

It is appropriate to appeal the benefit decision if you think the claim has not been properly adjudicated. When appealing a claim, it is important to follow the specific instructions provided by the particular carrier including the submittal of the appeal in writing within the time allowed by the carrier. It is important to send it to the specified department of the carrier and it must be in the required format. The word "appeal" should prominently appear in the title and text of the document, as well as in any cover letter that accompanies the appeal document.

Remember, the dentist consultant representing the carrier may only be looking at a dental claim form and you will want to provide the consultant as much information as possible so that he or she will agree with your treatment plan and approve the appropriate benefits for your patient.

A proper appeal involves sending the carrier a written request to reconsider the claim. Additional documentation should be included to give the carrier a clearer picture of why you recommended the treatment. For example, the following claim attachments may assist in getting consideration for core buildup claims – radiographic evidence of the need for a buildup, and a narrative description providing as much explanatory information as possible (even if this appears obvious to you). If you have further questions, it is best to give that carrier a call.

Remember, you are trying to have the dentist consultant understand the rationale for your recommended treatment plan so that your patient can receive the appropriate benefit from his or her plan.

It may help to ask the dentist consultant to call you if the claim is going to be denied. This way you can discuss the case with the dentist consultant on a professional level. You may want to leave a time and date when you will be available so that the consultant does not call while you are seeing patients.

Payers using the CDT Code must be licensed to do so – and abide by the copyright license. Any payer actions that do not adhere to contractual obligations may represent misuse, and be reason to seek redress. The copyright license does not dictate how a procedure code is to be reimbursed and cannot be used as a tool to force payers to use the CDT Code in a particular manner.

However, arbitrary payer action is an ongoing ADA concern and we ask that dentists report such actions so that staff can address recurring issues with the third-party payer involved. Also, it is appropriate to appeal the benefit decision if you think the claim has not been properly adjudicated, and ADA staff is prepared to assist in your understanding of the appeal process.

Even if an objectionable use of the CDT Code is not a license violation or illegal, ADA staff remains available to contact third-party payers, attempting to discuss the issues and to resolve potential conflicts. Dentist reports of concerns enable ADA staff to address individual issues with payers, as well as providing the means to determine, monitor and address patterns of payer actions.

Note: The ADA Member Service Center (MSC) is your first point of contact when you have questions about the CDT Code and its use, or to report possible third-party payer "misuse." Contact the MSC at 312.440.2500.

If you wish to simply alert the ADA to a concern, you can complete the downloadable form on *ADA.org* titled, "third-party payer complaint form," which gives dental offices the opportunity to provide information on the problems experienced with third-party payers.

This form was developed by the ADA Center for Dental Benefits, Coding and Quality to track industry trends and facilitate discussions with dental benefit plans and benefits administrators. The form is available online at: *https://success.ada.org/en/dental-benefits/online-third-party-form*.

The "Golden Rules" of Procedure Coding

Correct coding, part and parcel of the following rules, demonstrates a dentist's adherence to the ADA's Principles of Ethics and Code of Professional Conduct, particularly "5.A. Representation of Care" that states "Dentists shall not represent the care being rendered to their patients in a false or misleading manner."

- "Code for what you do" is the fundamental rule to apply in all coding situations.
- After reading the full nomenclature and descriptor, select the code that matches the procedure delivered to the patient.
- If there is no applicable code, document the service using an unspecified, by report ("999") code, and include a clear and appropriate narrative.
- The existence of a procedure code does not mean that the procedure is a covered or reimbursed benefit in a dental benefit plan.
- Treatment planning is based on clinical need, not covered services.

If you have difficulty finding an appropriate CDT code consider whether there may be another way to describe the procedure. The CDT Manual's alphabetic index, and the glossary of dental terms posted on *ADA.org* are likely to be helpful in these situations.

CDT Code Changes in 2021

The number and nature of annual CDT Code changes vary, as does their relevance to an individual dentist – primarily based on her or his type of practice. CDT 2021 incorporates a variety of CDT Code entry actions – 28 additions, seven revisions, four deletions, and 22 editorial – summarized in the following table.

Code	Change		Code	Change
I. Diagnostic			D5286	Editorial
D0120	Editorial		D5730	Editorial
D0150	Editorial		D5731	Editorial
D0604	Addition		D5740	Editorial
D0605	Addition		D5741	Editorial
D0701	Addition		D5750	Editorial
D0702	Addition		D5751	Editorial
D0703	Addition		D5760	Editorial
D0704	Addition		D5761	Editorial
D0705	Addition		D5820	Editorial
D0706	Addition		D5821	Editorial
D0707	Addition		**VII. Maxillofacial Prosthetics**	
D0708	Addition		D5994	Deletion
D0709	Addition		D5995	Addition
II. Preventive			D5996	Addition
D1110	Revision		**VIII. Implant Services**	
D1120	Revision		D6011	Revision
D1321	Addition		D6052	Deletion
D1355	Addition		D6091	Revision
D1557	Revision		D6098	Editorial
D1558	Revision		D6191	Addition
III. Restorative			D6192	Addition
D2928	Addition		**IX. Prosthodontics, fixed**	
D2960	Editorial		None	
D2961	Editorial		**X. Oral & Maxillofacial Surgery**	
D2962	Editorial		D7960	Deletion
IV. Endodontics			D7961	Addition
D3427	Deletion		D7962	Addition
D3471	Addition		D7993	Addition
D3472	Addition		D7994	Addition
D3473	Addition		**XI. Orthodontics**	
D3501	Addition		None	
D3502	Addition		**XI. Adjunctive General Services**	
D3503	Addition		D9971	Revision
V. Periodontics				
None				
VI. Prosthodontics (removable)				
D5225	Editorial			
D5226	Editorial			
D5282	Editorial			
D5283	Editorial			
D5284	Editorial			

Some of the CDT 2021 changes listed in this table are stand-alone and others – additions with associated revisions or deletions – are interrelated. These changes will be addressed in detail within the following chapters.

Substantive Changes: What and Why

D0100–D0999 Diagnostic

Tests and Examinations

D0604 **antigen testing for a public health related pathogen, including coronavirus**

D0605 **antibody testing for a public health related pathogen, including coronavirus**

Rationale for these additions (Ref: action request form; CMC discussion).

The need to identify patients who may be infected with SARS-CoV-2 (a.k.a., COVID-19) is important for the health of the patient as well as the dentist and other practice staff. Testing information is of value for epidemiological studies. The CPT and HCPCS medical procedure code sets, and the ICD-10-CM diagnosis code set, have been updated to enable reporting of testing procedures and diagnosis of COVID-19.

Image Capture Only

D0701 **panoramic radiographic image – image capture only**

D0702 **2-D cephalometric radiographic image – image capture only**

D0703 **2-D oral/facial photographic image obtained intra-orally or extra-orally – image capture only**

D0704 **3-D photographic image – image capture only**

D0705 **extra-oral posterior dental radiographic image – image capture only**
Image limited to exposure of complete posterior teeth in both dental arches. This is a unique image that is not derived from another image.

D0706 **intraoral – occlusal radiographic image – image capture only**

D0707 **intraoral – periapical radiographic image – image capture only**

D0708 **intraoral – bitewing radiographic image – image capture only**
Image axis may be horizontal or vertical.

D0709 **intraoral – complete series of radiographic images – image capture only**
A radiographic survey of the whole mouth, usually consisting of 14–22 images (periapical and posterior bitewing as indicated) intended to display the crowns and roots of all teeth, periapical areas and alveolar bone.

Rationale for these additions (Ref: action request form; CMC discussion):

The need for additional codes to document image capture only procedures was identified during the March 2019 CMC meeting discussion of such procedures. Image capture only procedures have the greatest applicability in teledentistry encounters where a locally licensed practitioner captures image(s) that are forwarded to a dentist for interpretation.

The image interpretation procedure is reported separately with CDT code **D0391 interpretation of diagnostic image by a practitioner not associated by capture of the image, including report**.

D1000–D1999 Preventive

Other Preventive Services

D1321 **counseling for the control and prevention of adverse oral, behavioral, and systemic health effects associated with high-risk substance use**
Counseling services may include patient education about adverse oral, behavioral, and systemic effects associated with high-risk substance use and administration routes. This includes ingesting, injecting, inhaling and vaping. Substances used in a high-risk manner may include but are not limited to alcohol, opioids, nicotine, cannabis, methamphetamine and other pharmaceuticals or chemicals.

Rationale for this addition (Ref: action request form; CMC discussion):

The CDT Code includes D1320 for tobacco counseling and D1310 for nutritional counseling. There currently is no code for counseling for high-risk substance use that may lead to adverse health effects.

Federal entities (e.g., CDC; U.S. Surgeon General) have issued warnings to the general public against use of all vaping devices, citing the risk of acute severe lung disease and the associated dangers of the "epidemic of teen vaping." Heavy alcohol use is a well-known risk factor for oral-pharyngeal cancer. Opioid use and abuse continues in the U.S.

Research reports show that more than 50% of people who have taken opioids for pain management received their first prescription from a dentist. The FDA, CDC and other organizations have called upon healthcare professionals to educate themselves and their patients on the dangers of high-risk substance use.

D1355 **caries preventive medicament application – per tooth**
For primary prevention or remineralization. Medicaments applied do not include topical fluorides.

Rationale for this addition (Ref: action request form; CMC discussion):

There is a gap in the current code. D1354 covers the application of medicaments for secondary (2°) prevention; that is, interim arrest of caries. But these same materials, particularly silver diamine fluoride, silver nitrate, and chlorhexidine, are used to prevent caries lesions on high-risk tooth surfaces, such as exposed root surfaces in older adults, deep fissures in permanent or primary teeth or around molar bands in fixed orthodontic treatment.

The procedure as described may not be documented with D1354 as there are no carious lesions, nor are D1206 or D1208 applicable as they are full-mouth procedures.

Space Maintenance

D1557   removal of fixed t space maintainer – maxillary
~~Procedure performed by dentist or practice that did not originally place the appliance.~~

D1558   removal of fixed bilateral space maintainer – mandibular
~~Procedure performed by dentist or practice that did not originally place the appliance.~~

Rationale for these revisions (Ref: action request form; CMC discussion):

The full CDT Code entries for D1557 and D1558 include a descriptor that limits who may report these procedures. These descriptors do not contain any information that clarifies the clinical aspects of these procedures. As written they create a CDT Code gap – these codes may only be used when the removal procedure is by a dentist or practice not involved in the original placement.

Without the requested revisions the only coding option for removal by the dentist or practice who placed the appliance is a "999" unspecified procedure by report code. A "999" code requires additional documentation to report the procedure delivered.

The requested deletion of the descriptors expands the utility of these codes for documentation and reporting purposes. There is no effect on the clinical aspects of the procedure's delivery.

There are many other changes in CDT 2021 as seen in the following list and they will be discussed further in their applicable *CDT 2021 Companion* category chapter.

Note: Some minor changes are highlighted for ready recognition.

Category	Change
	Clinical Oral Evaluations

D0120 **periodic oral evaluation – established patient**
An evaluation performed on a patient of record to determine any changes in the patient's dental and medical health status since a previous comprehensive or periodic evaluation. This includes an oral cancer evaluation ~~and~~, periodontal screening where indicated, and may require interpretation of information acquired through additional diagnostic procedures. Report additional diagnostic procedures separately.

D0150 **comprehensive oral evaluation – new or established patient**
Used by a general dentist and/or a specialist when evaluating a patient comprehensively. This applies to new patients; established patients who have had a significant change in health conditions or other unusual circumstances, by report, or established patients who have been absent from active treatment for three or more years. It is a thorough evaluation and recording of the extraoral and intraoral hard and soft tissues. It may require interpretation of information acquired through additional diagnostic procedures. Additional diagnostic procedures should be reported separately.

This includes an evaluation for oral cancer ~~where indicated~~, the evaluation and recording of the patient's dental and medical history and a general health assessment. It may include the evaluation and recording of dental caries, missing or unerupted teeth, restorations, existing prostheses, occlusal relationships, periodontal conditions (including periodontal screening and/or charting), hard and soft tissue anomalies, etc.

Diagnostic

Category	Change
Preventive	**D1110** **prophylaxis – adult** Removal of plaque, calculus and stains from tooth structures <u>and implants</u> in the permanent and transitional dentition. It is intended to control local irritational factors. **D1120** **prophylaxis – child** Removal of plaque, calculus and stains from tooth structures <u>and implants</u> in the primary and transitional dentition. It is intended to control local irritational factors.
Restorative	**D2928** **prefabricated porcelain/ceramic crown – permanent tooth** **D2960** **labial veneer (resin laminate) – ~~chairside~~ <u>direct</u>** Refers to labial/facial direct resin bonded veneers. **D2961** **labial veneer (resin laminate) – ~~laboratory~~ <u>indirect</u>** Refers to labial/facial indirect resin bonded veneers. **D2962** **labial veneer (porcelain laminate) – ~~laboratory~~ <u>indirect</u>** Refers also to facial veneers that extend interproximally and/or cover the incisal edge. Porcelain/ceramic veneers presently include all ceramic and porcelain veneers.
Endodontics	**~~D3427~~** **~~periradicular surgery without apicoectomy~~** **D3471** **surgical repair of root resorption - anterior** For surgery on root of anterior tooth. Does not include placement of restoration. **D3472** **surgical repair of root resorption – premolar** For surgery on root of premolar tooth. Does not include placement of restoration. **D3473** **surgical repair of root resorption – molar** For surgery on root of molar tooth. Does not include placement of restoration.

Category	Change
Endodontics	**D3501** **surgical exposure of root surface without apicoectomy or repair of root resorption – anterior** Exposure of root surface followed by observation and surgical closure of the exposed area. Not to be used for or in conjunction with apicoectomy or repair of root resorption.
	D3502 **surgical exposure of root surface without apicoectomy or repair of root resorption – premolar** Exposure of root surface followed by observation and surgical closure of the exposed area. Not to be used for or in conjunction with apicoectomy or repair of root resorption.
	D3503 **surgical exposure of root surface without apicoectomy or repair of root resorption – molar** Exposure of root surface followed by observation and surgical closure of the exposed area. Not to be used for or in conjunction with apicoectomy or repair of root resorption.
Prosthodontics, removable	**Partial Dentures (Including Routine Post-Delivery Care)**
	D5225 **maxillary partial denture - flexible base (including** ~~any clasps,~~ **retentive/clasping materials,** **rests, and teeth)**
	D5226 **mandibular partial denture – flexible base (including** ~~any clasps,~~ **retentive/clasping materials,** **rests, and teeth)**
	D5282 **removable unilateral partial denture – one piece cast metal (including** ~~clasps~~ **retentive/clasping materials,** **rests,** **and teeth), maxillary**
	D5283 **removable unilateral partial denture – one piece cast metal (including** ~~clasps~~ **retentive/clasping materials,** **rests,** **and teeth), mandibular**
	D5284 **removable unilateral partial denture – one piece flexible base (including** ~~clasps~~ **retentive/clasping** **materials, rests,** **and teeth) – per quadrant**
	D5286 **removable unilateral partial denture – one piece resin (including** ~~clasps~~ **retentive/clasping materials, rests,** **and teeth) – per quadrant**

Category	Change
	Denture Reline Procedures
	D5730 **reline complete maxillary denture (~~chairside~~ <u>direct</u>)**
	D5731 **reline complete mandibular denture (~~chairside~~ <u>direct</u>)**
	D5740 **reline maxillary partial denture (~~chairside~~ <u>direct</u>)**
	D5741 **reline mandibular partial denture (~~chairside~~ <u>direct</u>)**
	D5750 **reline complete maxillary denture (~~laboratory~~ <u>indirect</u>)**
	D5751 **reline complete mandibular denture (~~laboratory~~ <u>indirect</u>)**
Prosthodontics, removable	**D5760** **reline maxillary partial denture (~~laboratory~~ <u>indirect</u>)**
	D5761 **reline mandibular partial denture (~~laboratory~~ <u>indirect</u>)**
	Interim Prosthesis
	D5820 **interim partial denture ~~(maxillary)~~ <u>(including retentive/clasping materials, rests, and teeth), maxillary</u>** ~~Includes any necessary clasps and rests.~~
	D5821 **interim partial denture ~~(mandibular)~~ <u>(including retentive/clasping materials, rests, and teeth), mandibular</u>** ~~Includes any necessary clasps and rests.~~
	Carriers
Maxillofacial Prosthetics	~~**D5994**~~ ~~**periodontal medicament carrier with peripheral seal-laboratory processed**~~ ~~A custom fabricated, laboratory processed carrier that covers the teeth and alveolar mucosa. Used as a vehicle to deliver prescribed medicaments for sustained contact with the gingiva, alveolar mucosa, and into the periodontal sulcus or pocket.~~

Category	Change
Maxillofacial Prosthetics	**D5995 periodontal medicament carrier with peripheral seal – laboratory processed – maxillary** A custom fabricated, laboratory processed carrier for the maxillary arch that covers the teeth and alveolar mucosa. Used as a vehicle to deliver prescribed medicaments for sustained contact with the gingiva, alveolar mucosa, and into the periodontal sulcus or pocket. **D5996 periodontal medicament carrier with peripheral seal – laboratory processed – mandibular** A custom fabricated, laboratory processed carrier for the mandibular arch that covers the teeth and alveolar mucosa. Used as a vehicle to deliver prescribed medicaments for sustained contact with the gingiva, alveolar mucosa, and into the periodontal sulcus or pocket.

Surgical Services

D6011 <u>surgical access to an implant body (**second stage implant surgery**)</u>
~~Surgical access to an implant body for placement of a healing cap or to enable placement of an abutment.~~
<u>This procedure, also known as second stage implant surgery, involves removal of tissue that covers the implant body so that a fixture of any type can be placed, or an existing fixture be replaced with another. Examples of fixtures include but are not limited to healing caps, abutments shaped to help contour the gingival margins or the final restorative prosthesis.</u>

Supporting Structures

Implant Services

~~**D6052 semi-precision attachment abutment**~~
~~Includes placement of keeper assembly.~~

D6191 semi-precision abutment – placement
This procedure is the initial placement, or replacement, of a semi-precision abutment on the implant body.

D6192 semi-precision attachment – placement
This procedure involves the luting of the initial, or replacement, semi-precision attachment to the removable prosthesis.

Category	Change
	Other Implant Services
Implant Services	**D6091** replacement of <u>replaceable part of</u> **semi-precision or precision attachment (male or female component) of implant/abutment supported prosthesis, per attachment** ~~This procedure applies to the replaceable male or female component of the attachment.~~
	Other Repair Procedures
Oral & Maxillofacial Surgery	~~D7960~~ ~~frenulectomy – also known as frenectomy or frenotomy – separate procedure not incidental to another procedure~~ ~~Removal or release of mucosal and muscle elements of a buccal, labial or lingual frenum that is associated with a pathological condition, or interferes with proper oral development or treatment.~~
	D7961 **buccal / labial frenectomy (frenulectomy)**
	D7962 **lingual frenectomy (frenulectomy)**
	D7993 **surgical placement of craniofacial implant – extra oral** Surgical placement of a craniofacial implant to aid in retention of an auricular, nasal, or orbital prosthesis.
	D7994 **surgical placement: zygomatic implant** An implant placed in the zygomatic bone and exiting though the maxillary mucosal tissue providing support and attachment of a maxillary dental prosthesis.
	Miscellaneous Services
Adjunctive General Services	**D9971** **odontoplasty** ~~1-2 teeth; includes removal of enamel projections~~ **<u>– per tooth</u>** <u>Removal/reshaping of enamel surfaces or projections.</u>

 © American Dental Association

Section 2

Using the CDT Code: Definitions and Key Concepts, Coding Scenarios and Coding Q&A

Introduction

Individual chapters in this section, including one for each of the CDT Code's 12 categories of service, contain definitions of key terms, information on notable changes, clinical scenarios, and Q&A based on real-life situations. Answers to these questions and scenarios illustrate coding solutions for the situations described. These scenarios and solutions reflect common and accepted practices, but may not reflect the way your office would manage a given situation. The dentist who treats a patient is the person who can best determine appropriate treatment and the CDT codes that best describe it.

The scenarios and Q&A are the product of questions received from ADA members and developed by ADA staff, as well as based on the contributions of chapter authors. They are not to be considered legal advice or a guarantee that individual payer contracts will follow this assistance.

Use this information to get a better understanding of the principles of reporting using the CDT Code. Since it covers subjects from many different perspectives, it is likely that some will be more applicable to your particular situation than others. All the scenarios and Q&A, including those that involve procedures you may not usually report, are of value since the principles demonstrated can often be applied to areas of your practice.

Chapter 1: D0100–D0999 Diagnostic

By Ralph A. Cooley, D.D.S.

Introduction

Dentists and other dental health care providers dedicate years of their lives learning how to provide excellent oral health care to their patients. But just providing this quality of care is not enough. In today's world, one must have a complete and accurate record of the care that is delivered. That is why the *Code on Dental Procedures and Nomenclature* (CDT Code) was established. In CDT 2021, there are many changes in the Diagnostic Category of Service that involve diagnostic image capture, pathogen testing, and oral evaluations. In this chapter we will discuss key concepts and code changes, some common coding scenarios, and frequently asked questions about coding for diagnostic procedures.

Key Definitions and Concepts

Evaluation: The systematic determination or judgment about a condition, disease, or treatment.

Clinical oral evaluations: As with all ADA procedure codes, there is no distinction made between the evaluations provided by general practitioners and specialists. Report additional diagnostic and/or definitive procedures separately.

Imaging: Creating a visual representation of the interior of a body revealing inner structures that may have been blocked by skin or bone.

Intraoral image: A visual representation of the mouth derived by placing a film, plate, or sensor within the mouth.

Extraoral image: A visual representation of the mouth derived by placing a film, plate, or sensor outside the mouth.

Changes to This Category

There are thirteen changes to the codes in the Diagnostic Section in CDT 2021. Eleven of the changes are additions, and there are two editorial changes to commonly used diagnostic codes for oral evaluations. The following nine new codes relate to image capture:

D0701   **panoramic radiographic image – image capture only**

D0702   **2-D cephalometric radiographic image – image capture only**

D0703   **2-D oral/facial photographic image obtained intra-orally or extra-orally – image capture only**

D0704   **3-D photographic image – image capture only**

D0705   **extra-oral posterior dental radiographic image – image capture only**
Image limited to exposure of complete posterior teeth in both dental arches. This is a unique image that is not derived from another image.

D0706   **intraoral – occlusal radiographic image – image capture only**

D0707   **intraoral – periapical radiographic image – image capture only**

D0708   **intraoral – bitewing radiographic image – image capture only**
Image axis may be horizontal or vertical.

D0709   **intraoral – complete series of radiographic images – image capture only**
A radiographic survey of the whole mouth, usually consisting of 14–22 images (periapical and posterior bitewing as indicated) intended to display the crowns and roots of all teeth, periapical areas and alveolar bone.

These additions join the current suite of "image capture only codes" (D0380 – D0386). Image capture only procedures, especially the nine CDT 2021 additions, have the greatest applicability in teledentistry encounters where a locally licensed practitioner captures image(s) that are forwarded to a dentist for interpretation. The image interpretation procedure is reported separately with CDT code **D0391 interpretation of diagnostic image by a practitioner not associated with capture of the image, including report**.

These nine additions do not take the place of the current diagnostic imaging codes for full mouth series or periapicals or bitewings, etc. (e.g., D0210; D0220; D0270) when image capture with interpretation are delivered in the same setting.

In light of 2020's COVID-19 pandemic, two other new codes were added. They are:

D0604 **antigen testing for a public health related pathogen including coronavirus**

D0605 **antibody testing for a public health related pathogen including coronavirus**

These codes allow for testing of patients, both for antigens (indicating whether the patient is currently positive for the virus) or for antibodies (indicating that the patient has had the virus in the past and has recovered).

Two existing codes have editorial changes. They are:

D0120 **periodic oral evaluation – established patient**
An evaluation performed on a patient of record to determine any changes in the patient's dental and medical health status since a previous comprehensive or periodic evaluation. This includes an oral cancer evaluation ~~and~~, periodontal screening where indicated, and may require interpretation of information acquired through additional diagnostic procedures. Report additional diagnostic procedures separately.

D0150 **comprehensive oral evaluation – new or established patient**
Used by a general dentist and/or a specialist when evaluating a patient comprehensively. This applies to new patients; established patients who have had a significant change in health conditions or other unusual circumstances, by report, or established patients who have been absent from active treatment for three or more years. It is a thorough evaluation and recording of the extraoral and intraoral hard and soft tissues. It may require interpretation of information acquired through additional diagnostic procedures. Additional diagnostic procedures should be reported separately.

This includes an evaluation for oral cancer ~~where indicated~~, the evaluation and recording of the patient's dental and medical history and a general health assessment. It may include the evaluation and recording of dental caries, missing or unerupted teeth, restorations, existing prostheses, occlusal relationships, periodontal conditions (including periodontal screening and/or charting), hard and soft tissue anomalies, etc.

These oral evaluation codes were changed to make it clear that an oral cancer evaluation is always a part of these two oral evaluations, regardless of the timeline.

Clinical Coding Scenario #1:
Patient Age 11 – Evaluation, Preventive, and Orthodontic Services

A new patient, age 11, was seen for a first exam, cleaning, and fluoride varnish application. During the exam, the dentist noted that the erupting tooth #4 was impinging on the fixed space maintainer that spanned both the right and left side of the mouth. This space maintainer had been placed by another dentist but it was decided that the space maintainer needed to be removed now.

How might this visit be coded?

> **D0150** **comprehensive oral evaluation – new or established patient**
>
> **D1120** **prophylaxis – child**
>
> **D1206** **topical application of fluoride varnish**
>
> **D1557** **removal of fixed bilateral space maintainer – maxillary**

Note: If in this scenario, if the topical fluoride was a rinse or other appropriate in-office fluoride application other than a varnish, D1206 would not be correct. The appropriate CDT code would be:

> **D1208** **topical application of fluoride – excluding varnish**

But what if the same patient was not new and the doctor had placed the space maintainer two years ago? How would this encounter be coded?

> **D0120** **periodic oral evaluation**
>
> **D1120** **prophylaxis – child**
>
> **D1206** **topical application of fluoride varnish**
>
> **D1557** **removal of fixed bilateral space maintainer – maxillary**

The exam, in this case, would be periodic (D0120) because the patient was seen previously, but the prophylaxis and fluoride codes remain the same as would the code to remove the space maintainer. Codes D1557 and D1558 have both been modified to cover removal of a fixed bilateral space maintainer, regardless of who places it. D1557 is used for the maxillary arch and D1558 is used for the mandibular arch. In this case, D1557 is the appropriate code.

Clinical Coding Scenario #2:
Patient Seen After Office Hours with a Dental Accident

Andrew was hit in the mouth with a ball while playing catch with the coach. Fortunately, the team coach was also a dentist, so Andrew was seen in the office that night. The dentist did an oral evaluation and noticed that the patient had normal open and closing, no soft tissue injuries required any sutures, slight mobility of #8 and #9, and minimal bleeding of the lip. Two intra-oral periapical radiographs were taken to rule out root fractures with the maxillary anterior teeth. The dentist advised Andrew and his parents to return in two weeks for follow-up if there were no complications or discomfort.

How would the dentist code for this visit?

D0140 limited oral evaluation-problem focused

An evaluation limited to a specific oral health problem or complaint. This may require interpretation of information acquired through additional diagnostic procedures. Report additional diagnostic procedures separately. Definitive procedures may be required on the same date as the evaluation.

Typically patients receiving this type of evaluation present with a specific problem and/or dental emergencies, trauma, acute infections, etc.

D0220 intraoral-periapical first radiographic image

D0230 intraoral-periapical each additional radiographic image

Andrew was seen for a follow-up visit two weeks later and reported no problems. The dentist pulp tested teeth #7, #8, #9, and #10 and all tested normally. Andrew was advised to be seen in three months for his regularly scheduled dental visit, and that this area would be re-evaluated at that time.

What CDT codes were utilized for this visit?

D0170 re-evaluation – limited, problem focused (established patient; not post-operative visit)

Assessing the status of a previously existing condition. For example:
- a traumatic injury where no treatment was rendered but patient needs follow-up monitoring
- evaluation for undiagnosed continuing pain
- soft tissue lesions requiring follow-up evaluation

D0460 pulp vitality tests

Includes multiple teeth and contra lateral comparison(s), as indicated.

Clinical Coding Scenario #3:
New Patient with Diagnostic Gathering Challenges and Tobacco Use

A 21-year-old new patient is seen for a first exam. It is noted that he has numerous decayed anterior and posterior teeth but when an attempt to take a full mouth intraoral series of radiographs, the patient has a severe gag response. Only a panoramic image and two extra oral bitewings are able to be taken.

He is also a heavy chewing tobacco user so a tissue fluorescence oral cancer exam is performed and about 15 minutes is spent discussing his tobacco use, what it is doing to his mouth, and his options to try to quit.

How would this visit be coded?

D0150   comprehensive oral evaluation – new or established patient

D0330   panoramic radiographic image

D0251   extra-oral posterior radiographic image

Choosing the panoramic (D0330) and extra-oral bitewing (D0251) radiographs allowed you to get a preliminary understanding of his oral conditions. Note: this is not a "full mouth series" because these are not intraoral radiographic images. The dentist may consider utilizing some alternative methods to aid in capturing some intraoral images later.

Codes for the tissue fluorescence oral cancer exam and counseling the patient for his tobacco use are:

D0431   adjunctive pre-diagnostic test that aids in detection of mucosal abnormalities including premalignant and malignant lesions, not to include cytology or biopsy procedures

Note: Examples of adjunctive pre-diagnostic tests that aid in detection of mucosal abnormalities may include VELscope, OrallD, MicorLux DL, or VizLite Plus. This test is done in addition to your normal visual and palpation exam that is part of a comprehensive evaluation.

D1320   tobacco counseling for the control and prevention of oral disease

Clinical Coding Scenario #4:
Child Under Three – Evaluation and Parent Counseling, and Preventive Services

Note: The American Academy of Pediatric Dentistry (AAPD) and the ADA both advise that children should have their first dental visit within six months of the eruption of the first primary tooth.

The doctor performed an intraoral examination on a one-year-old patient while the mother restrained the child's forehead in her lap. The dentist determined that the child had maxillary and mandibular primary incisors and that they were caries free. The dentist also removed plaque using an ultra-soft toothbrush and applied fluoride varnish. The doctor explained to the parent how to use a washcloth or soft brush to remove plaque each day and the importance of getting the child to go to sleep without a bottle. They discussed foods that can "lead to decay" (caries) and recommended that she return in a year for an exam after most of the primary teeth have erupted.

Here is what occurred during the child's first dental visit:
- Oral examination
- Toothbrush deplaquing
- Fluoride varnish
- Discussion of diet and preventive care with the parent

How would you code this first visit?

D0145   **oral evaluation for a patient under three years of age and counseling with primary caregiver**

D1120   **prophylaxis – child**

D1206   **topical application of fluoride varnish**

Note: The evaluation and counseling code (D0145):
- has both diagnostic and preventive characteristics
- is specifically for children under three years of age
- includes an evaluation of oral conditions, history, and caries susceptibility
- includes development of an oral hygiene regimen
- always includes counseling the primary caregiver or parent

What evaluation code could be used on the next visit?

Either the same evaluation and counseling code (D0145) or the periodic evaluation code (D0120) could be used for the next visit. There is nothing in the D0145 nomenclature or descriptor that precludes its use for more than one visit, as long as the patient is still under three years of age and all the components of the procedure are completed. The periodic exam might be appropriate as the primary dentition develops and if the other criteria are not met. The prophylaxis and fluoride would remain the same.

Clinical Coding Scenario #5:
Radiographs – What Constitutes a Full Mouth Series?

The descriptor for procedure code D0210 defines a complete series of radiographic images, as seen in *CDT 2021: Current Dental Terminology's* entry:

D0210 intraoral – complete series of radiographic images
A radiographic survey of the whole mouth, usually consisting of 14–22 periapical and posterior bitewing images intended to display the crowns and roots of all teeth, periapical areas and alveolar bone.

Note: The descriptor was drawn from The Selection of Patients for X-Ray Examinations: Dental Radiographic Examinations published by the FDA in 2004.

With this in mind, consider how radiographs for patients A, B, C, and D are documented.

Patient A

The office takes periapical x-rays: three upper anterior, three lower anterior and one posterior in each quadrant.

Since the radiographs display the crowns and roots of all teeth, periapical areas and alveolar bone crest, the full mouth series procedure code D0210 would not be appropriate.

The correct procedure codes are:

D0220 intraoral – periapical first radiographic image

(Report D0220 one time.)

D0230 intraoral – periapical each additional radiographic image

(Report D0230 nine times.)

Patient B

The office takes a panoramic x-ray and four posterior bitewings.

D0330 panoramic radiographic image

D0274 bitewings – four radiographic images

Since a panoramic radiographic image is not intraoral, this combination could not correctly be reported as a full mouth series (D0210).

Note: The ADA Council on Dental Benefit Programs receives many calls stating that claims for D0330 and D0274 are downcoded by third-party payers to

D0210 for purposes of reimbursement. This term *downcoding* is defined in the Glossary published on *ADA.org* as:

> **downcoding**: A third-party payer claim adjudication process that uses a procedure code that is different from the one reported on the claim so that the reimbursement amount is less than would be allowed for the submitted code.

The ADA frowns upon such downcoding. The dentist should continue to document and report the procedure as described above instead of coding towards any third-party payers policies.

Patient C

The office takes four periapicals of the upper edentulous ridge, seven periapicals of the lower arch and four posterior bitewings. This situation, while not the most common scenario, does meet all the criteria for and is correctly coded as a full mouth series.

D0210 intraoral – complete series of radiographic images
A radiographic survey of the whole mouth, usually consisting of 14–22 periapical and posterior bitewing images intended to display the crowns and roots of all teeth, periapical areas and alveolar bone.

Patient D

A panoramic film and four periapicals were taken in the maxillary anterior region.

This situation would not be coded as a D0210 because there was not an intraoral radiographic image of the whole mouth. It would be coded as:

D0330 panoramic radiographic image

D0220 intraoral – periapical first radiographic image

(Report D0220 one time.)

D0230 intraoral – periapical each additional radiographic image

(Report D0230 three times.)

Regardless of the patient's dental benefit plan, the reporting of performed procedures should always reflect what treatment was provided. Alternate payment provisions may apply, but the third-party payer should send statements to patients and providers alike to explain why an alternate benefit was provided.

Dentists who have signed provider agreements with third-party payers should check their contracts to see if there are provisions that apply to this situation.

Clinical Coding Scenario #6:
Oral Cancer – An Enhanced Examination

An oral cancer evaluation is included in the descriptors of both the comprehensive oral evaluations (D0150 and D0180) and the periodic oral evaluation (D0120). Visual inspection using operatory lighting and palpation are the techniques that are frequently used in routine oral cancer evaluations. A dentist may decide that patients with increased cancer risk factors should also receive an enhanced oral cancer examination, one that is more extensive than a routine oral cancer screening and may include the use of additional diagnostic aids.

How could the dentist report use of additional diagnostic aids in the oral cancer examination?

There is not an independent code for an enhanced oral cancer examination, but there is a code that can be used when some type of staining or similar procedure is performed:

D0431 **adjunctive pre-diagnostic test that aids in detection of mucosal abnormalities including premalignant and malignant lesions, not to include cytology or biopsy procedures**

This code may be used to report the use of the following:

- Tissue reflectance (e.g., VizLite Plus, MicorLux DL)
- Autofluorescence (e.g. VELscope, OralID)
- Any intraoral vital staining technique (e.g., toluidine blue)

If the additional procedures are not described by D0431 the dentist could use:

D0999 **unspecified diagnostic procedure, by report**

D0999 can be used to report any diagnostic procedure which does not seem to be included in the CDT Code. A narrative that describes the service must be included on the claim when this code is used.

Clinical Coding Scenario #7:
Impression for an Appliance and Diagnostic Models

A 17-year-old patient of record is seen for a periodic oral exam and prophylaxis. Her radiographic images are up to date and the doctor notes that the patient has nearly perfect occlusion with no evidence of occlusal issues of wear, and had not received any orthodontic care in the past. The patient and her mother inquired about at home tooth whitening. This initial visit was coded as:

D0120   periodic oral evaluation – established patient

D1110   prophylaxis – adult

Two months later, the patient decided to request tooth whitening, and returned for impressions for maxillary and mandibular bleaching trays. She was seen a week later for the trays, instructions, and a follow up visit was scheduled. It was noted that there was no dental benefit reimbursement for bleaching trays, so the patient's mother inquired whether the models on which they were constructed could be considered diagnostic casts (D0470), and submitted as such after the fact.

Could these be considered "diagnostic casts" using code D0470 at this point?

Because these impressions were taken with the purpose of fabricating bleaching trays, the appropriate code is:

D9975   external bleaching for home application, per arch; includes materials and fabrication of custom trays

The dentist could have elected to take impressions for diagnostic models at the periodic exam appointment or any time after, and correctly coded for it, if indeed they were indicated to facilitate diagnosis and treatment planning. Diagnostic casts or models are extremely important for so many patients in diagnosis and treatment planning. However, in this case, the impressions were taken to serve another purpose, i.e., bleaching. Again, the purpose of coding is to show what treatment is actually performed and for what reason.

Clinical Coding Scenario #8:
Orthognathic Surgery Planning

An oral and maxillofacial surgery office recently installed a cone beam radiography machine. It was used to treatment plan some anticipated orthognathic surgery for a patient. Following image capture, several axial and lateral views were consulted to plan the surgery. A panoramic view was also produced to send to the patient's orthodontist.

After consultation with the orthodontist, the surgeon constructed a 3D virtual model, which they viewed together on the computer, to properly locate a temporary implant to anchor the orthodontic appliance. The virtual model could be manipulated on the screen to allow them to visualize other anatomical structures in the area and their relationship to the teeth to determine the ideal location to place the implant.

How could you code the initial treatment planning visit's diagnostic imaging procedures?

D0367   cone beam CT capture and interpretation with field of view of both jaws; with or without cranium

This code is used specifically to report procedures related to cone beam imaging technology. It replaced the separate cone beam data capture (D0360) and two-dimension reconstruction (D0362) codes. The image capture includes two-dimensional sectional (tomographic) views from the axial (coronal or frontal) and lateral (sagittal) planes, as well as the panoramic view.

How could you code the subsequent consultation? (3D virtual model)?

D0393   treatment simulation using 3D image volume

The 3D virtual model is a three-dimensional image reconstructed from data acquired during the treatment planning visit.

Clinical Coding Scenario #9:
Temporomandibular Joint (TMJ) Disorder Treatment

A patient, referred to the dental office by her ear, nose and throat (ENT) physician, has a history of constant headaches and facial pain. The ENT saw no sinus related issues after a thorough examination including radiographic images. After completing a comprehensive oral evaluation (D0150), the dentist recognized the patient's symptoms as a temporomandibular disorder of significant complexity. The patient exhibited limited opening and was in discomfort every morning.

Further evaluation was needed to diagnose this condition and that examination included listening to the joint with a stethoscope, detailed palpation of all the muscles of mastication, recording of occlusal relationships, ranges of motion, and areas of musculoskeletal tenderness.

The dentist did an extensive review of the patient's lifestyle, including stress coping mechanisms. She identified many potential contributing factors to the temporomandibular disorder (TMD) condition. Teeth #18 and #19 were missing and tooth #15 had super-erupted to the point where the patient could not close without moving his jaw to the right. A tongue thrust habit resulted in a severe anterior open bite, and there was extensive incisal wear on all anterior teeth.

The doctor decided that following extraction of #15, an orthotic TMJ appliance covering the mandibular occlusal surfaces would allow the patient to reposition her jaw to a more comfortable position. It would also protect those teeth from increasing wear due to oral habits. After the patient was more comfortable, the doctor believed that a comprehensive treatment plan could be made.

How would the recent diagnostic visit be coded?

Due to the limited scope, the doctor can choose one of two problem-focused evaluations:

> **D0140 limited oral evaluation – problem focused**

or

> **D0160 detailed and extensive oral evaluation – problem focused, by report**

In this case, the nature and complexity of the problems suggest that D0160 would be the most appropriate code for this evaluation. Use of this code requires submission of a narrative report.

Clinical Coding Scenario #10:
Treating a Patient Suffering From Swelling, Pain and Periodontal Disease

A patient presented in pain and complaining about swelling around one particular tooth. The doctor's emergency evaluation focused on the patient's complaint and included two periapical radiographic images and pocket measurements of the teeth in the area. The swelling was clearly adjacent to tooth #3 and there was bleeding and exudate upon probing.

The doctor treated the patient for a periodontal abscess by gross debridement and draining through the sulcus, irrigating the pocket with chlorhexidine and prescribing the patient an antibiotic.

How could this encounter be coded?

Since the evaluation was both problem-focused and limited to the patient's complaint, the appropriate codes for diagnostic procedures would be:

D0140   limited oral evaluation – problem focused

D0220   intraoral – periapical first radiographic image

D0230   intraoral – periapical each additional radiographic image

In this case there are several codes that might be used to document the operative services, alone or in combination. The procedure coding options are:

D9110   palliative (emergency) treatment of dental pain – minor procedure
This is typically reported on a "per visit" basis for emergency treatment of dental pain.

Note: D9110 is a "catch-all" code that covers a broad array of procedures.

D7510   incision and drainage of abscess – intraoral soft tissue
Involves incision through mucosa, including periodontal origins.

Note: Discussions at the Code Maintenance Committee (CMC) meetings indicated that D7510 was considered to be appropriate even when the incision is made through the gingival sulcus.

Clinical Coding Scenario #11:
A Partially Edentulous Patient with Bleeding Gums, Rampant Calculus, and White Lesions

Patient presented with massive accretion of calculus on teeth also covered by a dark brown veneer of coffee and tobacco residue. The calculus effectively cemented a lower partial in place that the doctor wished to remove. An ultrasonic scaler was the doctor's instrument of choice for calculus removal before a comprehensive oral evaluation, which would be delivered during a subsequent appointment.

After the full mouth debridement was completed there were additional diagnostic procedures: radiographs of the entire lower arch including four posterior and two anterior periapicals; two bitewings on the left and one on the right side; and a panoramic radiographic image.

Today's treatment included:

- initial evaluation that establishes the need for the gross removal of plaque and calculus
- gross removal of calculus and stain
- radiographs (6 PA, 3 BW, and 1 Panoramic)
- disaggregated transepithelial biopsy (brush) of white patch
- dispensing one 16 oz. bottle of chlorhexidine gluconate rinse

How would the services delivered during today's encounter be coded?

Initial evaluation:

D0191 assessment of a patient

> A limited clinical inspection that is performed to identify possible signs of oral or systemic disease, malformation, or injury, and the potential need for referral for diagnosis and treatment.

or

D0140 limited oral evaluation – problem focused

> An evaluation limited to a specific oral health problem or complaint. This may require interpretation of information acquired through additional diagnostic procedures. Report additional diagnostic procedures separately. Definitive procedures may be required on the same date as the evaluation.
>
> Typically, patients receiving this type of evaluation present with a specific problem or dental emergencies, trauma, acute infections, etc.

Gross removal of calculus and stain:

D4355 **full mouth debridement to enable a comprehensive oral evaluation and diagnosis on a subsequent visit**

Full mouth debridement involves the preliminary removal of plaque and calculus that interferes with the ability of the dentist to perform a comprehensive oral evaluation. Not to be completed on the same day as D0150, D0160, or D0180.

Note: This procedure is done prior to completing diagnosis when it is not possible to adequately access tooth surfaces and periodontal areas because of excessive plaque and calculus.

Radiographs (6 PA, 3 BW, and Panoramic):

These nine radiographs and the panoramic radiographic image do not match the CDT Code's definition of a "full mouth series" (D0210). Therefore, the radiographs in this scenario would be reported using the panoramic, periapical and bitewing codes:

D0220 **intraoral – periapical first radiographic image**

D0230 **intraoral – periapical each additional radiographic image**

Note: Report D0230 five times, once for each additional radiographic image.

D0273 **bitewings – three radiographic images**

D0330 **panoramic radiographic image**

Disaggregated transepithelial biopsy of white patch:

D7288 **brush biopsy – transepithelial sample collection**

Note: The brush biopsy samples disaggregated dermal and epithelial cells. A positive sample usually requires follow-up with an architecturally intact incisional or excisional sample.

Dispense one 16 oz. bottle of chlorhexidine gluconate rinse:

D9630 **drugs or medicaments dispensed in the office for home use**

Clinical Coding Scenario #12:
Preventive Resin Restorations

The patient arrived at the office for a recall visit. On the previous recall visit six months ago, this patient had nutritional counseling as well as several teeth that needed to be restored due to decay.

Before doing anything the doctor decided that a caries risk assessment should be completed, using the form posted on *ADA.org*. A look at the answers on the form – especially the combination of frequent consumption of soft drinks and energy drinks, past interproximal restorations, and two incipient carious lesions – led to the conclusion that the patient is at high risk of continuing caries development.

What is the appropriate CDT code to document the caries risk procedure?

D0603 **caries risk assessment and documentation, with a finding of high risk**
Using recognized assessment tools.

Note: Caries risk assessment information, including the updated tools, is available online at *ADA.org/en/member-center/oral-health-topics/caries-risk-assessment-and-management*. When a patient receives a caries risk assessment, the procedure is documented and reported with the CDT code whose nomenclature includes the identified level of risk:

D0601 **caries risk assessment and documentation, with a finding of low risk**

D0602 **caries risk assessment and documentation, with a finding of moderate risk**

D0603 **caries risk assessment and documentation, with a finding of high risk**

During the oral exam the doctor did indeed see what appeared to be small, carious, cavitated lesions on the occlusal surfaces of teeth #30 and #31. After opening the lesions using a handpiece and removing caries, both preparations were very slight, ending in enamel, and did not extend into the dentin.

The doctor concluded that a minimally invasive restorative technique would be appropriate for this situation. A composite resin would be used to restore tooth form and function along with an unfilled resin used afterwards to seal out all the radiating grooves.

What CDT code would be appropriate to document this minimally invasive procedure?

> **D1352   preventive resin restoration in a moderate to high caries risk patient – permanent tooth**

Note: The doctor knows that **D2391 resin-based composite – one surface, posterior** is not appropriate since the dentin was untouched. Likewise, **D1351 sealant – per tooth** isn't applicable since decay was present.

D1352 was added to the CDT Code to enable documentation of a conservative restorative procedure where caries, erosion or other conditions affect the natural form and function of the tooth. This procedure is part of many dental school curricula under names that vary by school and region (e.g., preventive resin restoration; conservative resin restoration; or minimally invasive resin restoration).

Clinical Coding Scenario #13:
Current Patient of Record with Substantial Increase in Carious Lesions on Exam

A 75-year-old patient is currently being seen every six months with preventive visits. This patient has periodontal probing depths of no greater than 3 mm in all four quadrants of the oral cavity, and has had no carious activity or replacement of restorations in the past five years. Upon current examination by the dentist, eight new carious lesions were noted, located on the facial or buccal surfaces of mandibular teeth. The patient shared that he had a change in his medical history, and is taking three new medications known to have "dry mouth" as a side effect. Before preceding further, the dentist decided to perform a caries risk assessment (as outlined in a previous scenario). In addition, the dentist decided to measure the amount of salivary flow for the patient. The patient was instructed to chew on unflavored gum and saliva was collected for five minutes. The patient had a saliva rate flow of 0.4 ml/min.

What are the appropriate CDT codes for this patient visit?

D0120 **periodic oral evaluation – established patient**

D0603 **caries risk assessment and documentation, with a finding of high risk**

D0419 **assessment of salivary flow by measurement**
This procedure is for identification of low salivary flow in patients at risk for hyposalivation and xerostomia, as well as effectiveness of pharmacological agents used to stimulate saliva production.

Note: Salivary assessment technique may vary by diagnosis and available equipment but generally can be evaluated by resting or stimulated saliva assessment.

Resting salivary flow is determined by asking the patient to let saliva accumulate in the floor of the mouth and, with the head tilted forward, let it drool into the collecting cup passively. After five minutes, volume collected is measured and divided by five to obtain the flow rate in mL/min. Rates lower than 0.1 mL/min are considered hyposalivation.

Stimulated salivary flow is determined by chewing paraffin wax or unflavored chewing gum (mechanical stimulation), or by dripping a few drops of citric acid on the tongue (chemical stimulation) and spitting for up to five minutes. Volume obtained is converted into mL/min. Rates lower than 0.7 mL/min are considered hyposalivation.

Clinical Coding Scenario #14:
Oral Evaluation and Prophylaxis with Natural Teeth and Implant Crowns

A 64-year-old patient of record had four implants placed in edentulous areas #18, #19, #30, and #31, and these implants were restored with single zirconia crowns, with all remaining dentition intact. The patient is being seen on a six month basis for examination and prophylaxis, but now has a "mixed" dentition of both natural teeth and implants that are restored.

How would you code for the visit which includes an oral evaluation and updated radiographic images?

D0120 **periodic oral evaluation – established patient**
An evaluation performed on a patient of record to determine any changes in the patient's dental and medical health status since a previous comprehensive or periodic evaluation. This includes an oral cancer evaluation, periodontal screening where indicated, and may require interpretation of information acquired through additional diagnostic procedures. Report additional diagnostic procedures separately.

D1110 **prophylaxis – adult**
Removal of plaque, calculus and stains from tooth structures and implants in the permanent and transitional dentition. It is intended to control local factors.

The code revision in CDT 2021 to both D1110 and D1120 added the terminology "and implants" to both descriptors to clarify that the prophylaxis procedure and code is properly reported when a patient's dentition includes natural teeth and implant restored areas, and no prosthesis is removed.

Clinical Coding Scenario #15:
Reactivated Recall Patient with Increased Periodontal Disease

A 51-year-old patient finally returns to the dental office after a two-year hiatus. Previously this patient (with a full complement of teeth) had been seen on a six-month basis with generalized 2–3 mm recession, periodontal pocket depths of 2–4 mm, and a propensity to build up supra-gingival calculus quickly. After performing a full mouth exam, including periodontal readings, most posterior teeth probe at 4–5 mm with some localized 6 mm and nearly 100 percent of the areas exhibit bleeding upon probing.

A full mouth radiographic series was taken two years ago, and the decision is made to take four bitewings. The patient reports increased fatigue and notes that all the nicks and scrapes received from being a mechanic "don't seem to heal as quickly this past year." The patient has not seen their MD in over two years but was previously informed that they were a borderline diabetic and provided nutritional counselling only. The rest of the medical history is unremarkable with no medications being taken, but the patient appears to weigh much more than when last seen.

Today, the dentist performs a finger prick blood glucose test which reads 180 mg/dl. Due to the elevation of the blood glucose and worsening periodontal condition, the patient is advised to see their physician for follow-up to diagnose, and manage, this chronic condition. The patient schedules two subsequent appointments for scaling and root planing for all four quadrants, and is informed that a blood glucose level test will be performed before the procedures are started. A third visit is scheduled for periodontal re-evaluation four to six weeks after the last SRP appointment and another glucose test.

How would you code today's appointment along with any subsequent treatment and follow up appointment?

Today: Initial Appointment

D0180	**comprehensive periodontal evaluation – new or established patient**
D0274	**bitewings – four radiographic images**
D0412	**blood glucose level test – in-office using a glucose meter**

Visit #1: SRP Two Quadrants

D0412   blood glucose level test – in-office using a glucose meter

Note: A dentist can determine, using the D0412 procedure, how the patient's blood glucose level, may affect treatment scheduled for the day's appointment.

- A glucose level below 70 mg/dl is the clinical definition of hypoglycemia alert level, which means the patient is at risk of a hypoglycemic event during the procedure. Therefore the procedure ought not to be initiated until the patient's blood sugar level is in the acceptable range.

- A glucose level over 300 mg/dl could lead to delayed healing of the surgical site and severe infection. This suggests that elective surgical procedures be rescheduled and delivered when the patient's circulating glucose level is in the acceptable range.

D4341   periodontal scaling and root planing – four or more teeth per quadrant

(Report D4341 two times.)

Visit #2: SRP Two Quadrants

D0412   blood glucose level test – in-office using a glucose meter

D4341   periodontal scaling and root planing – four or more teeth per quadrant

(Report D4341 two times.)

Visit #3: Four to Six Weeks After Completion of SRP and About Three Weeks After the First Visit

D0171   re-evaluation – post-operative office visit

D0412   blood glucose level test – in-office using a glucose meter

Note: D0412 does not include any guidance on frequency of delivery; third-party payer reimbursement will be based on benefit plan design.

Clinical Coding Scenario #16:
Off-site Radiographic Imaging and Teledentistry

A patient who is unable to travel because of current health concerns, calls the dentist's office with symptoms of slight non-localized dental pain. The patient was seen six months ago in the office for a periodic exam but has not had any radiographic images taken for two years. One of the hygienists who frequently visits patients in remote locations or those who are isolated, traveled to the home of the patient. The hygienist took four digital bitewing radiographic images, one periapical image with a portable unit, and two intra-oral photographs with the office camera. These images and photos were sent electronically to the dentist in the office to view. In real-time with the hygienist and the patient, the dentist viewed the images, spoke with the patient and the hygienist, and advised the patient to travel to the office as soon as it was feasible and safe to do so for a follow-up visit.

How are the procedures completed on this date of service coded?

For services delivered by the hygienist at the patient's home, use the following codes:

D0707   intraoral – periapical radiographic image – image capture only

Report code once with "1" in the claim service line Quantity (Qty.) field since only one periapical image was captured.

D0708   intraoral – bitewing radiographic image – image capture only

Report code once with "4" in the claim service line Quantity (Qty.) field since four separate bitewing images were captured.

D0703   2-D oral/facial photographic image obtained intra-orally or extra-orally – image capture only

Report code once with "2" in the claim service line Quantity (Qty.) field since two separate intra-oral photographic images were captured.

Note: Since the hygienist captured the images outside the office and transmitted the images for the dentist's interpretation the applicable codes from the CDT Code's "Image Capture Only" subcategory of service. In this scenario it is not appropriate to report codes from the "Image Capture with Interpretation" subcategory since interpretation of the transmitted images by the dentist occurred at the dentist's practice – and the separate interpretation is reported with its own unique CDT code.

For services delivered by the dentist at the practice office, use the following codes:

D0391 interpretation of diagnostic image by a practitioner not associated with capture of the image, including report

Report code once with "7" in the claim service line Quantity (Qty.) field since four separate bitewing images, two separate photographic images, and one periapical image were interpreted.

D0140 limited oral evaluation – problem focused

An evaluation limited to a specific oral health problem or complaint. This may require interpretation of information acquired through additional diagnostic procedures. Report additional diagnostic procedure separately. Definitive procedures may be required on the same date as the evaluation.

Typically, patients receiving this type of evaluation present with a specific problem and/or dental emergencies, trauma, acute infections, etc.

D9995 teledentistry – synchronous; real-time encounter

Reported in addition to other procedures (e.g., diagnostic) delivered to the patient on the date of service.

Note: For more information about teledentistry events and coding, the following ADA publication D9995 and D9996 – *ADA Guide to Understanding and Documenting Teledentistry Events* is available for download at *ADA.org/~/ media/ADA/Publications/Files/CDT_D9995D9996-GuideTo_v1_2017Jul17. pdf?la=en.*

1. *Is there a code to record tests for the Coronavirus for patients that I may see?*

    There are two new codes in CDT 2021 that would be used to document testing patients for the Coronavirus or other public health related pathogens. One code is for testing for antigens, which demonstrates that the person currently has the disease and is positive for the virus. This new code is:

    > **D0604 antigen testing for a public health related pathogen, including coronavirus**

    The other code for testing involves looking for the presence of antibodies, which means that the patient has had the virus in the past, and should not be currently infectious. This code is:

    > **D0605 antibody testing for a public health related pathogen, including coronavirus**

2. *I see there is a code for an immediate finding of a patient's blood glucose level in the dental office using a glucose meter. Does that mean that this is necessary for every diabetic patient at every visit in my office?*

    The code is:

    > **D0412 blood glucose level test – in-office using a glucose meter**
    > This procedure provides an immediate finding of a patient's blood glucose level at the time of sample collection for the point-of-service analysis.

    This code was adopted by the Code Maintenance Committee with a January 1, 2019 effective date. This enables the dental health care provider to code for this procedure but does not make any reference on when it should be done, and does not imply that it is necessary in every visit. The decision on whether to administer a glucose test is determined by the judgment of the treating health care provider for each individual circumstance. More information and guidance concerning the D0412 (and D0411) procedure is available on the ADA's Coding Education page linked to *www.ADA.org/cdt*.

3. *Is it possible to use **D0150 comprehensive oral evaluation – new or established patient** again within 90 days after the initial visit to our dental office?*

    Reading the full CDT Code entry for D0150 will help determine whether the code is appropriate for documenting and reporting the procedure delivered to a patient. The D0150 descriptor states, in part, that this procedure (comprehensive oral evaluation) is applicable "to new patients, established patients who have a significant change in health conditions or other unusual circumstances, by report, or established patients who have been absent from active treatment for three or more years."

Reporting the D0150 procedure would be appropriate if the patient had "a significant change in health conditions or other unusual circumstances." In that case, a narrative would accompany the code submission. If that were not the case with the patient, other oral evaluation codes such as **D0140 limited oral evaluation – problem focused** or **D0160 detailed and extensive oral evaluation – problem focused, by report** may be more appropriate.

4. *What is the difference between a patient screening procedure (D0190) and a patient assessment procedure (D0191)?*

Each procedure has a different scope and objective as indicated in their full CDT Code entries:

D0190 screening of a patient
> A screening, including state or federally mandated screenings, to determine an individual's need to be seen by a dentist for diagnosis.

A screening is a quick check of a child's mouth to determine if she or he needs a prompt exam and treatment. The oral examination is brief and usually requires only a tongue depressor and light source to check for decay, injury, pain, oral cancer, developmental problems, and other abnormal oral conditions or risk factors. Examples of screenings that can be documented using D0190 include the screening performed as part of the Head Start program.

D0191 assessment of a patient
> A limited clinical inspection that is performed to identify possible signs of oral or systemic disease, malformation, or injury, and the potential need for referral for diagnosis and treatment.

A dental assessment differs from a screening in that it includes a limited clinical examination (recording dental restorations and conditions that should be called to the attention of a dentist), and collection of other oral health data to assist in the development of a professional treatment plan.

5. *I sometimes go to assisted living homes to provide dental evaluations for some of the residents. The facility does not have any radiographic imaging equipment or a dental chair, so all of my evaluations take place in the resident's room. I do a visual inspection of the person's oral cavity and share any obvious findings with the family of the patient, and suggest that arrangements be*

made for transportation to a dental office for more information gathering and possible treatment. How can I code for these "evaluations"?

Doing this type of service would probably be best addressed under the CDT Code:

D0191   **assessment of a patient**
A limited clinical inspection that is performed to identify possible signs of oral or systemic disease, malformation, or injury, and the potential need for referral for diagnosis and treatment.

Using any of the clinical oral evaluation codes D0150, D0120, D0140 would not be appropriate due to the lack of a definitive diagnosis resulting from the preliminary visual inspection.

6. *My new panoramic imaging device enables me to acquire a single image that has the same, or more, diagnostic information than I see on multiple posterior bitewing images. I've always considered a bitewing as an intra-oral image since the film is placed in the patient's mouth. With my new imaging device, the receptor is outside the oral cavity. What CDT code should I use now?*

The ADA's online Glossary of Dental Clinical and Administrative Terms defines a bitewing radiograph as an "Interproximal radiographic view of the coronal portion of the tooth/teeth. A form of dental radiograph that may be taken with the long axis of the image oriented either horizontally or vertically, that reveals approximately the coronal halves of the maxillary and mandibular teeth and portions of the interdental alveolar septa on the same image." The CDT Code entry that most accurately describes the question's imaging procedure is:

D0251   **extra-oral posterior dental radiographic image**
Image limited to exposure of complete posterior teeth in both dental arches. This is a unique image that is not derived from another image.

7. *My patient needs several extra-oral images to help diagnose the problem, but I do not see any code for additional images. What do I do?*

When reporting multiple extra-oral images the applicable procedure code is D0250, as revised in CDT 2016, with the number of images acquired noted in the "Qty." (Quantity) field on the claim form.

D0250   **extra-oral – 2D projection radiographic image created using a stationary radiation source, and detector**

8. *Are bitewings and a panoramic radiographic image considered a full mouth series of radiographs?*

   No, these images are different from the **D0210 intraoral – complete series of radiographic images** procedure. According to the FDA's "The Selection of Patients for Dental Radiographic Examinations," published in 2004, a full mouth series is defined as "a set of intraoral radiographs usually consisting of 14–22 periapical and posterior bitewing images intended to display the crowns and roots of all teeth, periapical areas and alveolar bone crest." Effective January 1, 2009 this definition was incorporated into the D0210 descriptor.

   Further, a panoramic radiographic image cannot be considered a full mouth series as it is an extra-oral film and it does not reflect the FDA definition of a full mouth series. Different procedure codes are available to report a full mouth series of radiographs (D0210) and a panoramic radiograph (D0330). Please note that bitewings taken as part of a full mouth series are not reported separately.

9. *Is an oral cancer screening evaluation necessary for every comprehensive (D0150) and periodic (D0120) oral evaluation? The descriptor states that it is performed "where indicated"? What does that mean?*

   The descriptors you are reading are from a past CDT Code version. In CDT 2021 the descriptors for both a comprehensive oral evaluation (D0150) and a periodic oral evaluation (D0120) were edited to make it clear that an oral cancer screening examination is not a "where indicated" component of each procedure. Oral cancer screening is an integral part of both exams thorough a visual and hands on examination, and may also include any other diagnostic aids that the dentist may want to utilize.

10. *Our office has begun to use new technology that provides 3D or 2D images of a patient that are generated from a CT-like scan. How do we code this?*

    Several procedure codes (e.g., D0364–D0368) are available to document "cone beam CT" diagnostic images taken in the dentist's office. There are separate codes based on the field of view. For example, an initial scan that yields coronal, sagittal, and panoramic views would be documented with:

    D0367   cone beam CT capture and interpretation with field of view of both jaws; with or without cranium

    The entire "cone beam" nomenclature must be read to determine which describes the diagnostic image.

11. *I've used D0350 to document oral/facial photographic images, but now I'm able to create both two- and three-dimensional photographic images. How do I document what I do when my diagnosis and treatment planning makes use of one or both types of images?*

Changes effective with the publication of CDT 2015 enable you to document both 2D and 3D photographic images. There is a code for obtaining a 3D image as the procedure differs from acquiring a 2D image. D0350's nomenclature was revised to clarify that this procedure is applicable only to acquisition of 2D photographic images. The full CDT Code entries are:

D0350 **2D oral/facial photographic image obtained intra-orally or extra-orally**

D0351 **3D photographic image**
This procedure is for dental or maxillofacial diagnostic purposes. Not applicable for a CAD-CAM procedure.

12. *I took a digital panoramic image and my software was able to manipulate the captured data so that it produced the equivalent of one upper and one lower posterior bitewings on the left side of the patient's oral cavity. What it the correct procedure code to report – **D0273 bitewings – two radiographic images**?*

The applicable CDT code is **D0330 panoramic radiographic image** as that was the original image capture procedure – and as stated in this scenario the image data was manipulated after capture to create bitewing images.

However, if the panoramic imaging device was set up to capture only a single image whose content is the equivalent of upper and lower bitewing images, the correct coding from the Diagnostic Imaging section is:

D0251 **extra-oral posterior dental radiographic image**
Image limited to exposure of complete posterior teeth in both dental arches. This is a unique image that is not derived from another image.

Note: Include the number of D0251 images in the claim form's "Qty." field (e.g., "2" if one image captures the left side of the oral cavity and the other captures the right side).

13. *When is it appropriate to report a consultation versus an evaluation procedure?*

Typically, a consultation (D9310) is reported when one dentist refers a patient to another dentist for an opinion or advice on a particular problem encountered by the patient.

14. *Should the dentist who sees a patient referred by another dentist for an evaluation of a specific problem report a problem focused evaluation code (D0140; D0160), or the consultation code (D9310)? Also, does it matter if the dentist initiates treatment for the patient on the same visit?*

Both D0140 and D0160 are both problem focused evaluations and either may be reported if the consulting dentist believes one or the other appropriately describes the service provided. Please note that neither of these evaluation procedures' nomenclatures or descriptors contain language that prohibits the consulting dentist from initiating and reporting additional services. These services are reported separately by their own unique codes.

Code D9310 may be used if the consulting dentist believes it better describes the service provided when a patient is referred by another dentist for evaluation of a specific problem. According to this CDT code's descriptor, the dentist who is consulted may initiate additional diagnostic or therapeutic services for the patient, which are also reported separately by their own unique codes.

15. *When is it appropriate to report oral evaluation codes D0150, D0180, D0120 and D0140?*

These four commonly reported codes are from the CDT Code's series of clinical evaluation codes (D0120 through D0180). Each one is thoroughly explained by their respective nomenclature and descriptor. For example:

- The initial evaluation for a new patient may be reported using **D0150 comprehensive oral evaluation – new or established patient or by D0180 comprehensive periodontal evaluation – new or established patient**.

- If this patient becomes a patient of record returning after the initial evaluation, the service would be reported using **D0120 periodic oral evaluation – established patient**.

- An evaluation of a patient who presents with a specific problem or dental emergency may be reported using **D0140 limited oral evaluation – problem focused**.

Again, it is important to read the descriptor to distinguish what type of clinical oral evaluation is being coded for each particular patient visit.

16. **Can I submit a periodic evaluation (D0120) on the same day as a full mouth debridement to enable comprehensive periodontal evaluation and diagnosis (D4355)?**

According to its descriptor, D4355 is "not to be completed on the same day as D0150, D0160, or D0180." There is nothing in the descriptors of the oral evaluation code D0120 or D4355 that preclude reporting both on the same day. However, according to the ADA's Guide to Reporting Full Mouth Debridement, codes for patient assessment (D0191) or limited oral evaluation (D0140) procedures may be more appropriate depending on the clinical circumstances.

Note that benefit plans may have limitations or exclusions about paying for both D4355 and D0120 or D0140 procedures when delivered on the same day.

17. **We recently had a patient come in for a periodic oral evaluation. The doctor found signs and symptoms of periodontal disease and performed a complete periodontal evaluation. May I report both the periodic and periodontal evaluations since these are two separate procedures?**

The comprehensive periodontal procedure D0180 includes all the components of a periodic evaluation D0120, and adds additional requirements for periodontal charting and the evaluation of periodontal conditions. When a patient presents with signs or symptoms of periodontal disease, and all these components are performed, only D0180 would be reported.

18. **May I submit a limited oral evaluation (D0140) and another procedure on the same day?**

There is no language in the descriptor of D0140 that precludes the reporting of other procedures on the same date of service. However, some benefit plans have limitations or exclusions about paying for certain combinations of codes performed on the same day.

19. **If seven vertical bitewings and a panoramic image are taken to show the entire oral cavity, can it be coded as a full mouth series D0210?**

No. By definition of the descriptor of D0210, seven vertical bitewings and a panoramic radiographic image would not constitute a full mouth series (FMS) because the panoramic image is extra-oral and the intra-oral bitewings do not capture all of the structures of the entire mouth. It would be coded as:

D0330 panoramic radiographic image

D0277 vertical bitewings — 7 to 8 radiographic images
This does not constitute a full mouth intraoral radiographic series.

20. **Which CDT code could be used to document a periodontal re-evaluation, such as for monitoring post-operative tissue healing?**

The following CDT code, added in CDT 2015, enables documenting and reporting any type of post-operative office visit. Before this code's addition the only option was a "999" code:

D0171   re-evaluation – post-operative office visit

21. **Is reporting the "comprehensive periodontal evaluation" (D0180) limited to periodontists?**

D0180 is not limited to periodontists. All dental procedure codes are available to any practitioner providing service within the scope of her or his license.

22. **I have read the descriptors of the evaluation codes, but am confused as to which code should be reported when a very young child is evaluated in the office. None of them seem to apply. What should be reported?**

The procedure code for the evaluation of a child under age three and including counseling of the child's primary caregiver may be reported. This code is **D0145 oral evaluation for a patient under three years of age and counseling with primary caregiver**.

23. **Can code D0145 be reported every time the child comes into the office for an evaluation, or should we report a recall evaluation for subsequent visits?**

A separate evaluation code was added because of the unique procedures that are necessary when evaluating a very young child. Depending on the nature of the evaluation, a periodic evaluation (D0120) or an oral evaluation for a patient under three years of age (D0145) would be appropriate choices to consider.

24. **Must a caries risk assessment procedure be performed and submitted on a third-party claim that includes an oral evaluation code?**

The CDT code does not specify any joint reporting requirements for caries risk assessment procedures (D0601–D0603) and oral evaluation procedures (e.g., D0120, D0145 or D0150). These are unique procedures documented and reported separately with their own codes. Any requirement for concurrent delivery and reporting of a caries risk assessment procedure and an oral evaluation procedure comes from the payer's reimbursement policies, or benefit plan limitations and exclusions.

25. *Can I submit a code for pulp vitality tests or is this considered to be included in all endodontic procedures?*

Yes, you may submit this as a separate service (D0460) as it is a stand-alone code. This procedure includes multiple teeth and contra lateral comparison(s), as indicated. Note that separate payment for any submitted code is dependent on the benefit plan policies.

26. *Are radiographic images taken during endodontic procedures considered to be part of the procedure as well, or can they be coded for individually?*

Any image taken prior to the start (i.e., prior date of service) of endodontic therapy can be coded individually, but once the endodontic therapy begins, all intra-operative radiographs acquired as part of the treatment are considered part of the endodontic treatment.

27. *Are there rules or regulations regarding in office HbA1c testing?*

Yes, some states may consider this testing "outside the scope of the state's Dental Practice Act," which could make it unlawful to perform this test. Also, federal rules may limit the type or brand of device that may be used. Lastly a certificate of waiver may need to be in place prior to use of these tests. For a comprehensive guide on the D0411 procedure and its reporting visit the ADA's Coding Education web page *https://www.ADA.org/~/media/ADA/Publications/Files/CDT_D0411_D0412_Guide_v1_2019Jan02.pdf?la=en*.

28. *I use a laser caries detection device sometimes to help diagnose incipient decay. Is there a code for this?*

The following code, added in CDT 2017, would be applicable as the laser is considered part of the armamentarium that could be used to deliver the procedure.

D0600 non-ionizing diagnostic procedure capable of quantifying, monitoring, and recording changes in structure of enamel, dentin, and cementum

Note: A caries detection procedure is not the same as a caries susceptibility test procedure, which is reported with code "D0425 caries susceptibility tests".

29. *A patient was seen for a follow up visit after a car accident. No treatment was performed on the initial visit other than an evaluation and radiographic images on maxillary anterior teeth. What would be an appropriate code for the follow-up visit?*

>**D0170   re-evaluation – limited, problem focused (established patient; not post-operative visit)**

This descriptor allows for a patient to be seen for an oral evaluation in certain circumstances, including this one where there was a traumatic injury and at during the initial visit "no treatment was rendered but [the dentist determined that the] patient needs follow-up monitoring."

30. *What is the difference between the code for assessment of salivary flow by measurement D0419 and the other codes concerning saliva samples?*

D0419, added in CDT 2020, by its descriptor states that the procedure "is for identification of low salivary flow in patients at risk for hyposalivation and xerostomia, as well as effectiveness of pharmacological agents used to stimulate saliva production."

This in-office chairside procedure involves collecting saliva from a patient in a tube or cup for five minutes in either of the following two ways. The first way is to have the patient have a "stimulated salivary flow" by chewing on wax or unflavored gum. The second way is to allow the patient naturally to accumulate in the mouth and "drool" into a cup (resting saliva flow). Volume obtained is converted into mL/min. "Stimulated saliva flow" rates lower than 0.7 mL/min are considered hyposalivation. Also, rates lower than 0.1 mL/min for "resting salivary flow" are considered hyposalivation.

In contrast, codes **D0417 collection and preparation of saliva sample for laboratory diagnostic testing** and **D0418 analysis of saliva sample** require laboratory testing for chemical or biological analysis, not just simply flow rates.

31. *Our office uses "traditional" transillumination with a bright light to check for fractures and caries with anterior teeth. Can D0600 be used to report this?*

The full CDT Code entry for D0600 reads as follows:

>**D0600   non-ionizing diagnostic procedure capable of quantifying, monitoring, and recording changes in structure of enamel, dentin, and cementum**

As stated in the nomenclature, D0600 is specific to calibrated instruments capable of quantifying, monitoring and recording changes in enamel, dentin, and cementum. There are several modalities on the marketplace that use non-ionizing light, such as CariVu, DIAGNOcam, DIAGNOdent, and others. D0600 should not be used to report "traditional" transillumination alone.

32. *What is the difference between an adjunctive pre-diagnostic test procedure (D0431) and a brush biopsy procedure (D7288) for screening of patients for mucosal abnormalities and oral cancer?*

D0431 adjunctive pre-diagnostic test that aids in detection of mucosal abnormalities including premalignant and malignant lesions, not to include cytology or biopsy procedures may be used in addition to basic oral cancer screening that includes a visual and physical examination. This code defines the procedure, not the many products that can be utilized as part of its delivery. Some of these products' names are OralID, Identafi, Vizilite Plus, VELscope, Microlux DL, as well as staining with toluidine blue.

There is a definitive difference between the adjunctive test (D0431) and the oral brush biopsy (D7288). The adjunctive pre-diagnostic test specifically excludes "cytology or biopsy" when describing the procedure. D0431 typically includes steps that illuminate or stain the tissue to check for abnormalities. In contrast the complete CDT Code entry for D7288, noted below clearly indicates that this is a biopsy procedure where cells are collected.

> **D7288   brush biopsy-transepithelial sample-collection**
> For collection of oral disaggregated transepithelial cells via rotational brushing of the oral mucosa.

Summary

The Diagnostic Section of the *Code on Dental Procedures and Nomenclature* (CDT Code) deals with the gathering of data and cognitive skills necessary for patient evaluation. Although less than 100 in number, these diagnostic codes in CDT 2021 are the foundation of the CDT Code and are utilized for every patient throughout the course of care. Attention to detail of descriptors allows for correct coding in treatment, as explained in the scenarios and questions presented in this section. "Coding for what you do" does not mean that all procedures will be covered or reimbursed by third-party carriers. However, "coding for what you do" will mean that dental treatment is properly coded and reported, allowing for accuracy and transparency in patient record keeping.

Contributor Biography

Ralph A. Cooley, D.D.S. is a general dentist who was in private practice for more than 30 years and is currently the Assistant Dean for Admissions and Student Services at the UT Health School of Dentistry in Houston. He is a past member of the ADA Council on Dental Benefits and is currently a member of the Code Maintenance Committee.

Chapter 2: D1000–D1999 Preventive

By Jim Nickman, D.D.S., M.S.

Introduction

The dental procedure codes contained in CDT 2021's Preventive category of service are some of the most common used to provide care for children and adults. The type and frequency of preventive services should be based professional standards of care and the disease risks of the patient. Other services documented with codes in this category address preservation of space for the succedaneous tooth in the case of the early loss of a primary tooth and counseling for disease prevention. In order to assist patients in appropriately utilizing their dental benefits, it is important that the dental office understand the contractual obligations of the benefit plans that it accepts. It is not uncommon for dental benefit plans to contain service limitations, annual maximums, age restrictions, and limitation s based on the stage of the dentition.

This chapter will define key concepts of the codes contained within the preventive category. It also contains the CDT 2021 code changes, examples of coding scenarios, and a question and answer section of common issues.

Key Definitions and Concepts

Prophylaxis: Removal of plaque, calculus, and stains from the tooth structures or implants intended to control local irritational factors. Although the instruments used to remove plaque, calculus, or stains are different for implants (plastic) than natural dentition (metal), the procedure's techniques utilized are the same.

Prophylaxis is not a therapeutic procedure related to the healing of a disease or condition of the periodontium. These procedures are found under the periodontics codes (D4000–D4999).

The removal of local irritational factors may reduce transitory local gingival inflammation (gingivitis).

Topical application of fluoride varnish and **topical application of fluoride excluding varnish**: Professionally applied prescription topical fluoride products delivered separately from that contained in prophy paste (the mild abrasive compound used usually with rotary cup instrumentation to remove extrinsic stain and dental plaque from the enamel tooth surface).

Sealant: Dental sealants (also known as pit and fissure sealants) are materials placed in anatomically caries-susceptible tooth surfaces (usually posterior occlusal pits and fissures, posterior buccal or lingual pits or grooves, or incisor cingulum pits) after the adjacent tooth structure is mechanically or chemically prepared for enamel bonding. The material, after chemical or light curing, forms a mechanical barrier to the penetration of acid-producing cariogenic bacteria, thereby reducing the potential for caries initiation. The procedure is appropriate prior to dentin cavitation and is most effective when applied to enamel that has not undergone significant enamel demineralization.

Preventive resin restoration in a moderate to high caries risk patient – permanent tooth: Conservative restoration of an active cavitated lesion in a pit or fissure that does not extend into dentin; includes placement of a sealant in any radiating non-carious fissures or pits. This procedure differs from a sealant in that it involves mechanical removal (usually by rotary instrumentation) of demineralized, chalky enamel (enamel caries) and the restoration of the affected tooth surface with a restorative filling material such as a composite resin or glass ionomer cement. Dentin is not penetrated by caries or by instrumentation.

caries preventive medicament application – per tooth: The application of medicaments to prevent caries formation on high risk surfaces of the dentition. The procedure is different than D1354 interim caries arresting medicament application in that the medicament is applied prior to caries formation. The medicaments may be like those used in the caries arrest techniques but do not include the usage of topical fluoride. Examples of high-risk surfaces could include, but are not limited to, exposed root surfaces in elderly patients, deep fissures in primary and permanent teeth, and exposed enamel adjacent to a bonded or cemented orthodontic band or bracket.

interim caries arresting medicament application – per tooth: The treatment of an active, non-symptomatic carious lesion by the topical application of a medicament which arrests or inhibits caries progression. It is often (though not exclusively) intended as an interim measure in the medical management of dental caries in selected situations (such as a tooth nearing exfoliation) or populations (such as the frail elderly, the very young, or patients with special healthcare or developmental needs) to stabilize the tooth until it can later be treated in a conventional restorative manner. It is the appropriate code for the application of silver diamine fluoride or another similar **acting medicament.**

distal shoe space maintainer – fixed – unilateral: The fabrication and delivery of a fixed space maintaining appliance extending distally and subgingivally from the first primary molar immediately after extraction of the second primary molar to guide the eruption of the unerupted first permanent molar. While technically a type of fixed unilateral space maintainer (D1510), it differs importantly in that it is intended to be removed and replaced with another space maintenance appliance (usually a D1510) upon eruption of the first permanent molar.

D1510 space maintainer – fixed, unilateral – per quadrant specifically excludes the distal shoe space maintainer design.

Changes to This Category

CDT 2021 contains two additions and four revisions. The two additions address usage of caries preventive medicament application and counselling for the use of high-risk substances. Two of the revisions regard the inclusion of implants in the prophylaxis codes. The remaining two revisions address a gap in the code to allow reporting when space maintainers are removed. These changes are intended to provide greater specificity to the dental record and to smooth claims processing.

The two new additions are as follows:

D1355 **caries preventive medicament application – per tooth**
For primary prevention or remineralization. Medicaments applied do not include topical fluorides.

D1321 **counseling for the control and prevention of adverse oral, behavioral, and systemic health effects associated with high-risk substance use**
Counseling services may include patient education about adverse oral, behavioral, and systemic effects associated with high-risk substance and administration routes. This includes ingesting, injecting, inhaling and vaping. Substances used in a high-risk manner may include but are not limited to alcohol, opioids, nicotine, cannabis, methamphetamine and other pharmaceuticals or chemicals.

The four code revisions are as follows:

D1110 prophylaxis – adult
Removal of plaque, calculus and stains from tooth structures <u>and implants</u> in the permanent and transitional dentition. It is intended to control local irritational factors.

D1120 prophylaxis – child
Removal of plaque, calculus and stains from tooth structures <u>and implants</u> in the primary and transitional dentition. It is intended to control local irritational factors.

D1557 removal of fixed bilateral space maintainer – maxillary
~~Procedure performed by dentist or practice that did not originally place the appliance.~~

D1558 removal of fixed bilateral space maintainer – mandibular
~~Procedure performed by dentist or practice that did not originally place the appliance.~~

Note: The D1557 and D1558 revisions are significant as the descriptor's limitation on who may report the procedure is eliminated, without affecting the manner in which the procedure is delivered. These codes are now applicable to report removal by any dentist – the one who originally placed the appliance, or another dentist in the practice where the appliance was placed, or any other dentist in any practice location.

Clinical Coding Scenario #1:
Distal Shoe Space Maintainer

A four-year-old presents to your office in pain. After the emergency examination, you determine that the lower second molars are abscessed and not restorable. The first permanent lower molars are not erupted but can be visualized on the radiographs. After discussing the available treatment options with the child's parents, informed consent is obtained for extraction of the non-restorable molars and placement of two distal shoe space maintainers.

How would the space maintainers be coded?

In addition to the appropriate codes for the services provided at each visit, the appropriate code for the distal shoe space maintainers would be:

D1575 distal shoe space maintainer – fixed, unilateral – per quadrant
Fabrication and delivery of fixed appliance extending subgingivally and distally to guide the eruption of the first permanent molar. Does not include ongoing follow-up or adjustments, or replacement appliance, once the tooth had erupted.

Note: D1575 is reported twice on the claim as two separate appliances were placed. The applicable Area of the Oral Cavity code is also reported on each service line.

The same patient reports for a re-care appointment at age 7. You notice that the lower first molars are fully erupted and decide that it is appropriate to remove both of the lower distal shoe space maintainers and replace them with a bilateral lower lingual holding arch space maintainer to avoid potential issues with the development and eruption of the future lower second premolars. The correct code for the new space maintainer would be **D1527 space maintainer – fixed – bilateral, mandibular**.

Would the new bilateral lower lingual arch space maintainer be reimbursable under the patient's dental benefit plan?

Reimbursement by the patient's dental benefits carrier for the new appliance would depend upon the contractual limitations and policies governing covered benefits. Regardless of expected third-party payment, the dentist should record and code for the services provided.

Clinical Coding Scenario #2:
New 11-Year-Old Patient

An eleven-year-old female patient presents to your office for a new patient examination. Per the patient's parents, the child's last dental visit was several years ago in a different state. No current radiographs are available for the patient. Based on the clinical findings of a mixed dentition, you decide to expose and interpret two bitewing and panoramic radiographs. Other services provided at that visit are a prophylaxis and fluoride varnish treatment.

How would you code for this visit?
The appropriate codes that could be used are as follows:

D0150 **comprehensive oral evaluation – new or established patient**
D0272 **bitewings – two radiographic images**
D0330 **panoramic radiographic image**
D1120 **prophylaxis – child**
D1206 **topical application of fluoride varnish**

What would change if the patient was 12 years old?
Selection of the prophylaxis code is determined by how the dentist views the patient's dentition. Either the adult (D1110) or the child (D1120) code may be used for patients with transitional dentitions regardless of age. Patient age is not a part of either code's nomenclature or descriptor. ADA policy recommends that dental benefit determinations should be based on dental development rather than patient age. According to the ADA Policy "Age of 'Child'" adopted in 1991, benefits should be based on stage of dentition:

> "**Resolved**, that when dental plans differentiate coverage of specific procedures based on the child or adult status of the patient, this determination be based on the clinical development of the patient's dentition, and be it further
>
> **Resolved**, that for the sole purpose of eligibility for coverage, chronological age of at least 21 be used to determine enrollment status. "

The prophylaxis codes are dentition-specific rather than age-specific. Some third-party payers have in their contracts' policies that limit available benefits based on patient age, not stage of dentition. Most of these dental benefit plans specify an age between 12 and 21 as to when the patient is considered an adult.

What if the patient had only permanent teeth with eruption completed through the second permanent molars?
Regardless of age, patients with permanent dentition are appropriately coded using D1110.

Clinical Coding Scenario #3:
Silver Diamine Fluoride Palliative Treatment

A long-term patient of your practice has just entered hospice at home. She contacted your office regarding occasional dental pain and sensitivity. Although frail, she is well enough to visit your office for an emergency visit. After a thorough exam and a periapical radiograph of the tender area, you observe recurrent decay on the cervical margin of a crown clinically and radiographically. You discuss your clinical findings with the patient and her current medical status. Unsure of her prognosis and after a review of risks and benefits of possible treatment options, you propose palliative treatment of the recurrent decay using silver diamine fluoride.

What codes might be used to document this visit?

The appropriate codes that could be used are as follows:

D0140   **limited oral evaluation – problem focused**

D0220   **intraoral – periapical first radiographic image**

D1354   **interim caries arresting medicament application – per tooth**

Note: "D9110 palliative (emergency) treatment of dental pain – minor procedure" is not the appropriate code for documenting SDF delivery as the oral evaluation led the dentist to diagnose an active, non-symptomatic carious lesion (recurrent decay on the cervical margin of a crown).

Clinical Coding Scenario #4:
Silver Diamine Fluoride in Response to Trauma

During a recent re-care visit with a four-year-old male with a complete primary dentition and closed interproximal contacts, you perform a prophylaxis and bitewing radiographs. While taking the radiographs, the parents mention that their son had trauma several weeks ago to his maxillary anterior teeth. Based on the conversation, you decide to also expose and interpret a maxillary periapical radiograph. While interpreting the radiographs, you observe incipient interproximal decay in the lower first molars and widened periodontal ligament space for both central incisors.

After a thorough discussion of your findings and risks and benefits of the possible treatment options, the parents' consent to application of silver diamine fluoride to the incipient interproximal decay on the lower first molars. Based on the patient's caries risk, you also recommend the application of topical fluoride varnish.

How might this be reported using CDT codes?

The appropriate codes that could be used are as follows:

D0120 **periodic oral evaluation – established patient**

D0220 **intraoral – periapical first radiographic image**

D0272 **bitewings – two radiographic images**

D1206 **topical application of fluoride varnish**

D1354 **interim caries arresting medicament application – per tooth**

Note: For D1354 report the tooth numbers and number of teeth treated on the claim's service line that lists this procedure.

May the topical fluoride varnish be provided as a separate billable service on the same day as the application of a caries arresting medicament?

Yes. The two services are not mutually exclusive of each other and are not overlapping codes for the same procedure.

Due to the patient's trauma and radiographic findings, you discuss the signs and symptoms of possible future pulpal pathology with the parents. You also recommend that the patient have a follow-up visit in eight weeks to re-evaluate the status of the child's maxillary anterior teeth.

What codes could be used to report the follow-up visit?

This re-evaluation could be coded as follows:

D0170   re-evaluation – limited, problem focused (established patient; not post-operative visit)

D0220   intraoral – periapical first radiographic image

Six months later at a subsequent re-care visit, you observe no change in the size of the incipient lesions on the lower first molars. Due to the inconsistent oral hygiene habits and minor dietary changes that have occurred, you determine that the child still has a moderate caries risk. Following established protocols and best practice recommendations, you recommend the re-application of silver diamine fluoride to the affected interproximal areas.

What code could be used on subsequent silver diamine fluoride applications?

D1354   interim caries arresting medicament application – per tooth

Would these services be considered reimbursable under the patient's dental benefit plan?

Reimbursement by the patient's dental benefits carrier for these services would depend upon the contractual limitations and policies governing covered benefits. Regardless of expected third-party payment, the dentist should record and code for the services provided.

Clinical Coding Scenario #5:
Silver Diamine Fluoride Therapy for Root Caries

An elderly and frail adult presents to your office with multiple dental root caries and recurrent dental caries along the gingival margins of existing restorations adjacent to receding gingival tissues. You are aware of the efficacy of silver diamine fluoride in treating these lesions, but are unsure how to code for the procedure.

Does the per tooth application of an interim caries arresting medicament (D1354) apply only to carious lesions occurring on the crown?

This procedure is not limited to carious lesions on the crown. The tooth surface location and etiology of the asymptomatic active carious dental lesion is not relevant. does not change the definition of the service provided by the dentist, which is the. D1354 is the correct code to report application of an agent to arrest or inhibit caries progression on any part of a tooth.

Clinical Coding Scenario #6:
Re-cementing Bilateral Space Maintainer

An established ten-year-old patient reports for a re-care appointment. During the clinical examination, you observe that the patient's Nance appliance, a maxillary bilateral space maintainer, is loose in the upper left quadrant. Radiographs exposed at this visit demonstrate that the maxillary second premolars, whose space is being maintained, are not close to eruption. Based on this finding, you remove and immediately re-cement the loose bilateral space maintainer.

How may this be reported using CDT codes?

The appropriate code would be:

D1551   re-cement or re-bond bilateral space maintainer – maxillary

If the missing maxillary second premolars were erupting and the loose space maintainer was no longer indicated, what code could be used to report the removal procedure?

The appropriate code would be **D1557 removal of fixed bilateral space maintainer – maxillary**.

Note: D1557 is the applicable code to report removal by any dentist, who could be the one who originally placed the appliance, or another dentist in the practice where the appliance was placed, or a dentist in a different practice.

Reimbursement by the patient's dental benefits carrier for these services would depend upon the contractual limitations and policies governing covered benefits. Regardless of expected third-party payment, the dentist should record and code for the services provided.

Clinical Coding Scenario #7:
Sealant and Preventive Resin Restoration

An established seven-year-old patient reports for a re-care appointment. The first permanent molars are now fully erupted but have deep pits and fissures that contain staining and possible incipient decay. You decide to re-appoint the patient to apply sealants or possible restorations to the occlusal surfaces. At the follow-up visit, you remove the stain in the pits and fissures and find that one of the molars has decay that does not extend into dentin and requires mechanical removal of demineralized enamel. Based on the size of the affected area after the lesion has been removed, a sealant in that area is no longer appropriate. You place a small resin composite and seal the remaining groove structure.

What would be the appropriate CDT code for the tooth with the lesion that did not extend into dentin?

The appropriate code would be:

D1352   **preventive resin restoration in a moderate to high caries risk patient – permanent tooth**

If the lesion on the affected molar extended into the dentin, report the treatment using the **D2391 resin-based composite – one surface, posterior** would be the appropriate code.

D1351 sealant – per tooth would be the appropriate code for the three non-cavitated teeth to report sealant application.

Chapter 2: D1000–D1999 Preventive

Clinical Coding Scenario #8:
Sealant and Sealant Repair

An established thirteen-year-old patient reports for a re-care appointment and during the examination, you observe some missing sealant on several of the first permanent molars that had sealant placed in your office more than two years ago. The remaining sealant material on the affected first molars is not easily dislodged with an explorer and you are confident about the integrity of the residual marginal bond. The second permanent molars are now also fully erupted but have deep pits and fissures. Based on these findings, you recommend repair of the defective sealants on the first permanent molars and new sealants on the second permanent molars.

What would be the proper CDT codes for these procedures?

Because you are not removing the remaining sealant material on the first molars and are replacing only that which has been lost, you are accomplishing procedure **D1353 sealant repair – per tooth**. If, instead, you had removed all residual sealant material on the affected first molars and placed a completely new sealant across all occlusal pits, grooves and fissures you would be performing procedure **D1351 sealant – per tooth**.

Would either procedure be reimbursable service under the patient's dental benefit plan?

As with all other services, this would depend on benefit plan restrictions and limitations, such as time intervals after initial placement or if replacements are a benefit. Regardless, the dentist must code for the specific service provided.

Clinical Coding Scenario #9:
New Patient and Tobacco Counseling

A 12-year-old patient reports for an initial oral evaluation appointment in your practice and no current radiographs are available. The adolescent has a late-mixed dentition with full eruption of the lower second permanent molars. The bitewing radiographs show no signs of interproximal decay, but the lower second primary molars are present and you are unable to visualize the lower second premolars. A panoramic radiograph is exposed and confirms that the lower second premolars are congenitally missing.

During the examination, you detect signs that the patient has been smoking. A conversation with the patient about the potential long-term problems with tobacco use and its impact on the adolescent's oral and systemic health. The patient is receptive to the information and methods of tobacco cessation are discussed in detail. At this visit, the patient receives a prophylaxis, four bitewing radiographs, a panoramic image, and due to patient preference, a fluoride gel treatment.

What would be the proper CDT codes for these procedures?
The appropriate codes to report this visit are:

D0150	**comprehensive oral evaluation – new or established patient**
D0274	**bitewings – four radiographic images**
D0330	**panoramic radiographic image**
D1110	**prophylaxis – adult**
D1208	**topical application of fluoride – excluding varnish**

D1110 prophylaxis – adult is appropriate as the patient's current dentition represents the full and complete natural permanent dentition.

The oral cancer screening completed during the oral evaluation revealed no changes in tissue structure related to the tobacco usage.

What would be the proper code to report the counseling on tobacco use and cessation?
The appropriate code would be **D1320 tobacco counseling for the control and prevention of oral disease**. Other procedures and referral may be necessary if changes to the tissue were noted during the oral cancer screening.

Would the tobacco counseling service be considered reimbursable under the patient's dental benefit plan?
Reimbursement by the patient's dental benefits carrier for these services would depend upon the contractual limitations and policies governing covered benefits. Regardless of expected third-party payment, the dentist should record and code for the services provided.

Clinical Coding Scenario #10:
Periodontal Maintenance Therapy and Prophylaxis Visits

Following either surgical or non-surgical periodontal therapy the patient is placed by the treating dentist on a program of scheduled periodic periodontal maintenance (D4910) visits, which could be at various intervals (e.g., 2, 3, 4, or 6 months) depending on the patient's clinical condition. The **D4910 periodontal maintenance** procedure includes removal of bacterial plaque and calculus (mineralized deposits) from subgingival and supragingival tooth surfaces, site-specific scaling and root planing, and coronal tooth polishing. Between these scheduled periodontal maintenance visits the patient is also seen by the dentist for routine dental prophylaxis (tooth cleaning procedures).

May the dentist code and bill for the prophylaxis procedure (D1110 or D1120) or is this prohibited as a duplication of existing services under D4910?

Nothing in the D4910 or the D1110 (or D1120) code nomenclatures or descriptors make these procedures mutually exclusive. If the dentist determines that the patient's periodontal health can be augmented with periodic routine prophylaxis procedures (removal of plaque, calculus and stains from the tooth structures for the purpose of controlling local irritational factors), then this service should be performed and reported as D1110 or D1120, depending on the state of the dentition.

Does it make any difference if the reporting dentist for prophylaxis (D1110 or D1120) is the same dentist providing periodontal maintenance (D4910)?

No. The dentist should code and report for the services provided regardless of the provision of other services by the same or a different dentist.

Will both procedures be reimbursed by the patient's dental benefit carrier?

Reimbursement will depend upon the dental benefit plan language and the contractual policies governing covered benefits.

Clinical Coding Scenario #11:
Use of Caries Preventive Medicament in an Elderly Patient

Mrs. Johnson is a long-term patient of Dr. Meyers and has recently transitioned into a long-term care facility from her home. Fortunately, the long-term care facility has a rudimentary dental clinic that allows for limited dental services and Dr. Meyers has provided care for other residents in that setting. During a recent visit with Mrs. Johnson, Dr. Meyers noted that her oral care has noticeably worsened placing her at risk for caries formation. After completion of the oral evaluation and caries risk assessment procedures, and a thorough informed consent discussion of the findings with the patient or the patient's legal guardian, Dr. Meyers applies a caries preventive medicament to the most at-risk tooth surfaces at that visit.

How would Dr. Meyers document and report that patient encounter (e.g., examination, caries risk finding and medicament application) using CDT procedure codes?

Since the encounter occurred in a long-term care facility and not in the doctor's office it is appropriate to report **D9410 house/extended care facility call** in addition to any other services provided. The following codes would be used to report and document the other services provided.

> **D0120** **periodic oral evaluation – established patient**
>
> **D0603** **caries risk assessment and documentation, with a finding of high risk**
>
> **D1355** **caries preventive medicament application – per tooth**

Will the procedures be reimbursed by the patient's dental benefit carrier?

Reimbursement will depend upon the dental benefit plan language and the contractual policies governing covered benefits. Regardless of any expected benefit payment, the dentist should provide and code for medically necessary services that are determined by community standards and the patient's informed consent for these services.

Clinical Coding Scenario #12:
High Caries Risk Orthodontic Patient

Dr. Hemann is an orthodontist who has noted that several of her patients have extremely poor oral hygiene and poor diet habits that could contribute to caries formation. An avid learner, Dr. Hemann has recently read several studies about the effectiveness of using medicaments to prevent dental caries in patients who are in orthodontic appliances. One of her patients, Billy, a healthy 12-year-old, presented for an orthodontic appointment with extremely poor oral hygiene. This led the doctor to perform a caries risk assessment, which led to a conclusion that Billy is at high risk for caries.

After discussing her findings with Billy and Billy's mother, which included nutritional counseling and oral hygiene instructions, Dr. Hemann recommended applying a caries preventive medicament to the at-risk areas adjacent to his brackets and bands. Billy's mother agrees and gives written consent for the procedure. To document the discussion and procedure, Dr. Hemann sends a letter to Billy's parents and his general dentist.

What CDT procedure codes would Dr. Hemann use to report what services were provided today?

D0140 **limited oral evaluation – problem focused**

D0603 **caries risk assessment and documentation, with a finding of high risk**

D1310 **nutritional counseling for control of dental disease**

D1330 **oral hygiene instructions**

D1355 **caries preventive medicament application – per tooth**

Will the procedures be reimbursed by the patient's dental benefit carrier?

Reimbursement will depend upon the dental benefit plan language and the contractual policies governing covered benefits. Regardless of any expected benefit payment, the dentist should provide and code for medically necessary services that are determined by community standards and the patient's informed consent for these services.

Clinical Coding Scenario #13:
Prophylaxis Usage with a Patient Who Has Dental Implants

Marge, a long-term patient of your practice presents for a re-care examination. In the past, she had several dental implants placed to replace congenitally missing mandibular second premolars. During the routine visit, she had four bitewing radiograph images exposed and interpreted. Two periapical radiograph images were also obtained to evaluate the bone structure supporting the implants. Minor supra- and sub-gingival calculus was removed, and a prophylaxis was completed uneventfully. A routine oral examination was also completed. Although a low caries risk patient, Marge opted to have a fluoride varnish treatment.

What CDT codes would be reported to document the services provided today?

In addition to the clinical notes, the following CDT codes could be utilized:

> **D0120**   **periodic oral evaluation – established patient**
>
> **D0220**   **intraoral – periapical first radiographic image**
>
> **D0230**   **intraoral – periapical each additional radiographic image**
>
> **D0274**   **bitewings – four radiographic images**
>
> **D1110**   **prophylaxis – adult**
>
> **D1206**   **topical application of fluoride varnish**

Will the procedures be reimbursed by the patient's dental benefit carrier?

Reimbursement by the patient's dental benefits carrier for these services would depend upon the contractual limitations and policies governing covered benefits. Regardless of expected third-party payment, the dentist should record and code for the services provided.

Clinical Coding Scenario #14:
Teenage Patient Who Is Currently Vaping

A 13-year-old female patient presents to your office for a re-care appointment. During a conversation with her parent/guardian, nothing remarkable was reported during the update of the patient's medical history and chief complaint. The hygienist engaged in a conversation with the patient during the appointment and the patient let it slip that she had started vaping with friends. The patient reported that she has been doing this regularly and now feels that she may have trouble stopping vaping. The conversation also revealed that the patient has been purchasing the off-market vaping refills from her friends as she is unable to legally purchase vaping supplies.

With concern, the hygienist spends a considerable amount of time discussing the dangers of vaping on her oral and physical health. During the examination, the dentist also discusses the long-term danger of vaping and strategies of cessation. Luckily, the teen is interested in stopping due to her vaping experiences and concern over possible addiction. The dentist has the hygienist follow-up with the patient in the upcoming weeks to check on the patient's progress with vaping cessation.

What CDT code would be used to report what the counseling that occurred today?

In addition to the clinical notes and coding for other services provided, the following CDT code applies to the vaping discussion and guidance:

D1321 **counseling for the control and prevention of adverse oral, behavioral, and systemic health effects associated with high-risk substance use**

Will the procedures be reimbursed by the patient's dental benefit carrier?

Reimbursement will depend upon the dental benefit plan language and the contractual policies governing covered benefits. Regardless of any expected benefit payment, the dentist should provide and code for medically necessary services that are determined by community standards and the patient's informed consent for these services.

Coding Q&A

1. **What is the definition of prophylaxis?**

   A prophylaxis is removal of plaque, calculus and stains from the tooth structures and implants, and is intended to control local irritational factors. It is a preventive and not a therapeutic procedure, and the applicable CDT code is determined by the clinical state of the patient's dentition as determined by the dentist.

2. **Does the patient's age dictate whether a child or adult prophylaxis is reported?**

   Patient age is not the code selection criterion; the clinical state of dentition determines which procedure code is appropriate to report the service. For a patient with permanent or transitional tooth structures or implants **D1110 prophylaxis – adult** is the correct code. For another patient who has primary and transitional tooth structures and implants, the correct code is **D1120 prophylaxis – child**.

   Although the prophylaxis codes are dentition specific rather than age specific and should be reported in this manner, some third-party payers may have restrictions in their contracts that limit available benefits or benefit levels based on age and not stage of the dentition.

   According to the ADA Policy "Age of 'Child'" adopted in 1991, benefits should be based on stage of dentition:

   "**Resolved**, that when dental plans differentiate coverage of specific procedures based on the child or adult status of the patient, this determination be based on the clinical development of the patient's dentition, and be it further

   Resolved, that for the sole purpose of eligibility for coverage, chronological age of at least 21 be used to determine enrollment status."

   Nonetheless, prophylaxis claims may be rejected by third-party carriers as not meeting plan age specifications for this service. It is appropriate to appeal such claim rejection. It is not appropriate for a dental benefit plan to ask that the claim be resubmitted with a different prophylaxis code solely for reimbursement.

3. **What code is appropriate for a difficult prophylaxis?**

   There is no separate procedure code that reflects a greater degree of difficulty of a dental prophylaxis. The available prophylaxis codes are **D1110 prophylaxis – adult** and **D1120 prophylaxis – child**.

   However, if the patient's clinical condition reveals moderate to severe gingival inflammation without bone loss, it may be that the patient's condition may more appropriately be treated by the **D4346 scaling in the presence of generalized moderate or severe gingival inflammation – full mouth, after oral evaluation** procedure.

Chapter 2: D1000–D1999 Preventive

4. *When might a patient have benefits coverage for more than the usual two prophylaxis procedures in a 12-month period or in a calendar year?*

Some dental benefit plans may allow more frequent prophylaxis procedures based on medical risk or other factors (e.g., diabetic; immunosuppressed; pregnancy).

Other patients in the same plan who are not deemed "at risk" would be subject to standard frequency limitations. If the dentist determines medical necessity for more frequent cleanings not provided under plan parameters, the dentist or the patient may explore the plan's appeal process or that appeal process provided under state regulation.

5. *What code is used to report a scaling and root planing in the presence of generalized moderate or severe gingival inflammation?*

When the dentist's oral evaluation reveals generalized moderate to severe gingival inflammation with no loss of attachment or bone, the appropriate procedure is **D4346 scaling in the presence of generalized moderate or severe gingival inflammation – full mouth, after oral evaluation**. D4346 is delivered and reported as a separate procedure and not in conjunction with a prophylaxis.

When any inflammation present is localized and there is no loss of attachment or bone, a prophylaxis procedure is appropriate and would be reported with the applicable CDT Code (D1110 or D1120).

6. *After a full mouth gross debridement (D4355) for the purpose of enabling a later comprehensive periodontal evaluation is delivered, may the patient receive a prophylaxis procedure on the next visit?*

A dental prophylaxis (cleaning) may be delivered on the next visit, if indicated. The appropriate sequence of services would be D4355 followed after an appropriate interval, by an oral evaluation. The oral evaluation findings may indicate that a prophylaxis is the next appropriate periodontal service.

7. *Can **D1110 prophylaxis – adult** and **D4342 scaling and root planing – one to three teeth per quadrant** be reported on the same date of service?*

There is no language in the descriptor of an adult prophylaxis that precludes the reporting of any other procedure on the same date of service and no language in the descriptor of D4342 which precludes at the same visit the provision of a dental prophylaxis. However, third-party reimbursement for these procedures is dependent on the specific dental benefit plan provisions. Some plans may pay for both services when delivered at the same time, while others might impose a specified interval.

8. *Could the CDT code **D1206 topical application of fluoride varnish** be used when applying fluoride varnish to desensitize a tooth?*

No. When fluoride varnish is utilized to desensitize a tooth, the appropriate CDT Code is **D9910 application of desensitizing medicament**. CDT code **D1206 application of topical fluoride varnish** is exclusive to the use for caries prevention.

9. *When resin is applied to a tooth's pit and fissure area, what distinguishes a sealant (D1351) from a preventive resin restoration (D1352)?*

Application of an unfiled resin or glass ionomer cement limited to the enamel surface is a sealant procedure and would be documented using D1351. When a filled resin or glass ionomer cement is applied to an area of an active cavitated lesion that does not extend into the dentin, this procedure is a preventive resin restoration and the applicable procedure code is D1352.

Note: Should the lesion extend into the dentin, the procedure code for a one surface composite resin restoration (D2391) would be used to document the service.

10. *I have several questions concerning the caries arresting medicament application procedure reported with CDT code D1354:*

a. *I've heard this code referred to as the Silver Diamine Fluoride application procedure; is this implied limitation correct?*

No. D1354's CDT Code entry describes a discrete procedure for delivery "of a caries arresting or inhibiting medicament." The dentist providing this service would determine the appropriate medicament to be applied, and the choice is not limited to Silver Diamine Fluoride.

b. *Is the procedure reported with this code limited to primary teeth?*

No. There are no words in either the nomenclature or descriptor that limits the procedure to primary dentition. This is a per-tooth procedure that may be delivered to any type of dentition – primary, succedaneous and permanent.

c. *Does the delivery of the D1354 procedure preclude a subsequent restorative procedure at a later time?*

No. A subsequent restorative procedure may be needed some time after application of a caries arresting medicament. Caries is a disease that is treated with the medicament. The lesion in the tooth resulting from the disease (i.e., the cavity) may need a subsequent restoration to restore function.

Chapter 2: D1000–D1999 Preventive

d. *Must there be a specific interval between the D1354 procedure and a restorative procedure on the same tooth?*

No. As noted in the answer to question 10.c, the clinical condition of a patient's tooth is affected by a variety of factors and can change over time. The patient's dentist is in the best position to evaluate the need for restorative services, and when such services should be delivered.

e. *May other preventive procedures be delivered to the tooth on the same day it receives the D1354 treatment?*

Yes. Other preventive procedures may be delivered as there is no such exclusionary language in D1354's nomenclature or descriptor. Individual circumstances would affect the order in which preventive services are delivered (e.g., prophylaxis before medicament application).

11. *Sometimes dental sealants fail completely (i.e., no sealant material remains bonded to the tooth surface), but most often failure is incremental with a partial loss of sealant material. The fix is to reapply sealant material only to the unprotected caries-susceptible pits and fissures. This is a much more limited procedure than D1351, which applies when the entire tooth surface is re-sealed. What CDT code applies to a sealant repair?*

The correct CDT code for this application is **D1353 sealant repair – per tooth**.

12. *What code should be used to report the removal of a fixed space maintainer?*

When the dentist determines that the space maintainer has served its useful purpose, the appropriate codes depending on type are as follows:

For unilateral space maintainers, the appropriate code is:

> **D1556   removal of fixed unilateral space maintainer – per quadrant**

For bilateral space maintainers, the appropriate codes are:

> **D1557   removal of fixed bilateral space maintainer – maxillary**

> **D1558   removal of fixed bilateral space maintainer – mandibular**

Dental health care professionals should use the CDT code set to report what was done, not what would be reimbursed. Reimbursement will depend upon the dental benefit plan language and the contractual policies governing covered benefits. Regardless of any expected benefit payment, the dentist should provide and code for medically necessary services that are determined by community standards and the patient's informed consent for these services.

13. Can a practice post a fee for a space maintainer appliance at the time that the impression is taken and sent to a dental lab for appliance fabrication?

    Historically, the dentist has preferred to post the cost of the service at the time of tooth preparation in the case of indirect restorations or at the time of impression in the case of dental appliances. Likewise, third-party payers adjudicate claims and make reimbursements based on the dental benefit plan coverage provisions. What prevails are the legally enforceable provisions of the dental benefit plan and the provisions of an applicable participating provider agreement.

14. What is the difference between the **D1355 caries preventive medicament application – per tooth** and **D1354 interim caries arresting medicament application – per tooth**? It appears that some of the same medicaments are recommended for both applications.

    The difference is in the intent of the usage of the medicament. D1355 is intended to prevent the development of a caries lesion in a high-risk area. D1354 is appropriate with the intent of arresting an active carious lesion.

15. There currently are two CDT codes that could be used for patients that are using tobacco products. Which code is recommended?

    D1320 tobacco counseling for the control and prevention of oral disease is used when counselling a patient on the adverse oral health effects of tobacco products and cessation.

    Patients that we serve may use other harmful substances in addition to tobacco. **D1321 counseling for the control and prevention of adverse oral, behavioral, and systemic effects associated with high-risk substance use** has a broader application potential for those individuals.

16. There are several counseling codes within the CDT Code's Preventive category of service. What determines whether the usage of these codes will be reimbursed?

    Dental health care professionals are constantly striving to improve the oral and overall health of the patients that they serve. The CDT code set is available to assist the practitioner in documenting what services are provided. Reimbursement by the patient's dental benefits carrier for these services would depend upon the contractual limitations and policies governing covered benefits. Regardless of expected third-party payment, the dentist should record and code for the services provided.

Summary

The 27 codes which comprise the preventive category are straightforward and easy to understand because some of these procedures are among the most common services in dental practice, especially in the care of infants and children. Prevention of dental disease is the cornerstone of the profession and procedures such as professional removal plaque and calculus, application of prescription strength topical fluoride, nutritional counseling, oral hygiene instruction, and sealant placement help ensure optimal oral health.

Contributor Biography

Jim Nickman, D.D.S., M.S. is a practicing pediatric dentist in St. Paul, Minnesota, and a Clinical Associate Professor of the Division of Pediatric Dentistry at the University of Minnesota School of Dentistry. He serves as chair of the American Academy of Pediatric Dentistry Committee on Dental Benefit Programs and is a voting member of the American Dental Association's Code Maintenance Committee, representing the AAPD.

By Fred L. Horowitz, D.M.D.

Introduction

Restorative codes continue to represent the majority of dental procedures done in a general dental practice on a day-to-day basis. Selection of the applicable code, or codes, for restorative services is generally straightforward when the user understands the CDT Code's underlying organization and concepts. However, the advent of new technology can present some challenges.

Key Definitions and Concepts

Direct Restorations

Direct refers to a restoration that is fabricated completely in the mouth without the use of an impression, physical or digital, to create a model outside the mouth for fabrication.

> The ADA Glossary definition of **direct** is "A procedure where the service is delivered completely in the patient's oral cavity and without use of a dental laboratory."

Amalgam restorations include the tooth preparation, all adhesives (including amalgam bonding agents), as well as liners and bases. If pins are used, they are reported separately using the applicable procedure code (see D2951).

The amalgam codes are used to report procedures performed on primary or permanent dentition, with no differentiation between anterior and posterior teeth.

> The ADA Glossary definition of **amalgam** is "An alloy used in direct dental restorations. Typically composed of mercury, silver, tin and copper along with other metallic elements added to improve physical and mechanical properties."

Resin-based composite restorations include tooth preparation, acid etching, adhesives, liners and bases and curing of the material. There is no differentiation based on the various composite resin materials utilized. If pins are used, they are reported separately (see D2951).

The resin-based composite codes are used for reporting procedures performed on the primary or permanent dentition. However, unlike amalgam codes the resin-based codes differentiate between procedures performed on anterior and posterior dentition.

The ADA Glossary definition of **resin-based composite** is "A dental restorative material made up of disparate or separate parts (e.g., resin and quartz particles)."

All **glass ionomers**, when used as restorations, are reported using the resin-based composite codes.

The ADA Glossary definition of glass ionomer is "A restorative material listed as a "resin" in *CDT 2021: Current Dental Terminology's* "Classification of Materials" that may be used to restore teeth, fill pits and fissures, lute and line cavities."

Indirect Restorations

Indirect refers to a restoration that is fabricated outside of the mouth through use of impressions, physical or digital, and creation of the either physical or digital reproductions of the mouth or area of the mouth to be restored.

The ADA Glossary definition of **indirect** is "A procedure that involves activity that occurs away from the patient, such as creating a restorative prosthesis. An indirect procedure is also known as a **laboratory** procedure, and the laboratory's location can be within or separate from the dentist's practice."

Inlay restorations are intra-coronal restorations made outside the mouth. They conform to a prepared cavity and do not restore any cusp tips.

The ADA Glossary definition of **inlay** is "A fixed intracoronal restoration; a fixed dental restoration made outside of a tooth to correspond to the form of the prepared cavity, which is then luted to the tooth. (*Glossary of Prosthodontic Terms*, 9th Edition; ©2019 Academy of Prosthodontics)."

Onlay restorations are made outside the mouth. They cover one or more cusp tips and adjoining occlusal surfaces, but not the entire external surface.

The ADA Glossary definition of **onlay** is "A partial coverage restoration that restores one or more cusps and adjoining occlusal surfaces or the entire external surface and is retained by mechanical or adhesive means. (Glossary of Prosthodontic Terms, 9th Edition; ©2019 Academy of Prosthodontics)."

Crown restorations are made outside the mouth. They cover all of the cusps on posterior teeth, extend beyond the height of contour on all covered surfaces and restore all four proximal surfaces.

The ADA Glossary definition of **crown** is "An artificial replacement that restores missing tooth structure by surrounding the remaining coronal tooth structure, or is placed on a dental implant. It is made of metal, ceramic or polymer materials or a combination of such materials. It is retained by luting cement or mechanical means. (American College of Prosthodontics; The Glossary of Prosthodontic Terms)."

¾ crown restorations are made outside the mouth. They cover all of the cusps on posterior teeth, extend beyond the height of contour on the covered surfaces and restore three of the four proximal surfaces.

Explanation of Restorations

Please note that "Facial" and "Labial" as used in this table are synonymous terms when describing surfaces involved in a restoration.

Location	Number of Surfaces	Characteristics
Anterior	1	Placed on one of the following five surface classifications – Mesial, Distal, Incisal, Lingual, or Facial (or Labial)
	2	Placed, without interruption, on two of the five surface classifications – e.g., Mesial-Lingual
	3	Placed, without interruption, on three of the five surface classifications – e.g., Lingual-Mesial-Facial (or Labial)
	4 or more	Placed, without interruption, on four or more of the five surface classifications – e.g., Mesial-Incisal-Lingual-Facial (or Labial)
Posterior	1	Placed on one of the following five surface classifications – Mesial, Distal, Occlusal, Lingual, or Buccal
	2	Placed, without interruption, on two of the five surface classifications – e.g., Mesial-Occlusal
	3	Placed, without interruption, on three of the five surface classifications – e.g., Lingual-Occlusal-Distal
	4 or more	Placed, without interruption, on four or more of the five surface classifications – e.g., Mesial-Occlusal-Lingual-Distal

Note: Tooth surfaces are reported on the HIPAA standard electronic dental transaction and the ADA Dental Claim Form using the letters in the table on the right.

Surface	Code
Buccal	B
Distal	D
Facial (or Labial)	F
Incisal	I
Lingual	L
Mesial	M
Occlusal	O

Changes to This Category

There are four changes in this category for CDT 2021, one additional code and three editorial changes.

The addition is:

D2928   prefabricated porcelain/ceramic crown – permanent tooth

This addition is for crowns that are manufactured in advance of the procedure and fitted in the mouth by utilizing a substrate, occlusion adjustment and a form of adhesive.

The editorial changes are listed below. For these three codes the last word of their nomenclatures was changed from "chairside" to "direct" or from "laboratory" to "indirect" – changes that do not affect the nature or scope of these procedures.

D2960   labial veneer (resin laminate) – direct

Refers to labial/facial direct resin bonded veneers.

D2961   labial veneer (resin laminate) – indirect

Refers to labial/facial indirect resin bonded veneers.

D2962   labial veneer (porcelain laminate) – indirect

Refers also to facial veneers that extend interproximally and/or cover the incisal edge. Porcelain/ceramic veneers presently include all ceramic and porcelain veneers.

Clinical Coding Scenario #1:
Fractured Tooth – After Hours Visit and the Final Restoration

The patient presents with a broken front tooth on Saturday, a day the office was usually closed. On examination, tooth #8 appeared to have a fractured mesial-incisal angle and lost a mesial composite restoration, with no pain reported. The doctor removed enough tooth structure to fit and cement a polycarbonate crown. The patient was told that the tooth would need a porcelain-fused-to-metal crown (PFM), but this could be done at a scheduled appointment during regular office hours.

How could you code for this after hours visit?

> **D0140** **limited oral evaluation – problem focused**
>
> **D2799** **provisional crown – further treatment or completion of diagnosis necessary prior to final impression**
>
> **D9440** **office visit – after regularly scheduled hours**

Note: The after-hours office visit code (D9440) is from the CDT Code's Adjunctive General Services category and can be reported in addition to the other services performed at that appointment. This service may not be covered or reimbursed by some dental benefits plans.

When the patient returned to the office, the doctor removes the polycarbonate crown. Following caries excavation, the doctor determines that the tooth required some replacement of lost structure to achieve proper strength and retention for the crown. One threaded titanium pin and a bonded resin core material were used to restore the tooth, followed by a preparation and an impression for a PFM. The PFM was fabricated using an alloy containing gold 15%, Palladium 25% and Platinum 10%.

How would this visit during regular office hours be coded?

> **D2950** **core buildup, including any pins, when required**

Replacement of tooth structure that is more than simply filling undercuts is appropriately reported using the code for a core buildup (D2950). The retentive pin that was placed is included in the procedure documented with this code.

Note: D2950 would not be appropriate if the material is used only to eliminate undercuts or to yield a more ideal form for a subsequent indirect restoration. In this situation the procedure would be documented as **D2949 restorative foundation for an indirect restoration**.

D2752   crown – porcelain fused to noble metal

The code for a PFM crown utilizing a noble metal (D2752) was selected instead of the high noble metal PFM code (D2750) because of the alloys used in fabrication. The noble metal percentage of the alloy was 50%, which is under the 60% high noble metal (gold + palladium + platinum) threshold specified in the CDT Code's Classification of Metals table that is published in the CDT manual.

Note: A porcelain fused to titanium crown procedure is reported with its own unique code – **D2753 crown – porcelain fused to titanium and titanium alloys**. According to the Classification of Metals titanium and titanium are not considered noble or high noble metals from the coding perspective.

Clinical Coding Scenario #2:
Indirect Restorations – Veneers

Doctor A has a CAD/CAM machine in his office. It is now being used to mill an esthetic ceramic veneer for tooth #8. A 3D scanner is utilized to capture the details of the prepared tooth and entered into the milling machine. When completed, the veneer is bonded in place.

Doctor B uses a dental lab to prepare ceramic veneers. Today's treatment involves restoring tooth #8 with a porcelain veneer created from an impression taken after the tooth is prepared. The impression is made utilizing a 3D scanner and sent to the lab after the doctor approves the image and design. The laboratory fabricates the porcelain veneer by first making a model of the prepared tooth from the scanned image. Upon receipt from the lab, the veneer is bonded in place.

What CDT codes are appropriate for these procedures?

Doctor A and Doctor B use the same CDT code.

D2962   labial veneer (porcelain laminate) – indirect

Although the fabrication of the veneer occurred in two different types of laboratory locations the same code is used as the place of fabrication for both is outside the oral cavity and away from the patient.

Clinical Coding Scenario #3:
Labial Veneer (Resin Laminate)

<u>Patient #1</u>

The patient presents for the fabrication of a labial veneer on tooth #9. The doctor will prepare the tooth and fabricate the restoration directly on the tooth on the same day. The veneer is bonded in place.

<u>Patient #2</u>

The patient presents for the fabrication of a labial veneer on tooth #9. The doctor prepares the tooth and makes an impression utilizing a 3D scanner. The scanned image is then transferred to a milling machine wherein the veneer is created. The doctor then fits and bonds the veneer in place on the same day as the tooth was prepared.

For Patient #1, the doctor will record the procedure as **D2960 labial veneer (resin laminate) – direct**, and for patient #2 the doctor will record the procedure as **D2961 labial veneer (resin laminate) – indirect**.

Although both restorations were created on the same day and in the office they are recorded differently as the veneer fabrication locations differed – Patient #1 inside the oral cavity and Patient #2 outside the oral cavity.

Clinical Coding Scenario #4:
Modifying an Existing Partial Denture After an Extraction

The patient presented complaining that he could not wear his upper partial because of some loose, painful teeth. After clinical evaluation the doctor determined that a well-designed maxillary removable partial denture had been placed and that it could be reused. This partial replaced teeth #2, #3, #4, and #14, with clasps on teeth #5, #13, and #15. The doctor's examination indicated that tooth #13 had Class III mobility due to advanced periodontal bone loss; #12 was fractured and decayed so that only a small piece of root remained exposed; and #15 had a fractured MOBL silver amalgam restoration with a fair amount of recurrent decay.

These findings led to a treatment plan that contained several separate procedures, coded as follows:

Extractions involving teeth #12 (residual root) and #13 (entire tooth)

> **D7140   extraction, erupted tooth or exposed root (elevation and/or forceps removal)**

Both the routine extraction of #13 and the root tip removal of #12 are coded using D7140. If #12's root tip removal required the laying of a mucoperiosteal flap and bone removal, the appropriate code for surgical extractions is D7210.

Addition of teeth #12 and #13 to the partial

> **D5650   add tooth to existing partial denture**

This procedure is reported twice in this scenario, one time for each tooth added, and generally requires reporting the tooth number added (based on its anatomy).

Additional clasp to the partial for retention on tooth #11

> **D5660   add clasp to existing partial denture – per tooth**

There is a single code for the addition of a clasp to a partial, whether it is wrought wire and processed or cast and soldered.

Full cast noble metal crown (tooth #15) to fit the existing clasp

> **D2792   crown – full cast noble metal**

> **D2971   additional procedures to construct new crown under existing partial denture framework**

When a crown is constructed to fit an existing partial denture the code for a regular crown is selected based on the material from which it is fabricated. The additional procedures required to allow the crown to accommodate the existing clasp are coded using D2971.

Clinical Coding Scenario #5:
A Child Who Needs Endodontic Treatment and a Crown

It was a sad story that the doctor had heard too often. The three-year-old patient had early childhood caries and was in pain. Treatment consisted of three pulpectomies followed by a resorbable filling and four esthetic-coated stainless steel crowns cemented on the maxillary incisors.

How would you code for this encounter?

Endodontic procedure

> **D3230   pulpal therapy (resorbable filling) – anterior, primary tooth (excluding final restoration)**

"Pulpal therapy" with a resorbable filling is a typical pulp treatment for primary teeth that have carious pulp exposure. It is <u>reported three times</u> in this case, once for each treated tooth.

Primary crowns

> **D2934   prefabricated esthetic coated stainless steel crown – primary tooth**

There are three types of stainless steel crowns for primary teeth: the standard stainless steel crown, one with a resin window and the esthetic coated stainless steel crown. The esthetic coated crown was used in this case and it is reported four times on the claim.

Clinical Coding Scenario #6:
Treating Acute Pulpitis

The patient's diagnosis was acute pulpitis of tooth #5. During the first appointment, the dentist opened tooth #5 to gain access to the pulp chamber and removed the tissue with a broach. Tooth closure was a temporary filling.

Ten days later the patient returned to have the root canal completed. The canal was opened, thoroughly flushed and cleaned, then obturated with gutta percha and an appropriate sealer.

What codes are applicable to the endodontic treatment on each appointment?

Visit #1

D3221   pulpal debridement, primary and permanent teeth

D2940   protective restoration

These procedures describe the simple removal of acutely inflamed pulp tissue and closure with a temporary restoration, for the relief of pain. This is not a definitive endodontic treatment.

Visit #2

D3320   endodontic therapy, premolar tooth (excluding final restoration)

This is a completed root canal therapy using an appropriate endodontic therapy procedure code.

Note: Language in the descriptor of D3221 pulpal debridement precludes the same provider from reporting this procedure on the same date as an endodontic therapy (D3320) procedure. Since the date of completion of the root canal is different from the date of initiation of the procedure, and the patient presented with an emergency, both codes may be reported.

Clinical Coding Scenario #7:
Failed Endodontically Treated Tooth with Post, Core and Crown

The patient complained of "a bad taste" in their mouth at a routine recall exam and prophylaxis. Upon examination the doctor found a draining fistula between teeth #28 and #29. After reviewing the chart and taking a periapical radiographic image, the doctor determined that #28's root canal therapy was failing and there was decay evident at the distal margin of the tooth's existing PFM crown. In addition to treating the failed root canal therapy the dentist replaced the PFM crown with a prefabricated post and core followed by placement of a new titanium crown.

How would you code to treat this situation?

D1110	prophylaxis – adult
D0120	periodic oral evaluation – established patient
D0220	intraoral – periapical first radiographic image
D3347	retreatment of previous root canal therapy – bicuspid
D2954	prefabricated post and core in addition to crown
D2794	crown – titanium and titanium alloys

Clinical Coding Scenario #8:
Patient with Fractured Tooth and Uncertain Diagnosis

A patient comes to the dental office at the end of the day, presenting with a fractured clinical crown that occurred earlier that same day. The tooth is somewhat sensitive to cold, and there appears to be a potential horizontal fracture of the root 5 mm below the crestal bone. But you cannot definitively determine that there is a fracture, and there are no other symptoms. You decide to fabricate a provisional crown and re-evaluate at a later date if symptoms intensify or new symptoms develop.

How would you code this encounter's treatment?

D2799 **provisional crown – further treatment or completion of diagnosis necessary prior to final impression**

Clinical Coding Scenario #9:
Porcelain Fused to Titanium and Titanium Alloys

The patient requires a crown to restore tooth #30. Based on occlusal analysis and considering cost to the patient and longevity of the restoration, the dentist chooses to fabricate a porcelain fused to titanium alloy crown.

How would you code this particular restoration?

D2753 **crown – porcelain fused to titanium and titanium alloys**

Coding Q&A

1. *How may I document and report local anesthesia as a separate procedure when restorative (or any other operative or surgical) services are being delivered?*

   D9215 local anesthesia in conjunction with operative or surgical procedures is the available code if you wish to document and report this procedure separately. Benefit plan limitations may preclude separate reimbursement for local anesthesia.

2. *I prepared tooth #7 for a porcelain laminate veneer, made a digital impression, and sent it to my lab for fabrication. Do I code that as a lab created veneer?*

   Yes, using CDT code **D2962 labial veneer (porcelain laminate) – indirect**. In CDT 2021 the last word of the nomenclature was changed from "laboratory" to "indirect" – a change that does not affect the nature or scope of the procedure.

3. *How do I report two separate two-surface restorations on the same tooth? Carriers advise me to report a MO amalgam and a DO amalgam as a MOD restoration. Is this correct?*

   The carriers' advice is incorrect. Dentists must document the procedures performed, and in this scenario there are two separate two-surface restorations, an MO and a DO. Guidance applicable to reporting procedures on a single tooth is found in the CDT manual's "Explanation of Restorations".

   Following the carriers' advice and reporting a single MOD procedure instead of properly reporting the two separate procedures will lead to a discrepancy between your accurate patient records and the carrier's claim records. Such a difference may become a problem during any audit or other review of services rendered.

   Note: Some dental plans may have clauses that restrict coverage on the same surface twice on the same date of service. This is why the carriers may apply an alternate benefit provision that leads to reimbursement of the two separate two-surface restorations as a single three-surface restoration.

4. *I recently purchased a laser and have been unable to find any "laser" codes in the CDT Manual. Where are the "laser" codes?*

   CDT codes are procedure based rather than instrument based. You would report the appropriate code based on the actual procedure that was performed without regard to the armamentarium used to deliver the procedure.

5. *A 17-year-old patient required the placement of a crown on tooth #18. Clinically, the tooth has not quite fully erupted. I wanted to place a crown on the tooth that would last a few years, but understood it will need to be replaced. I did not feel that either an acrylic or stainless steel crown would have a good prognosis. Instead I used prefabricated ceramic crown. How do I code this?*

A CDT code just for this type of crown – **D2928 prefabricated porcelain/ ceramic crown for a permanent tooth** – was added in CDT 2021.

6. *Should single crowns that are splinted together be coded as single crowns (in the D2700 series of codes) or as a bridge (in the D6700 series)?*

Single crowns that are splinted together are appropriately reported as single crowns using the applicable code(s) from the "Crowns – Single Restorations Only" (D2700) series of codes.

7. *What procedure code should I report for a porcelain fused to a zirconium substrate crown?*

This question contains a commonly made error, using the word zirconium when describing the crown's material. Dental crowns use zirconia, which is an oxide and considered chemically to be a ceramic.

With this in mind, the applicable procedure code is **D2740 crown – porcelain/ ceramic**.

8. *How do I code a porcelain fused to titanium crown? I only see a code for titanium code **D2794 crown – titanium**.*

Beginning with CDT 2020, there is code, **D2753 crown – porcelain fused to titanium and titanium alloys** available to report a porcelain fused to titanium crown.

9. *Is there a code for retrofitting a new crown to an existing partial denture?*

The code is **D2971 additional procedures to construct new crown under existing partial denture framework** and should be reported in addition to the crown.

10. *Is there a procedure code for re-cementing an onlay?*

D2910 re-cement or re-bond inlay, onlay, or partial coverage restoration includes the re-cementation of an onlay, as well as inlays and any other partial coverage restorations such as a veneer.

11. *If I place an IRM (intermediate restorative material) restoration, do I report this as sedative restoration or a palliative procedure?*

    Delivery and reporting placement of IRM may be reported as either a protective restoration (D2940) or palliative (e.g., emergency) treatment of dental pain (D9110). Selection of one or the other is based on the dentist's clinical judgment as to which most appropriately describes the service delivered to the patient. However, both codes would not be reported simultaneously for the same procedure on the same date of service.

12. *With all the restorative codes published in the CDT manual, when may it be necessary to consider using **D2999 unspecified restorative procedure, by report** to document and report services rendered?*

    No matter how many definitive CDT codes exist exceptional situations arise, sometimes due to widespread adoption of a new procedure, the CDT Code's maintenance timetable, or due to limited frequency or scope of occurrence there is a need to use D2999. Some examples of situations where D2999 would be applicable follow:

    - The restorative procedure was started but was not completed due to clinical complications requiring a referral (e.g., extensive decay necessitating surgical extraction instead of direct restoration) or patient compliance (e.g., patient does not return for placement of permanent crown).
    - The patient's treatment plan includes placement of a prefabricated post and core under an existing crown.
    - The patient's treatment plan includes placement of a prefabricated post without a core.
    - Single crowns are splinted together.

13. *An access cavity was made through a crown for endodontic treatment. What procedure code is appropriate to report sealing an endodontic access cavity?*

    There is no code that specifically addresses the procedure for sealing an endodontic access cavity. Sealing the access cavity is a procedure reported with the appropriate single surface direct restoration code e.g., **D2391 resin-based composite – one surface, posterior**.

14. *My patient had a fractured tooth and I placed a temporary crown solely to protect the remaining tooth structure and space. I usually document this procedure with D2970 but do not see this code in the current CDT manual. What procedure code should I use instead?*

"D2970 temporary crown (fractured tooth)" was deleted when CDT 2016 was published as the Code Maintenance Committee determined: 1) that this entry was limiting by specifying "fractured tooth" in the nomenclature; and 2) there are other codes that more accurately describe the procedure and its intended outcome. In this case the appropriate procedure is placement of a protective restoration (**D2940 protective restoration**) a procedure that protects the tooth and prevents further deterioration.

15. *I placed a temporary restoration to protect my patient's tooth structure and surrounding tissues. Would **D2940 protective restoration** be appropriate for reporting this procedure?*

Yes, D2940 is appropriate based on the code's descriptor, which follows:

Direct placement of a restorative material to protect tooth and/or tissue form. This procedure may be used to relieve pain, promote healing, or prevent further deterioration. Not to be used for endodontic access closure, or as a base or liner under restoration.

16. *There are post and core codes only in the restorative category, but not in the fixed prosthodontics category. What is the correct code to use when the final restoration will be a multiple unit fixed bridge?*

The codes in the restorative category may be used when a single crown or a multiple unit fixed prosthesis is the final restoration. Remember the placement of codes within categories is to enable ease of navigation through the CDT Code and does not limit use of codes across specialties:

> **D2952**   **post and core in addition to crown, indirectly fabricated**
>
> **D2954**   **prefabricated post and core in addition to crown**

17. What code should be reported for placement of a composite restoration in a non-carious cervical lesion or an erosive lesion in a cusp tip or other surface of a tooth?

    Such lesions are treated with resin materials, which include glass ionomers, and the appropriate code depends on tooth position: anterior or posterior. The applicable code for an anterior tooth is:

    D2330   resin-based composite – one surface, anterior

    For a posterior tooth the applicable code is:

    D2391   resin-based composite – one surface, posterior
    > Used to restore a carious lesion into the dentin or a deeply eroded area into the dentin. Not a preventive procedure.

    Note: Non-carious cervical lesions commonly extend into the dentin due to thin enamel at this portion of a tooth's anatomy. In an exceptional situation where the lesion does not extend into a posterior tooth's dentin the available procedure code is:

    D2999   unspecified restorative procedure, by report

18. I repaired a porcelain "chip" on a PFM crown. What procedure code would I use?

    D2980   crown repair necessitated by restorative material failure

19. A college student presented with a "chip" on #10. The patient had an enamel fracture of the disto-incisal of #10. She had the chipped piece of enamel. I bonded the fractured enamel piece back on the tooth until the patient could get back to her hometown dentist. What procedure code should I use?

    D2921   reattachment of tooth fragment, incisal edge or cusp

20. A child became uncooperative as I was removing the decay on a primary molar. I was able to remove all the decay but unable to place a permanent restoration due to the patient's behavior. Eventually the primary molar will need a stainless steel crown. However I placed glass ionomer in the cavity to aid in healing prior to definitive treatment. How should I code this?

    D2941   interim therapeutic restoration – primary dentition

21. I had to remove a post and core on tooth #9. What code should I use to document this?

    D2955   post removal

22. *The periodontal diagnosis suggests the fabrication of two adjacent PFM single crowns that are splinted for additional strength to oppose masticatory forces. Appropriate individual crown codes should be utilized, as there is no CDT coding mechanism to indicate the crowns are splinted. How should I code this?*

D2750   porcelain fused to high noble metal

This procedure is reported twice, and the patient's record should note that the individual crowns were splinted for additional strength. The splint may be reported with D2999 unspecified restorative procedure, by report.

23. *A patient presented with a fractured gold inlay. The doctor placed a provisional inlay, anticipating a final restoration. What code should be used to report this treatment?*

D2999   unspecified restorative procedure, by report

24. *A patient presented with a partial fracture of a fixed partial denture. The doctor believes this can be repaired without complete replacement. What code should be used to report the repair?*

D6980   fixed partial denture repair necessitated by restorative material failure

25. *What is a strip crown and how do I record it?*

A "strip crown" is a direct procedure that involves: 1) placing a form on the tooth; 2) filling the form with composite resin that bonds directly to the tooth in the shape of a crown; 3) removal of the form from the tooth after the composite resin cures (i.e., the form is "stripped away" from the tooth and composite resin crown); and 4) finishing and final polishing as necessary.

The ADA's position is that a "strip crown" procedure would be reported with a CDT Code listed within the "Resin-Based Composite Restorations — Direct" subcategory of service. Further, the dentist who delivers this procedure would consider the full CDT Code entry when determining the code that appropriately describes the service she or he delivered. Should a dentist be delivering a direct composite resin restoration, selection of the appropriate CDT Code is affected by the preparation —

a. If the restoration is full coverage with no visible original enamel, this is a crown procedure documented with the following CDT Code.

D2390   resin-based composite crown, anterior
Full resin-based composite coverage of tooth.

Note: Should a dentist elect to deliver such a direct crown to a posterior tooth, the applicable CDT Code is **D2999 unspecified restorative procedure, by report**.

b. If some of the original enamel is preserved on any of the surfaces, this is a multi-surface restoration procedure documented with one of the following CDT Codes.

D2335 resin-based composite – four or more surfaces or involving incisal angle (anterior)
Incisal angle to be defined as one of the angles formed by the junction of the incisal and the mesial or distal surface of an anterior tooth.

D2394 resin-based composite – four or more surfaces, posterior

There is no question that a "strip crown" procedure is a direct resin-based composite restoration procedure. All the clinical steps occur inside the patient's mouth, which meets the ADA Glossary of Dental Clinical and Administrative Terms definition of direct restorations ("A restoration fabricated inside the mouth."). The "strip" is simply a form that enables creation of the artificial crown in-situ.

Summary

Restorative procedures are an integral part of treatment that patients receive every day. Because we use the restorative codes so frequently, we must make sure that over time we are indeed using the correct code. It is important for the dentist and the coder to be familiar with any CDT Code changes that enable them to more accurately document and report the procedure delivered to a patient.

Remember, "Code for what you do and do what you code for."

Contributor Biography

Fred L. Horowitz, D.M.D. is president of Primecare Benefits, Inc., a dental insurance holding company based in Nevada. Following graduation from Washington University School of Dental Medicine, Dr Horowitz completed a general practice residency at Sinai Hospital of Detroit. He practiced full time for ten years and has since had executive level positions with dental benefits companies across the country. He is also a three-term board member of the National Association of Dental Plans (NADP), and served on the Board of the National Dental EDI Council, and the National Association of Specialty Health Organizations. He represented the United States dental payer industry to the International Health Terminology Standards Development Organization (now SNOMED), serving as the Vice-Chairman of the International Dental SIG component. He also currently serves on the Joint Operating Committee of the Culinary Health Center, and the Board of Directors of Access Health Dental, a DSO based in Las Vegas, NV.

By Elizabeth Shin Perry, D.M.D.

Introduction

The Endodontics category of service describes procedures which involve treatment of the dental pulp, root canals, and the tissues surrounding the roots of the tooth. These codes describe nonsurgical procedures related to debridement and disinfection of the root canal space, maintenance and regeneration of the pulp, removal of previously placed materials within the root canal space (including root canal filling, posts, and broken instruments), and obturation of the root canal space. In addition, endodontic surgical codes describe periradicular surgical procedures such as apicoectomy and root amputation, root repair due to perforation or resorptive defects, exploratory curettage to examine for root damage, placement of retrograde filling materials, intentional re-implantation, and placement of bone grafting and regeneration materials.

Some of the main challenges typical to endodontics involve coding for procedures which require multiple appointments. Other concerns relate to what should be coded separately from an endodontic therapy procedure such as D3331 (root canal obstruction treatment) or D2955 (post removal). Another question often encountered is which radiographs are considered part of the endodontic therapy procedure. Separately, CDT code entries for procedures that involve pulpal regeneration are clear, but they are less commonly used and can be confusing unless the process has been studied by the office coding specialist.

It is important to understand that procedure codes are meant to describe the treatment rendered, not the means that are used to accomplish the treatment. For example, disinfection of a root canal during endodontic therapy can be accomplished using different techniques, including irrigation with multiple irrigating solutions and devices. The code used for the procedure, however, is the same.

Key Definitions and Concepts

Root canal: This term is used both for the passage or channel in the root of the tooth extending from the pulp chamber to the apical foramen, and also to describe the endodontic therapy procedure which involves cleaning, shaping and obturating the canals with a dental material. Thus, it has two different definitions, as a noun and also as a verb as in "to root canal." Some teeth have a single root canal space, while others have multiple. A root canal procedure for a given tooth treats all of the root canal spaces within the tooth. The root canal therapy procedure is referred to as "endodontic therapy" in the CDT code set.

> The ADA Glossary definition of **root canal** is "The portion of the pulp cavity inside the root of a tooth; the chamber within the root of the tooth that contains the pulp."

> The ADA Glossary definition of **root canal therapy** is "The treatment of disease and injuries of the pulp and associated periradicular conditions."

Endodontic therapy: The procedure which involves the cleaning, shaping, and obturating the root canals of a tooth. Also known as root canal therapy.

Pulpectomy: The process of removal of the pulp entirely from the root canal space.

> The ADA Glossary definition of **pulpectomy** is "Complete removal of vital and non-vital pulp tissue from the root canal space."

Pulpotomy: The process of removal of the pulp from the pulp chamber only, but not the root canal spaces within a tooth. A pulpotomy may be used as a temporary solution to relieve symptoms or as a permanent solution for a tooth which may be able to maintain pulp vitality despite exposure of the pulp.

> The ADA Glossary definition of **pulpotomy** is "Removal of a portion of the pulp, including the diseased aspect, with the intent of maintaining the vitality of the remaining pulpal tissue by means of a therapeutic dressing."

Irrigation: Part of the endodontic therapy procedure in which a disinfectant fluid is used to flush and disinfect the root canals.

Obturation: The process of filling the root canal space (where the dental pulp normally resides) with some type of dental material. This process must be performed for endodontic therapy to be complete. After obturation a tooth must be permanently restored with a coronal restoration.

> The ADA Glossary definition of **obturate** is "With reference to endodontics, refers to the sealing of the canal(s) of tooth roots during root canal therapy

procedure with an appropriately prescribed material such as gutta percha in combination with a suitable luting agent."

Dental dam: A rubber-like sheet used to isolate a tooth from the oral environment and to prevent migration of fluids or foreign objects into or out of the operative field. Dental dams are considered standard operating procedure per the American Association of Endodontist's Position Statement entitled, "Dental Dams" found at:

www.aae.org/specialty/wp-content/uploads/sites/2/2017/06/ dentaldamstatement.pdf

There are endodontic therapy procedures which involve surgical manipulation prior to rubber dam placement. In these cases rubber dam placement is documented using CDT code **D3910 surgical procedure for isolation of tooth with rubber dam**.

Pulpal regeneration: A biologically-based procedure designed to physiologically replace damaged tooth structures, including dentin and root structures, as well as cells of the pulp-dentin complex of an incompletely formed root in teeth with necrotic pulps.

Apexification: A method to induce a calcified barrier in a root with an open apex or the continued apical development of an incompletely formed root in teeth with necrotic pulps.

> The ADA Glossary definition of **apexification** is "The process of induced root development to encourage the formation of a calcified barrier in a tooth with immature root formation or an open apex. May involve the placement of an artificial apical barrier prior to nonsurgical endodontic obturation."

Apexogenesis: A vital pulp therapy procedure performed to encourage continued physiological development and formation of the root end.

> The ADA Glossary definition of **apexogenesis** is "Vital pulp therapy performed to encourage continued physiological formation and development of the tooth root."

Chapter 4: D3000–D3999 Endodontics

Changes to This Category

Six codes were added to the Endodontics category to enable differentiation and more accurate documentation of procedures that would have been reported with a single code until CDT 2021 became effective. These new codes replace one deleted code.

The six new codes are:

D3471 **surgical repair of root resorption – anterior**
For surgery on root of anterior tooth. Does not include placement of restoration.

D3472 **surgical repair of root resorption – premolar**
For surgery on root of premolar tooth. Does not include placement of restoration.

D3473 **surgical repair of root resorption – molar**
For surgery on root of molar tooth. Does not include placement of restoration.

D3501 **surgical exposure of root surface without apicoectomy or repair of root resorption – anterior**
Exposure of root surface followed by observation and surgical closure of the exposed area. Not to be used for or in conjunction with apicoectomy or repair of root resorption.

D3502 **surgical exposure of root surface without apicoectomy or repair of root resorption – premolar**
Exposure of root surface followed by observation and surgical closure of the exposed area. Not to be used for or in conjunction with apicoectomy or repair of root resorption.

D3503 **surgical exposure of root surface without apicoectomy or repair of root resorption – molar**
Exposure of root surface followed by observation and surgical closure of the exposed area. Not to be used for or in conjunction with apicoectomy or repair of root resorption.

The one deleted code is:

~~**D3427**~~ ~~**periradicular surgery without apicoectomy**~~

Clinical Coding Scenario #1:
Root Canal Started in Another State

A patient presents for endodontic treatment of tooth #29, having had a root canal started on this single rooted tooth in another state while on vacation. The patient is not in any pain. An exam is performed and diagnostic, preoperative radiographs (a periapical and a bitewing) are taken and evaluated. The radiographs shows evidence of a large periapical radiolucency as well as radiopaque evidence that calcium hydroxide has likely been placed in the root canal space. A treatment plan is made to complete root canal therapy and restore the tooth with a buildup and crown.

During the patient's second visit, the appointment during which the root canal was intended to be completed, it is found that ninety minutes was insufficient to complete the case. A significant amount of purulence was seen actively exuding into the tooth from the periapical tissues. The tooth was dressed with calcium hydroxide and temporized. A third treatment visit was scheduled.

During the third visit the root canal was completed and a core buildup was placed. An intraoperative radiograph and two post-operative radiographs were taken during this appointment. A crown preparation appointment was scheduled for a later date.

What procedure codes would be used to document and report the services provided during each of the three encounters?

Visit #1: Initial Appointment

    D0140 **limited oral evaluation – problem focused**

    D0220 **intraoral – periapical first radiographic image**

    D0270 **bitewing – single radiographic image**

Visit #2: Root Canal Begun, But Not Completed

    D2940 **protective restoration**

    D3999 **unspecified endodontic procedure, by report**
        [to indicate that the root canal was not completed]

Visit #3: Root Canal Completed and Core Buildup Placed

    D3320 **endodontic therapy, premolar (excluding final restoration)**

    D2950 **core buildup, including any pins when required**

Note: The third visit's radiograph would be documented in the patient's record but not included in the claim submission as the "Endodontic Therapy" subcategory descriptor states that the procedures "...includes intra-operative radiographs..." Any radiographs taken for diagnostic purposes, during visit #1 in this scenario, are appropriately included separately on the claim for that date of service.

Clinical Coding Scenario #2:
Pulpectomy

A patient of record calls the office with a severe toothache. He did not sleep well the previous night and needs to be seen by a dentist immediately. The schedule is already fully committed, but accommodations are made to see the patient during the office lunch hour.

The patient presents to the office and periapical and bitewing radiographs are taken. A problem-focused examination is performed and the patient is diagnosed with symptomatic irreversible pulpitis and symptomatic apical periodontitis of tooth #30. Definitive treatment is recommended to relieve the patient's pain.

A complete pulpectomy was performed and a temporary restoration was placed as emergency treatment. Three weeks later, the patient returns for completion of the root canal and the access opening closed by placement of composite resin restorative material.

What procedure codes would be used to document and report the services provided during each of the two encounters?

Visit #1

D0140   **limited oral evaluation – problem focused**

D0220   **intraoral – periapical first radiographic image**

D0270   **bitewing – single radiographic image**

D3221   **pulpal debridement, primary and permanent teeth**

D2940   **protective restoration**

Visit #2

D3330   **endodontic therapy, molar (excluding final restoration)**

D2391   **resin-based composite – one surface, posterior**

Note: **D2391** is the procedure often used when sealing the access opening in the tooth's crown requires a relatively uncomplicated restoration. When sealing the access opening is more complicated core buildup (**D2950**) and crown (e.g., **D2740**), procedures are more likely to be delivered and reported.

Clinical Coding Scenario #3:
Patient Referral for Apicoectomy

A patient is referred by a friend who is a general dentist. The general dentist referred this patient for an "apico" of tooth #3 since the referring dentist prefers not to do this type of procedure in her practice. It is determined that periapical radiographs and a cone beam computed tomography (CBCT) image are needed to evaluate the complex case prior to determining the treatment plan.

A problem-focused examination was performed, along with capture and evaluation of a CBCT image of a portion of the upper jaw and two periapical radiographs. A diagnosis of chronic apical periodontitis was made and a treatment plan for apicoectomy was confirmed. Included in the plan is a bone graft, which will be used due to the presence of the large lesion that appears to have eroded both the buccal and palatal cortical plates of bone. Consent is received and an appointment is scheduled.

Note: A surgery of this nature is not usually done on an emergency basis and often the examination is done on a day separate from the procedure.

The surgery is performed for tooth #3 on both the MB and DB roots. 3 mm of each root end was resected and a root-end filling was placed in each root end. A confirmation periapical radiograph was taken. Non-autogenous bone graft material was placed. There was no sinus perforation in the surgical field and it was determined that no barrier would be needed in this situation.

Sutures were placed and post-operative instructions given. The patient returned for suture removal after a few days. This follow-up appointment was uneventful and sutures were removed.

What procedure codes would be used to document and report the services provided during each of the three encounters?

Visit #1: Initial Appointment

D0140 **limited oral evaluation – problem focused**

D0220 **intraoral – periapical first radiographic image**

D0230 **intraoral – periapical each additional radiographic image**

D0364 **cone beam CT capture and interpretation with limited field of view – less than one whole jaw**

Visit #2: Endodontic Procedures Delivered

D3425 **apicoectomy – molar (first root)**

D3426 **apicoectomy (each additional root)**

D3430 **retrograde filling – per root**

D3430 **retrograde filling – per root**

Note: Root-end fillings are coded per root. For a tooth #3, often there are two roots, which is why D3430 is reported twice.

D3428 **bone graft in conjunction with periradicular surgery – per tooth, single site**

D3431 **biologic materials to aid in soft and osseous tissue regeneration in conjunction with periradicular surgery**

Visit #3: Post-operative Follow Up, Sutures Removed

D0171 **re-evaluation – post-operative office visit**

Note: Visit #3 is the suture removal appointment that is considered part of the patient's routine follow-up care. There is no CDT code for the post-operative suture removal procedure.

 © American Dental Association

Clinical Coding Scenario #4:
Emergency Root Canal Patient

A patient of record presents with a dental emergency of severe pain in tooth #9. Clinical examination is performed and radiographs are taken. A diagnosis of symptomatic irreversible pulpitis with symptomatic apical periodontitis is made and root canal therapy is recommended as emergency treatment.

The following codes would be utilized for what would be a typical and straight forward procedure that is completed in the same day, with the access opening restored with composite resin material:

D0140   limited oral evaluation – problem focused
D0220   intraoral – periapical first radiographic image

Note: If more than one periapical is taken cite number of additional images with:
D0230 intraoral – periapical each additional radiographic image

D3310   endodontic therapy, anterior tooth (excluding final restoration)
D2330   resin-based composite – one surface, anterior

What if I see them for a root canal appointment on emergency basis, then have to refer it out to a specialist?

In this case, if a general dentist opens a tooth on an emergency basis due to pain and then feels the need to refer the case, the following codes could be utilized to document the situation:

D0140   limited oral evaluation – problem focused
D0220   intraoral – periapical first radiographic image

Note: If more than one periapical is taken cite number of additional images with:
D0230 intraoral – periapical each additional radiographic image

D3221   pulpal debridement, primary and permanent teeth
D2940   protective restoration

Notes: The pulpal debridement, also known as pulpectomy, (D3221) is done to alleviate acute pain. A protective restoration (D2940) is placed for temporary protection of the pulp chamber until the necessary endodontic therapy can be performed.

A referral is then made to an endodontist for specialty care. The endodontist would then perform and code for the following procedures – a limited oral evaluation; new diagnostic preoperative radiographs to establish the present condition; endodontic therapy; restore the access opening. The procedures and coding for access opening restoration would depend upon the restorative situation (e.g., simple closure; crown placement).

Clinical Coding Scenario #5:
Pulpal Regeneration

Visit #1: Initial Appointment

A 12-year-old patient presents with a somewhat painful tooth #29. The parent noticed that the child avoids chewing on the tooth.

Clinical examination is performed and radiographs (one bitewing and one periapical) are taken. There is mild swelling in the vestibule, buccal to tooth #29. It is percussion sensitive, palpation sensitive, slightly mobile (class I) and there are no probing depths over 3 mm. The tooth is sensitive to biting on the Tooth Slooth® and is non-responsive to pulp vitality testing. The tooth has never been restored and no caries is present, radiographically or clinically. Radiographically a moderately-sized periapical radiolucency is present. There is a very tall pulp chamber, making the enamel look like a thin shell, rather than a thick band over the occlusal area of the pulp chamber. The apex of the tooth has an immature foramen with no apical constriction and the apical opening is over 1 mm wide. The tooth appears 3–5 mm shorter than adjacent tooth #28.

A diagnosis of pulpal necrosis and acute apical abscess is made. The etiology is determined to be that a dens evaginatus tubercle had previously fractured and led to ingress of bacteria and eventual pulpal necrosis. A treatment plan for pulpal regeneration is discussed, and with the parent's consent, treatment is initiated.

Local anesthetic is administered, a rubber dam is placed, and an access opening is made. The canal is appropriately instrumented and irrigated according to established protocols. Calcium hydroxide or antibiotic paste is placed as an intracanal medicament and a temporary restoration is placed.

What CDT Codes are applicable for the procedures delivered during this visit?

- **D0140**   **limited oral evaluation – problem focused**
- **D0220**   **intraoral – periapical first radiographic image**
- **D0270**   **bitewing – single radiographic image**
- **D0460**   **pulp vitality tests**
- **D3355**   **pulpal regeneration – initial visit**
- **D2940**   **protective restoration**

Visit #2

The patient is asymptomatic at the second visit, three weeks after initiation of treatment. There is no swelling, the tooth is not abnormally mobile, but the patient is unable to chew normally upon tooth #29. Local anesthetic is administered, a rubber dam is placed, the tooth is re-instrumented, re-irrigated and re-medicated and a temporary restoration is placed.

The CDT code for the second visit is:

D3356   pulpal regeneration – interim medication replacement

D2940   protective restoration

Visit #3

Three weeks have passed since the second visit. The tooth is now completely normal; all symptoms have resolved. Local anesthetic is administered, a rubber dam is placed, and the canal space is re-irrigated to remove all intracanal medicament. Apical bleeding is initiated, a bioceramic barrier is placed in the cervical area of the root canal, and a composite restoration is placed in the access opening. A final radiograph is taken for documentation and to be used as a baseline for future follow up. Regular follow-up visits are recommended to monitor the maturation of the root of tooth #29.

The CDT codes for this third visit are:

D3357   pulpal regeneration – completion of treatment

D2391   resin-based composite – one surface, posterior

Clinical Coding Scenario #6:
Apicoectomy with Bony Defect

A 36-year-old patient presents complaining of pain on tooth #9. The tooth is very dark and the soft tissues buccal to the tooth exhibit swelling and fluctuance. Radiographic examination (two periapical images, and a CBCT image of a portion of the lower jaw, were captured and interpreted) reveals a very large periapical radiolucency associated with tooth #9. The patient reports a history of a traumatic injury involving the tooth when he was a child. An antibiotic was prescribed.

The next morning the patient returns and endodontic therapy of tooth #9 is performed. Later that same day, surgical exposure of the area is performed, with an incision extending from the distal of #8 to the distal of #10 to reveal the a large area of perforation of the buccal cortical plate. Curettage of the bony defect was performed to reveal the lesion extends to the palatal cortical plate. Apicoectomy of tooth #9 was completed, the bony defect was irrigated, and 2 gm of bone graft material was placed.

How would these procedures be documented?

Visit #1: Initial Appointment

Radiographs

D0220 intraoral – periapical first radiographic image

D0230 intraoral – periapical each additional radiographic image

D0364 cone beam CT capture and interpretation with limited field of view – less than one whole jaw

Oral Evaluation

D0140 limited oral evaluation – problem focused

Prescribe antibiotic – No applicable CDT code

Note: D9630 drugs or medicaments dispensed in office for home use is not applicable since the nomenclature states this procedure applies to drugs or medicaments dispensed in the office for home use, and its descriptor specifically excludes writing prescriptions.

Visit #2 – Morning

Root canal on #9

> **D3310 endodontic therapy, anterior tooth (excluding final restoration)**

Visit #2 – Afternoon

Apicoectomy on #9

> **D3410 apicoectomy – anterior**

Curettage and irrigation of the bony defect require no separate CDT code; these actions are considered a component of D3410.

Placement of 2 gm of bone graft material to preserve the bone around teeth #8 and #9.

> **D3428 bone graft in conjunction with periradicular surgery – per tooth, single site**

> **D3429 bone graft in conjunction with periradicular surgery – each additional contiguous tooth in the same surgical site**

Note: "D7955 repair of maxillofacial soft and/or hard tissue defect" could apply depending on how much the defect that requires bone grafting extends beyond the treated tooth, But D7955 should not be reported in addition to D3428 or D3429.

Clinical Coding Scenario #7:
Non-carious Cervical Resorption Lesion

A patient presents with invasive cervical resorption on the buccal of tooth #18. It was discovered during a routine hygiene appointment when a periapical and a bitewing radiograph were taken. The tooth has no symptoms. It is clear that this lesion is not caries, as a cavitated lesion cannot be detected with any type of explorer. There is no periapical radiolucency.

When areas of resorption are suspected, the American Association of Endodontics and the American Association of Oral and Maxillofacial Radiography recommend the following: "Limited field of view CBCT is the imaging modality of choice in the localization and differentiation of external and internal resorptive defects and the determination of appropriate treatment and prognosis."

The CBCT scan is taken and a diagnosis of a Heithersay Class II external invasive cervical resorption on the buccal surface of the tooth #18 is made. The treatment plan includes surgical exposure of the resorptive defect followed by external repair of the resorptive lesion.

A full thickness mucoperiosteal flap is reflected and the area of resorption is identified and excavated. There is no exposure of the pulp in the excavation of the resorptive defect. The area of resorption is then treated with 90% trichloracetic acid to arrest the progression of the resorption. The defect is restored with a resin-modified glass ionomer. The area is surgically closed and sutures are placed. The patient is instructed to return for suture removal and continued follow up to monitor the pulpal status and to identify any onset of pulpitis.

How would you code for this scenario?

> **D0140**   limited oral evaluation – problem focused
>
> **D0220**   intraoral – periapical first radiographic image
>
> **D0270**   bitewing – single radiographic image
>
> **D0364**   cone beam CT capture and interpretation with limited field of view – less than one whole jaw
>
> **D3473**   surgical repair of root resorption – molar
>
> **D2391**   resin-based composite – one surface, posterior

Note: D3473 is a CDT code for surgical repair of root resorption effective January 1, 2021. It is one of three additions, parsed by tooth type (anterior, premolar, molar) that would previously be reported with **D3427 periradicular surgery without apicoectomy**.

Clinical Coding Scenario #8:
Surgical Exposure of Root Surface for Exploration

A patient presents for evaluation and treatment of tooth #10 which has a persistent sinus tract. The tooth has a history of root canal therapy two years previously. Radiographic examination with a periapical radiograph reveals a small periapical radiolucency. Clinically, no significant periodontal probing defects are seen and the sinus tract can be traced to the apex of tooth #10.

When evaluating a previously endodontically treated tooth with a non-healing lesion, the American Association of Endodontics and the American Association of Oral and Maxillofacial Radiography recommend the following:

> "Limited field of view CBCT should be the imaging modality of choice when evaluating the non-healing of previous endodontic treatment to help determine the need for further treatment, such as nonsurgical, surgical or extraction."

A CBCT scan is taken and a diagnosis of chronic apical abscess of previously endodontically treated tooth #10 is made. The treatment plan includes surgical exposure of the periapex of tooth #10 followed by apicoectomy, if indicated.

An Ochsenbein-Luebke mucoperiosteal flap is reflected and a perforating defect is seen in the buccal cortex over the periapex of tooth #10. Curettage of the apical lesion is performed and the root surface can be visualized to reveal a 6 mm vertical root fracture from the mid-root to the apex of the tooth. At this point the prognosis of the tooth is determined to be guarded and extraction is indicated. Due to treatment planning and esthetic considerations, the extraction will be done at a later date. The area is surgically closed and sutures are placed.

How would you code for this scenario?

D0140 **limited oral evaluation – problem focused**

D0220 **intraoral – periapical first radiographic image**

D0364 **cone beam CT capture and interpretation with limited field of view – less than one whole jaw**

D3501 **surgical exposure of root surface without apicoectomy or repair of root resorption – anterior**

Note: D3501 is a code effective January 1, 2021 to report surgical exposure of root surface without apicoectomy or repair of root resorption. This code's descriptor describes the procedure as exposure of the root surface followed by observation and surgical closure of the exposed area, and this procedure is not used for or in conjunction with apicoectomy or repair of root resorption. D3501 is one of three additions, parsed by tooth type (anterior, premolar, molar) that would previously be reported with **D3427 periradicular surgery without apicoectomy**.

Remember, the existence of a code does not mean that this code will be covered by a given patient's dental benefits, despite recommendations by a dental professional.

 © American Dental Association

Clinical Coding Scenario #9:
Emergency Incision and Drainage and Endodontic Therapy

A patient presents with significant facial swelling and pain in the upper right quadrant. She reports that she had multiple crowns placed in this quadrant and that her dentist told her that she may need a root canal in the future. Clinical examination is performed and a periapical and bitewing radiographs are taken. In addition, a CBCT scan is taken to aid in the diagnosis. A diagnosis of pulpal necrosis with acute apical abscess of tooth #2 is made and a treatment plan for incision and drainage of the facial swelling followed by endodontic therapy of tooth is discussed.

Incision and drainage is performed with significant purulent drainage. Root canal therapy of tooth #2 is initiated at the same visit; the root canals are instrumented completely and the tooth is medicated with calcium hydroxide followed by the placement of a temporary restoration.

The patient returns two weeks later and the swelling and discomfort has resolved completely. Root canal therapy of tooth #2 is completed with re-instrumentation followed by obturation of the canals. The access opening is permanently restored with composite.

How would you code for this scenario?

Visit #1

> **D0140** limited oral evaluation – problem focused
>
> **D0220** intraoral – periapical first radiographic image
>
> **D0270** bitewing – single radiographic image
>
> **D0364** cone beam CT capture and interpretation with limited field of view – less than one whole jaw
>
> **D7510** incision and drainage of abscess – intraoral soft tissue
>
> **D3999** unspecified endodontic procedure, by report

Note: Root canal procedure was initiated but not completed. Record should note that pulpal debridement was performed on this date of service.

> **D2940** protective restoration

Visit #2

> **D3330** endodontic therapy, molar (excluding final restoration)
>
> **D2391** resin-based composite – one surface, posterior

Coding Q&A

1. *I worked really hard on a tooth that had six root canals in it and it seems like I should be able to have a code to express the difficulty of the case.*

   CDT codes for documenting and reporting endodontic therapy procedures by tooth type or location (e.g., anterior, premolar, molar) were established with CDT-1, effective January 1, 1990. This change replaced dental procedure codes based on number of canals per tooth (2, 3 or 4), plus a separate code for "each additional canal" that is used when needed. The rationale was that tooth anatomy or location better reflects the degree of difficulty most often encountered in clinical situations.

2. *I want to use an expensive adjunct irrigant or irrigating device, instead of, or in addition to, the traditional sodium hypochlorite that is commonly used. What code can I use to reflect the additional expertise and expense?*

   Irrigation as well as other aspects of endodontic therapy are considered part of the procedure itself and are included in the code set for the type of tooth for which the root canal is performed. Separating out what is generally considered part of the procedure is often called "unbundling." From an ethical perspective intentional unbundling by a dentist to increase reimbursement and intentional bundling by a third-party payer to decrease reimbursement, are both considered inappropriate.

3. *How can I use the CDT Code to describe that I have done an endodontic therapy in two visits instead of one visit? It costs the dentist more to do it in two visits, and I think that should be reflected.*

   This is a common inquiry made to the American Association of Endodontists that has multiple considerations. One question is about how to document the two visits. The first visit, when the need for RCT is diagnosed and then started, may be recorded with D3999 for record-keeping purposes. Then, at the second appointment, the typical D3330 code is used to reflect the completion of the treatment.

   The second, implied question seems to be more about how to charge more for the procedure than the dentist's established full D3330 fee. There is not a simple answer, as every dentist is responsible for determining their fee and when doing so must consider the legal and ethical ramifications of having different full fees for the same procedure. This consideration should include a review of your participating provider contracts in effect and discussion with your legal counsel.

 © American Dental Association

In addition, coding for a root canal that was never actually finished is a recurring issue. If the code for the root canal is submitted, but the procedure has not been completed, corrections must be made with the dental benefits company involved, and explanations must be made to the patient and any other dentist or specialist who becomes involved in the completion of the treatment. Clear communication using the codes as the language and descriptor for treatment performed is helpful for all parties involved.

4. *What is the difference between using the apexification codes and the pulpal regeneration codes?*

The procedures are very different in their intentions.

Apexification is a procedure which had previously been the only option to treat teeth that had necrotic pulp and open apices and immature root formation. Long-term calcium hydroxide treatment was used until a hard tissue bridge formed over the apex. Gutta-percha could then be safely condensed against that bridge, in a manner that prevented the root filling material from extruding into the periapical tissues.

In contrast, pulpal regeneration is a different way to treat these teeth with necrotic pulp and open apices and immature root formation. Pulpal regeneration involves disinfection of the root canal system and using stem cell technology to stimulate ingrowth of pulp-like tissue into the root canal. This process promotes maturation of the root, including closure of the open apex, and increased length and width of the root canal walls.

5. *When is it appropriate to use* **D3331 treatment of a canal obstruction; non-surgical access?**

This code is to document a procedure that is delivered infrequently and for extremely difficult cases, such as one where the root canal is more than 50% calcified. Another example of when a dentist separates a file in the canal and then refers the case to a new dentist or specialist who is able to remove it using their expertise and specialized equipment.

6. *When retreating a root canal that had a post and core I had to spend a significant amount of time removing the post prior to performing the retreatment. I submitted the codes for post removal and retreatment and the dental benefits company denied benefits for the post removal. What should I do?*

Coding for this scenario is straightforward as there are two separate procedures – **D2955 post removal** and **D3346 (or D3347 or D3348) retreatment of previous root canal therapy**. In cases when the procedure requires more than one visit D2955 (post removal) is usually completed and posted on the first visit, and the root canal retreatment (e.g., D3346) is posted on the second or final visit when this separate procedure is completed.

While post removal is clearly a distinct procedure separate from retreatment of previous root canal therapy, some dental benefit companies "bundle" the post removal into the retreatment. According to the ADA, bundling, or the "the systematic combining of distinct dental procedures by third-party payers that results in a reduced benefit for the patient/beneficiary" is frowned upon. Dentists who have signed participating provider agreements with third-party payers may be bound to plan provisions that limit or exclude coverage. Submission of a short narrative with the original claim or appeal, explaining the complexity of the post removal along with radiographs and/or photographs, may be helpful in obtaining full available reimbursement for both procedures.

7. *A patient was referred to me after a dentist attempted endodontic treatment and perforated the furcation of tooth #19. I repaired the perforation with bioceramic putty internally and completed the endodontic therapy. How do I code for the placement of the bioceramic putty?*

D3333 internal root repair of perforation defects is used for the perforation repair procedure. The use of bioceramic putty is not relevant as the CDT code entry does not specify (i.e., limit) the material that the dentist may select to repair the perforation defect.

Summary

Dental procedure codes that are applicable and from the CDT Code version effective on the date of service are integral to a complete patient record as they describe the endodontic treatment that has been performed. "Code for what you do" is the fundamental rule in all coding situations. The existence of a procedure code does not necessarily mean that it is a covered service of a given dental benefit plan. Unless a code is used appropriately and submitted, dental benefit plans will not have a history of the frequency of use or fees associated with the procedures performed. By consistently coding for endodontic procedures as they are performed, we may influence third-party payers for consideration of coverage in the future.

Contributor Biography

Elizabeth Shin Perry, D.M.D. is a board certified endodontist and has been in private practice in Westfield, Massachusetts since 1995. She is a graduate of the University of Pennsylvania and the Harvard School of Dental Medicine. She completed her post-doctoral residency in endodontics at the University of Connecticut. Dr. Perry is past chair of the Practice Affairs Committee of the American Association of Endodontists and serves as District I Director on the AAE's Board of Directors. She has been active in code maintenance nationally since 2016 and also represents the AAE as a voting member of the American Dental Association's Code Maintenance Committee.

Chapter 5: D4000–D4999 Periodontics

By Marie Schweinebraten, D.M.D.

Introduction

Periodontal treatment has seen many changes over time. For example, different types of grafting material, both autogenous and non-autogenous, are more common. Dental implants are often included in periodontal treatment planning. Bone regeneration has become more predictable with the availability of new products and techniques. Periodontal procedure coding has grown with these changes as has the knowledge base required to code correctly and obtain reimbursement for the treatment completed.

Periodontics has always been a unique category because it has included both non-surgical and surgical procedures. What complicates matters is that some of the codes are site specific while others are tooth, quadrant (four or more teeth), or area (one to three teeth) specific. Adding to the confusion is that procedure codes have become differentiated as to the type of material used as well as to whether the procedure is performed on a tooth or implant. There are also many periodontal codes that overlap with codes from other categories.

Thus, for a given outcome there could be a number of separate procedures involved, each documented with its individual CDT code. Grafts are an example of such "á la carte" coding. Bone graft materials are listed separately from the procedure for achieving access – osseous surgery (D4260 or D4261) or gingival flap (D4240 or D4241). There are separate codes for other procedures that may be required in a graft case, including placement of barrier membranes or biologic materials to aid in regeneration.

It is especially important in the Periodontics category to realize that procedure codes are meant to describe the treatment rendered, not the means that are used to accomplish the treatment. For example, a gingivectomy can be done by several techniques, including utilizing a blade, a periodontal knife or a laser. The code for the procedure, however, is the same.

With attention to detail and a basic understanding of periodontal treatment and the codes, a dental office can prevent confusion for the patient and misunderstanding of plan coverage while at the same time obtaining reimbursement as effectively and efficiently as possible.

Key Definitions and Concepts

Full quadrant: The mouth is divided into four quadrants. A full quadrant is defined for coding purposes as four or more teeth.

> The ADA Glossary definition of **quadrant** is: "One of the four equal sections into which the dental arches can be divided; begins at the midline of the arch and extends distally to the last tooth."

Partial quadrant: One to three contiguous teeth, when present within the same quadrant, is defined as a partial quadrant.

Site: The term site is used to describe a single area, or position. "Site" is frequently used to describe an area of recession on a single tooth or an osseous defect adjacent to a single tooth. It can also apply to soft tissue or osseous defects in an edentulous area.

For example:

- If two contiguous teeth have areas of recession, each tooth is considered a single site.
- If two contiguous teeth have adjacent but separate osseous defects, each defect is a single site. If these defects communicate, however, they would be considered a single site.
- Up to two contiguous tooth positions in an edentulous area may be considered a single site.

> The ADA Glossary definition of **site** is: "A term used to describe a single area, position, or locus. For periodontal procedures, an area of soft tissue recession on a single tooth or an osseous defect adjacent to a single tooth; also used to indicate soft tissue defects and/or osseous defects in edentulous tooth positions."

Autogenous soft tissue graft: Donor graft material is taken from the patient's mouth resulting in a second surgical site.

> The ADA Glossary definition of **autogenous graft** is: "Taken from one part of a patient's body and transferred to another."

Non-autogenous: There is no second surgical site in the patient's mouth. The graft material comes from another source. Example are (trade names) AlloDerm, Fibro-Gide and OrACELL.

> The ADA Glossary definition of **non-autogenous** is: "A graft from donor other than patient."

Changes to This Category

There are no changes to the Periodontics category in CDT 2021.

Clinical Coding Scenario #1:
Periodontal Abscess

A patient presented in pain and complained about swelling around one tooth. The doctor's emergency evaluation included two periapical radiographic images and pocket measurements of the teeth in the area. The swelling was clearly adjacent to tooth #3 and a purulent mixture of blood and pus was present when the sulcus was probed.

The doctor treated the patient for a periodontal abscess by debridement and draining through the sulcus, irrigating the pocket with chlorhexidine and prescribing the patient an antibiotic.

How could this encounter be coded?

Since the evaluation was problem-focused, the appropriate codes for diagnostic procedures would be:

D0140   limited oral evaluation – problem focused

D0220   intraoral – periapical first radiographic image

D0230   intraoral – periapical each additional radiographic image

In this case there are a number of codes that might be used to document the operative services, alone or in combination. Possible procedure coding options are:

D9110   palliative (emergency) treatment of dental pain – minor procedure

Use of this code to document the service provided may require a narrative to describe the exact treatment rendered. It may be the most appropriate code to use in this case. The following code may also be considered:

D7510   incision and drainage of abscess – intraoral soft tissue
Involves incision through mucosa, including periodontal origins.

Clinical Coding Scenario #2:
Periodontitis

A 49-year-old male patient presents for periodontal examination with a chief complaint of sore and bleeding gums. Medical history is significant for type II diabetes being treated with Metformin (glucophage), and hypertension which was being treated with a calcium channel blocker (nifedipine-adalat). He smokes one pack of cigarettes a day. His last dental appointment was five years ago and there are heavy accumulations of plaque and calculus, both supra-gingival and sub-gingival.

Since the amount of calculus and plaque prevented a periodontal evaluation from being performed adequately, the patient was seen by the hygienist that same day. Without using any anesthesia, she utilized an ultrasonic scaler to debride supragingival calculus and plaque in all four quadrants. After reviewing home care instructions and giving the patient chlorhexidine rinse, provided by the office, the patient was scheduled to return in two weeks for a periodontal evaluation and appropriate radiographic images.

How would these visits be coded?

Visit #1: Assessment and Debridement

> **D0191** **assessment of a patient**
>
> **D4355** **full mouth debridement to enable a comprehensive oral evaluation and diagnosis on a subsequent visit**
>
> **D1330** **oral hygiene instructions**
>
> **D9630** **drugs or medicaments dispensed in the office for home use**

Visit #2: Evaluation, Diagnosis and Treatment Planning

Two weeks later, the patient returned for radiographic images and a complete periodontal evaluation.

The diagnosis is Stage III Grade C periodontitis with pocket depths ranging from 4 to 9 millimeters, furcation involvement, mobility, and localized recession. There are interproximal papillae that exhibit swelling with a "granulated" surface appearance to the soft tissue resembling hyperplasia possibly caused by the calcium channel-blocking drug. Consultation with the patient's internist to evaluate possibility of changing the high blood pressure medication was done by the dentist.

A complete oral evaluation with full mouth periapical radiographic images were taken. The diagnostic findings were:

1. Missing teeth #1, #5, #12, #16, #17, #21, #28 and #32. The premolars were extracted for orthodontic reasons when he was a teenager.

2. Bone loss of up to 40 percent around the posterior teeth with pocket depths ranging from 5 to 9 mm in the posterior.

3. Heavy accumulations of plaque and calculus supra and sub-gingival

4. Moderate generalized gingival overgrowth probably related to his calcium channel medication

5. Furcation involvement on the molars

6. Mobility of teeth

7. Inadequate oral hygiene

The evaluation and diagnosis led to a multiple appointment treatment plan for this patient – four quadrants of scaling and root planing spread across two appointments, and a third appointment four to six weeks after the SRP for a post-operative visit to assess the outcome.

Note: Some dental benefit plans will not cover four quadrants of SRP delivered at one appointment.

CDT codes for the services delivered and planned during the second visit follow:

D0150   comprehensive oral evaluation – new or established patient

or

D0180   comprehensive periodontal evaluation – new or established patient

Note: Some dental benefit plans will deny benefits for a second D0180 procedure when the first is reported by a general dentist who then refers the patient to a periodontal practice where the second D0180 is reported.

D0210   intraoral – complete series of radiographic images

D1330   oral hygiene instructions

D9311   consultation with a medical health care professional

Visit #3: SRP – Two Quadrants

D4341   periodontal scaling and root planing – four or more teeth per quadrant

Note: This procedure is reported twice and the two quadrants treated (e.g., maxillary right and mandibular right) are identified by entering the applicable area of the oral cavity code on the claim.

Visit #4: SRP – Two Quadrants

D4341   periodontal scaling and root planing – four or more teeth per quadrant

This procedure is reported twice and the two quadrants treated (e.g., maxillary left and mandibular left) are identified by entering the applicable area of the oral cavity code on the claim.

Visit #5: Four to Six Weeks After SRP Completed

D0171   re-evaluation – post-operative office visit

Post-scaling and root planing, re-charting was done at this appointment, noting that significant pocket depth with bleeding on probing in the posterior areas was evident. The dentist felt that the patient would benefit from osseous surgery in the posterior quadrants (D4260) at a later date. The medical consultation from the first appointment was returned and the physician plans to change the patient's hypertension medication.

Clinical Coding Scenario #3:
Treatment to Eliminate Periodontal Pocketing

A 60-year-old female has been under care since having scaling and root planing done eight months ago, followed by periodic periodontal maintenance (D4910) every three months. The patient decided she is ready to proceed with planned treatment to eliminate periodontal pocketing, but is very anxious about the surgery. Before proceeding, the doctor completed a new periodontal chart to assess her current situation. Since the full mouth radiographs were less than a year old, no additional radiographs were necessary.

Note: If additional radiographs are deemed necessary for a better diagnosis there may not be reimbursement by the dental benefit plan if coverage provisions have diagnostic imaging frequency limitations.

The diagnostic findings are as follows:
1. Missing teeth #1, #2, #16, #17, #18, and #32
2. Bone loss is generalized and ranges from 10–50 percent with periodontal pocket depths up to 5 to 9 mm
3. Furcation involvement in the molar areas
4. Vertical defects on the distal of tooth #19 and the mesial of tooth #21
5. Tooth mobility
6. Periodontal bleeding on probing in the periodontal pocket areas
7. Patient apprehension to dental treatment

What CDT code is used to report the periodontal charting completed at this appointment?

Charting is considered to be a part of a comprehensive periodontal evaluation (D0180), which also should include details such as bleeding on probing, furcation involvement, mobility, recession, and clinical attachment loss. These findings may also be part of a comprehensive oral evaluation (D0150). It is recommended that periodontal charting and evaluation be completed annually for patients with a history of periodontitis.

The patient's next appointment was for four quadrants of osseous surgery and bone grafts to address the defects on teeth #19 and #21. These procedures would be delivered with the patient under conscious sedation due to her anxiety.

Services delivered during this appointment would be coded as follows:

For four quadrants of osseous surgery:

> **D4260 osseous surgery (includes elevation of a full thickness flap and closure) – four of more contiguous teeth or tooth bounded spaces per quadrant**

Note: This procedure is reported four times as it is a "per quadrant" service and all four quadrants were involved (maxillary right and left; mandibular right and left) by entering the applicable area of the oral cavity code on the claim on this date of service.

For tooth #19 (distal):

> **D4263** **bone replacement graft – retained natural tooth – first site in quadrant**
>
> **D4265** **biologic material to aid in soft and osseous tissue regeneration**
>
> **D4266** **guided tissue regeneration – resorbable barrier, per site**

For tooth #21 (mesial):

> **D4264** **bone replacement graft – retained natural tooth – each additional site in quadrant**
>
> **D4265** **biologic material to aid in soft and osseous tissue regeneration**
>
> **D4266** **guided tissue regeneration – resorbable barrier, per site**

For 2.5 hours of anesthesia:

> **D9239** **intravenous moderate (conscious) sedation/analgesia – first 15 minutes**
>
> **D9243** **intravenous moderate (conscious) sedation – each subsequent 15 minute increment**

Note: Since the anesthesia procedure took 2.5 hours (150 minutes) and these codes are reported in 15-minute increments, the patient record and claim would document the first 15 minutes of sedation, D9239, once and then document the additional 135 minutes with D9243 and a "Quantity" of nine.

The patient returned for a post-surgery check two weeks later for suture removal, light cleansing of the affected areas, and oral hygiene instructions. At that time, the doctor determined that the patient would benefit from an antimicrobial mouth rinse (chlorhexidine), which the office provided.

CDT Codes for this visit are:

> **D0171** **re-evaluation – post-operative office visit**
>
> **D1330** **oral hygiene instructions**
>
> **D9630** **drugs or medicaments dispensed in the office for home use**

Clinical Coding Scenario #4:
Orthodontic Patient with Gingival Inflammation

A patient, who is a teenager in active orthodontic treatment, comes in for a prophylaxis every three to four months. She struggles with homecare and, as a result, the gingiva is bleeding and tender with enlarged tissue, actually covering some of the brackets. Her medical history is unremarkable. There is no bone loss as determined by a panoramic radiograph taken six months ago. In addition, scaling is difficult with brackets and appliances present. This is a three-appointment scenario.

How would the appointments be coded?

Visit #1: Initial Appointment

An examination was done with periodontal charting that included notation of bleeding points and pocketing. Homecare instructions were reinforced, and all tissues were irrigated with chlorhexidine rinse. Extra-oral photographs were taken to document the hyperplastic tissue. The patient was scheduled for a gingivectomy in four full quadrants.

CDT codes for the first appointment's procedures are:

D0180 comprehensive periodontal evaluation – new or established patient

D0350 2D oral/facial photographic image obtained intra-orally or extra-orally

Note: As D0350 is, according to its nomenclature wording, a single image capture procedure the code is reported one time and the number of images captured is recorded in the service line's "Quantity" field.

D1330 oral hygiene instructions

D4921 gingival irrigation – per quadrant

Note: D4921 is reported four times as all quadrants of the mouth received gingival irrigation with the applicable Area of the Oral Cavity code recorded on each claim service line.

Visit #2: Gingivectomy

The patient received a gingivectomy in each quadrant. These procedures were completed using local anesthesia for patient comfort and with a laser for the instrumentation.

CDT codes for the second appointment's procedures are:

D4210 gingivectomy or gingivoplasty – four or more contiguous teeth or tooth bounded spaces per quadrant

Note: D4210 is reported four times as all quadrants of the mouth received a gingivectomy, along with recording the applicable Area of the Oral Cavity code on each claim service line. Use of a laser in this procedure is not relevant from the coding perspective as the code documents the treatment done, not the specific instrument or technique used to perform the gingivectomy.

Visit #3: Follow Up

The patient was seen a month later for follow-up, with no services provided, and the CDT code for this encounter is:

D0171 re-evaluation – post-operative visit

The patient should then be placed on a periodontal maintenance schedule since active periodontal treatment was rendered. It is important to remember, however, that carriers have plan limitations, which may reimburse only a limited number of prophylaxes or periodontal maintenance visits per year. This may also apply to comprehensive examinations. In unusual cases, a narrative may explain the need for additional treatment outside the plan limitation.

Clinical Coding Scenario #5:
Scaling in the Presence of Mucositis around an Implant

A patient of record who has been on a periodontal maintenance (D4910) treatment plan presents for this visit with the complaint of soreness around the implant for tooth #5. Examination revealed bleeding with probing around the implant accompanied by swelling and some suppuration. Resulting pocket depths were 4–5 mm. A periapical radiograph was taken, which indicated bone height comparable to that seen previously.

The doctor treated this area with debridement and curettage of the area. The periodontal maintenance procedure is not done at this appointment.

How would this encounter be coded?

Visit #1: Initial Appointment

D0140   **limited oral evaluation – problem focused**

D0220   **intraoral – periapical first radiographic image**

D6081   **scaling and debridement in the presence of inflammation or mucositis of a single implant, including cleaning of the implant surfaces, without flap entry and closure**

The D6081 procedure is not performed in conjunction with D1110, D4910, or D4346.

Subsequent Visits

Continuation of periodic periodontal maintenance plan, each reported with:

D4910   **periodontal maintenance**

Clinical Coding Scenario #6:
Ailing Failing Implant

Visit #1: Initial Appointment

The patient presents with the chief complaint of soreness and bleeding associated with a restored implant #19. Evaluation of the area reveals a 7 mm pocketing surrounding the implant with bleeding on probing. No mobility in the implant is detected. A periapical radiographic image reveals circumferential bone loss increasing from previous radiographs. It was determined that the implant was treatable. The patient was placed on an appropriate antibiotic and scheduled to return for treatment.

How would this encounter be coded?

> **D0140   limited oral evaluation – problem focused**
>
> **D0220   intraoral – periapical first radiograph image**

Visit #2: Treatment of Implant

The patient returned in 10 days and the swelling had subsided. Under oral sedation and local anesthesia, full thickness mucoperiosteal flaps were elevated and the implant surface was debrided with saline, scaled with an ultrasonic implant tip, cleaned with an air polisher, and then treated with chlorhexidine solution. The site was grafted with bone and covered with a resorbable barrier and closed with sutures.

How would this encounter be coded?

This encounter would be coded as:

> **D9248   non-intravenous conscious sedation**
>
> **D6101   debridement of a peri-implant defect or defects surrounding a single implant, and surface cleaning of the exposed implant surfaces, including flap entry and closure**
>
> **D4921   gingival irrigation – per quadrant**
>
> **D6103   bone graft for repair of peri-implant defect – does not include flap entry and closure**
>
> **D4266   guided tissue regeneration – resorbable barrier, per site**

Note: Should there be a need for a post-operative evaluation that procedure would be recorded with **D0171 re-evaluation – post-operative office visit**.

Clinical Coding Scenario #7:
Overdue Patient with Gingivitis

A patient of record in the office has not been seen for over two years. When they arrive for a routine prophylaxis, the evaluation reveals heavy plaque, some supra- and sub-gingival calculus, with moderate stain. Bleeding on probing is noted on most teeth accompanied by edema and swelling. No bone loss is seen on the four bitewing radiographs that are taken. From the clinical evaluation, a diagnosis of generalized moderate to severe gingivitis is made. The hygienist proceeds with a full mouth scaling treatment, not a prophylaxis, noting that this scaling procedure requires more time than needed for a prophylaxis.

How should this appointment be coded for reimbursement?

Since the patient has not been seen in the office for over two years, a comprehensive evaluation should be done. This includes both dental and periodontal charting, with pocket depths, bleeding points, and any additional findings such as suppuration and edema.

D0180   comprehensive periodontal evaluation – new or established patient

As mentioned, bitewing radiographs were also taken, so you would also use the following code:

D0274   bitewings – four radiographic images

It is recommended that patients have a panoramic radiograph or full mouth radiographs every five years. If this patient does not have either in the last five years, then most likely a panoramic radiograph would also be taken in addition to the bitewings and reported separately with **D0330 panoramic radiographic image**.

In this case, a comprehensive oral evaluation has been done and treatment will be done at the same visit. Since the diagnosis is generalized moderate to severe gingivitis a routine adult prophylaxis is not appropriate – but the applicable procedure is:

D4346   scaling in the presence of generalized moderate or severe gingival inflammation – full mouth, after oral evaluation

This scenario emphasizes that an evaluation can be done the same day as treatment when scaling is coded as D4346. The D4346 procedure differs from **D4355 full mouth debridement to enable a comprehensive oral evaluation and diagnosis on a subsequent visit** as the full mouth debridement procedure addresses removal of accumulations and inflammation present that do not allow a comprehensive evaluation to be done. For example, pocket depths cannot be recorded due to the amount of calculus present both supra- and sub-gingivally. These cases require a healing period to accurately do the evaluation and make a diagnosis.

Also note that D4346 is a full mouth procedure. It cannot be coded multiple times by quadrant.

Many times a second procedure of scaling may be necessary to accomplish adequate debridement for patients who have had the D4346 procedure. For example, a re-evaluation (**D0171 re-evaluation – post-operative office visit**) might be appropriate, or a second appointment for a prophylaxis (D1110) if inflammation and pocket depths have decreased.

As with all codes, carriers differ as to the benefit allowed for D4346. A clinician should code for what they do, not code for reimbursement. Also remember that unless a code is used appropriately and submitted, carriers will not have a history of the frequency of use or the dentist's full fee for the procedure.

Note: The procedure documented with D4346 is intended to treat patients who have widespread gingival inflammation but no bone or attachment loss. Patients with generally healthy periodontium receive preventive care, and those with periodontal disease involving bone and attachment loss receive therapeutic care. Code D4346 documents the procedure that lies between a prophylaxis and a scaling and root planing. The ADA has published a separate document that contains a detailed discussion of the nature, scope and decision-making process that leads to delivery of the D4346 procedure. This guidance document, and its related webinar, are found on the "Coding Education" web page linked to the ADA's *Code on Dental Procedures and Nomenclature* (CDT Code) web page – *ADA.org/en/publications/cdt/coding-education*.

Clinical Coding Scenario #8:
Foreign Object Stuck Between Teeth

A patient comes in for an emergency visit. Something is "stuck" between teeth #19 and #20 and is causing some swelling and pain. The patient has not been able brush or floss the area and resolve the issue. After examining the area and taking a periapical radiograph, you decide the problem has not caused any bone loss or is endodontically related. Infiltrating the interproximal area and scaling, you find a husk from popcorn, which is removed. After giving post-operative instructions, the patient is dismissed.

How should this be coded?

In this case, the exam should be coded:

D0140   limited oral evaluation – problem focused

A periapical radiograph was taken.

D0220   intraoral – periapical first radiographic image

Treatment of the swelling and pain can be coded in various ways depending on what procedures have been delivered, using a code's nomenclature and descriptor as the guide. D9110 would be the most likely one to describe the service (infiltrating the interproximal area and scaling) provided. At times, carriers request a narrative to explain the rationale for the procedure.

D9110   palliative (emergency) treatment of dental pain – minor procedure
This is typically reported on a "per visit" basis for emergency treatment of dental pain.

In cases where D7510 is appropriate, the lesion will not only exhibit swelling and bleeding on probing, but will also have suppuration or exudate when scaled. This occurs frequently when periodontal pockets are present.

D7510   Incision and drainage of abscess – intraoral soft tissue
Involves incision through mucosa, including periodontal origins.

Clinical Coding Scenario #9:
Scaling and Root Planing of Only Three Quadrants

A new patient presents at the office and during the evaluation which accompanied the prophylaxis, it was determined that three quadrants of scaling and root planing are needed. The fourth quadrant has no periodontal disease, but does require a prophylaxis. All treatment is completed after two appointments.

How could these visits be coded?

Visit #1: Evaluation, Diagnosis and Treatment Planning

It would be correct to code for an evaluation and the adult prophylaxis.

D0150   comprehensive oral evaluation – new or established patient

or

D0180   comprehensive periodontal evaluation – new or established patient

Note: Periodontal charting including pocket depths and current radiographs will be necessary to support the need for scaling and root planing.

D1110   prophylaxis – adult

Visit #2: SRP – Three Quadrants of Scaling and Root Planing

At a subsequent appointment, the scaling and root planing can be performed. In some instances, performing a prophylaxis prior to scaling and root planing can decrease the inflammation and allow a more thorough debridement during scaling and root planing since bleeding will be less and access to subgingival calculus and toxins is improved.

Note: It is always advisable to request a pre-treatment estimate prior to any periodontal therapy since carriers may have plan limitations that may affect reimbursement. For example, some carriers will only reimburse a maximum of two quadrants of scaling and root planing per appointment.

The bottom line is that you submit for what you do. A prophylaxis was performed at the first visit and should be dated differently than the three quadrants of scaling and root planing completed on a different date.

D4342   periodontal scaling and root planing – one to three teeth per quadrant

Note: D4342 is reported three times and claim service line includes the applicable area of the oral cavity code to identify the specific quadrant treated.

Clinical Coding Scenario #10:
Recession

During a prophylaxis the patient complains of sensitivity and soreness in the lower anterior area. A comprehensive periodontal evaluation is completed. Findings include three to four millimeters of recession with either no attached gingiva or one millimeter of attached gingiva on teeth #22–25, and tooth #28, as well as the implant in the area of #29. The threads of the implant are visible on the facial where recession has occurred. Pocketing is two to three millimeters, but the tissue bleeds easily and edema is present. There is no mobility present, but the incisors exhibit slight fremitus with occlusion.

During this initial appointment there were several other procedures in addition to the routine prophylaxis and oral evaluation. Periapical radiographs were taken of teeth #22–25 and #28–29, the teeth with recession. Two intraoral photographs were also taken to visually document the amount of recession, lack of attached gingiva, and the inflammation present. The occlusion is adjusted on the mandibular incisors and homecare (oral hygiene) instructions were provided. This visit concluded discussion of the treatment plan that addressed the oral evaluation findings.

How could these visits be coded?

Visit #1: Initial Appointment Procedure Coding

D1110   prophylaxis – adult

D1330   oral hygiene instructions

D0180   comprehensive periodontal evaluation – new or established patient

D0220   intraoral – periapical first radiographic image

D0230   intraoral – periapical each additional radiographic image

(Report the number of additional periapical images in the claim service line's "Quantity" field.)

D0350   2D oral/facial photographic image obtained intra-orally or extra-orally

(Report "2" in the "Quantity" field of the claim service line where D0350 is posted.)

D9951   occlusal adjustment – limited

Treatment Plan Notes

Evidence of clinical attachment loss with recession and lack of keratinized tissue accompanied by inflammation indicates that soft tissue grafts should be performed on teeth #22–25 and #28–29. The patient prefers that all grafts be completed at the same appointment with a local anesthetic.

Non-autogenous connective tissue grafts using AlloDerm are to be completed at one appointment. Suture removal is done two weeks after the surgery and a final check of the surgical areas is completed six weeks later. Homecare is stressed during all subsequent appointments.

It is important to obtain a pre-treatment estimate in this case so that the patient clearly understands coverage for the soft tissue grafts, which varies between plans. Some plans may request additional attachments such as radiographs or photographs for soft tissue grafts. Once the pre-treatment is obtained, the date of surgery only is the additional information required to receive benefits.

Visit #2 – Graft Procedures Delivered

Codes for the procedures to be delivered at this scheduled appointment are listed by teeth being treated.

Teeth #22–25

D4275 non-autogenous connective tissue graft (including recipient site and donor material) first tooth, implant, or edentulous tooth position in graft

D4285 non-autogenous connective tissue graft procedure (including recipient surgical site and donor material) – each additional contiguous tooth, implant or edentulous tooth position in same graft site

(Repeat D4285 three times.)

Tooth #28 and Implant #29

D4275 non-autogenous connective tissue graft (including recipient site and donor material) first tooth, implant, or edentulous tooth position in graft

D4285 non-autogenous connective tissue graft procedure (including recipient surgical site and donor material) – each additional contiguous tooth, implant or edentulous tooth position in same graft site

For soft tissue grafts, each separate tooth or implant is considered a site. When they are contiguous, meaning adjacent and the graft site is only one surgical area, then the coding includes the first tooth and then each additional tooth in that surgical area is listed with a separate code. As a result, in this case, for tooth #22 one D4275 is needed, and for teeth #23–25 the D4285 is reported three times.

Tooth #28 and the implant for #29 are coded separately since they are not adjacent to the other surgical site. That is, there are several teeth between the areas treated. Therefore the same codes for soft tissue grafts apply for both teeth and implants. As a result, the coding for these teeth is very similar, with tooth #28 coded with D4275 and the implant D4285.

D1330   oral hygiene instructions

Visit #3: Suture Removal

At the suture removal appointment:

D0171   re-evaluation – post-operative office visit

D1330   oral hygiene instructions

Visit #4: Post-surgery Appointment

At the final check appointment six weeks after surgery:

D0171   re-evaluation – post-operative office visit
or
D9430   office visit for observation (during regularly scheduled hours) – no other services performed

D1330   oral hygiene instructions

Both Visit #3 and #4 are considered post-operative visits after the surgical treatment. Since sutures are removed during the third visit, D0171 is appropriate. At the fourth (final) visit either D0171 can be used or D9430, depending on whether there is additional treatment performed. It is important to code for what you do whether or not the procedure is reimbursed. Precise documentation is necessary for both medical and legal reasons.

Clinical Coding Scenario #11:
Post-orthodontic Treatment

After completion of orthodontic treatment and removal of appliances, a 30-year-old woman is seen for a routine prophylaxis to remove any residual cement and polish. She states she is not satisfied with the way her teeth look. Her teeth are straight but appear short and she sees too much gum when she smiles. A periodontal evaluation reveals excellent homecare with healthy gingival tissues including probing depths in the range of one to three millimeters, no bleeding on probing, and minimal recession with adequate attached gingiva.

Since the appliances have been removed, a full mouth series of radiographs is taken. No decay is found either clinically or radiographically. Six intraoral photos are taken. After evaluation, it is determined that clinical crown length is short, with the CEJ subgingival, which results in a compromised smile line and gingival contour.

Recommended treatment includes crown lengthening to increase the clinical crown length, provide correct biologic width between the CEJ and the height of bone, and improve the contour of the gingiva in both the maxilla and mandible, including the anterior teeth and bicuspids in four quadrants. The patient will have the maxilla completed at the first appointment, and the mandibular addressed at a second appointment six weeks later. Suture removal appointments will be scheduled one week after surgery and a final evaluation six weeks after the last surgery appointment.

How could these visits be coded?

Visit #1: Initial Appointment

> **D1110** **prophylaxis – adult**
>
> **D0180** **comprehensive periodontal evaluation – new or established patient**
>
> **D0210** **intraoral – complete series of radiographic images**
>
> **D0350** **2D oral/facial photographic image obtained intra-orally or extra-orally**

(Report D0350 six times.)

The initial appointment is straightforward, with an adult prophylaxis, followed by a periodontal evaluation since the patient has had orthodontic appliances removed. A full mouth series of radiographs determined not only was the patient caries free, but also established that no bone loss was evident. Photographs documented her current smile and length of the teeth.

Visit #2: Upper Left and Upper Right Quadrants

D4230 anatomical crown exposure – four or more contiguous teeth or bounded tooth spaces per quadrant

(upper right quadrant)

D4230 anatomical crown exposure – four or more contiguous teeth or bounded tooth spaces per quadrant

(upper left quadrant)

In this case, four or more teeth per quadrant were treated (central incisor through second bicuspid), so the quadrant code is applicable reported with the applicable area of the oral cavity code on the claim.

Visit #3: Suture Removal

D0171 re-evaluation – post-operative office visit

This is appropriate for the appointment one week later to remove sutures. If oral hygiene instructions are also given, D1330 would be added.

Visit #4: Lower Right Quadrant and Lower Left Quadrant

D4230 anatomical crown exposure – four or more contiguous teeth or bounded tooth spaces per quadrant

(lower right quadrant)

D4230 anatomical crown exposure – four or more contiguous teeth or bounded tooth spaces per quadrant

(lower left quadrant)

Visit #5: Suture Removal

D0171 re-evaluation – post-operative visit

These appointments are duplicates of the treatment completed in the maxilla. Again, if home care instructions are included a D1330 would be reported.

Visit #6: Suture Removal

D0171 re-evaluation – post-operative office visit

or

D9430 office visit for observation (during regularly scheduled hours) – no other services performed

Either code can be used for the last visit when the patient is evaluated and treatment is complete – depending on whether there is additional service(s) performed.

Clinical Coding Scenario #12:
Treatment and Maintenance of Hybrid Appliance

Visit #1

A new patient was scheduled for a prophylaxis and evaluation. Once in the office, a medical history was taken, and a comprehensive oral evaluation was performed. Previous treatment included periodontal surgery in the mandibular arch five years ago, and placement of a hybrid restoration in the maxilla with six implants placed in the arch. The patient did not have any radiographs from his previous dentist, so a panoramic radiograph was taken with vertical bitewings to include the maxillary implants. Some inflammation was noted surrounding the implants.

It was decided that at the next visit a periodontal maintenance procedure was necessary rather than a routine prophylaxis. Another appointment would be indicated if the inflammation surrounding the implants did not resolve after the maintenance appointment. If so, at a subsequent visit it would be necessary to remove the appliance due to the mucositis surrounding the implants. The second appointment was scheduled.

How would this initial appointment be coded?

D0150   comprehensive oral evaluation – new or established patient
or
D0180   comprehensive periodontal evaluation – new or established patient

D0330   panoramic radiographic image

D0277   vertical bitewings – 7 to 8 radiographic images
>   This does not constitute a full mouth intraoral radiographic series.

Visit #2

The patient was delayed returning for his periodontal maintenance and was seen two months later. Treatment included supra and subgingival plaque and calculus removal. Implants in the maxillary arch were debrided using air abrasion as well as hand instrumentation. The patient received homecare instructions and was scheduled for a re-evaluation in four weeks.

How could visit #2 be coded?

D4910   periodontal maintenance

D0120   periodic oral evaluation – established patient

D1330   oral hygiene instructions
>   This may include instructions for home care. Examples include tooth brushing technique, flossing, and use of special oral hygiene aids.

In this case, a periodic evaluation is necessary to determine if any additional changes had occurred in the two months since the last appointment. If the patient had been seen a week after the evaluation, D4910 would be the only code necessary. In some cases, state law requires an examination at a maintenance appointment, so a D0120 would also be used in this situation. The primary goal of the evaluation is to determine if further treatment is needed in the maxillary arch. In this case, a re-evaluation is scheduled to permit the tissues to heal and then determine if further treatment is necessary.

Visit #3

Periodontal charting is done, and it is determined that the patient will require further therapy, removing the appliance and treating the mucositis present around the implants in the maxillary arch.

How could visit #3 be coded?

> **D0171   re-evaluation – post-operative office visit**

Visit #4

The hybrid appliance is removed, resulting in the implants being more accessible to address the mucositis. Using local anesthesia, scaling and debridement is completed. The appliance is replaced after being examined and cleaned. Instructions for post-operative and daily care of the implants are given. The patient is then placed on a three month maintenance schedule.

How could visit #4 be coded?

> **D6080   implant maintenance procedure when prostheses are removed and reinserted, including cleansing of prostheses and abutments**
> This procedure includes active debriding of the implant(s) and examination of all aspects of the implant system(s), including the occlusion and stability of the superstructure. The patient is also instructed in thorough daily cleansing of the implant(s). This is not a per implant code, and is indicated for implant supported fixed prostheses.

> **D6081   scaling and debridement in the presence of inflammation or mucositis of a single implant, including cleaning of the implant surfaces without flap entry and closure**
> This procedure is not performed in conjunction with D1110, D4910, or D4346.

Note: D6081 is a code for treatment of a single implant. In this case, six implants are present, so it should be coded six times.

Clinical Coding Scenario #13:
Generalized Periodontitis Treatment

How could the following visits be coded?

Visit #1

A 55-year-old patient presents with a maxillary denture and natural teeth in the mandible. A cursory examination reveals periodontal disease to be her primary problem, so a comprehensive evaluation is performed. A panoramic radiograph and seven periapical radiographs are taken to determine a diagnosis and develop a treatment plan.

The evaluation reveals isolated pocket depths of 5–6 millimeters generally, with 7 millimeters between teeth #24 and #25. Bone loss is primarily horizontal in the coronal third of the root except in the central incisor area where it is approximately 50% of the root, with a moderate crater. Mobility is noted on the incisors. Except for the third molars, all teeth are present in the mandible. Oral hygiene is fair, with some supra- and sub gingival calculus. Medical history includes medication for high blood pressure, which is controlled. The patient smokes four to five cigarettes per day. Further questioning reveals that the maxillary teeth were not lost from periodontal disease but rather from extensive caries. Diagnosis: Periodontitis: Stage III, Grade B.

> **D0180** **comprehensive periodontal evaluation – new or established patient**

or

> **D0150** **comprehensive oral evaluation – new or established patient**
> **D0330** **panoramic radiographic image**
> **D0220** **intraoral – periapical first radiographic image**
> **D0230** **intraoral – periapical each additional radiographic image**

Note: D0230 should be recorded six times as a total of seven periapical images were acquired and interpreted.

Visit #2

During the second visit, the treatment plan included scaling and root planing, as well as splinting the mandibular anterior teeth. The mandible was anesthetized with local anesthetic, two quadrants of scaling and root planing were completed. A splint was placed from teeth #22–27, using orthodontic archwire and composite on the lingual of these anterior teeth to reduce mobility. Oral hygiene instructions were given, particularly for the teeth included in the splinting.

> **D4341** **periodontal scaling and root planing – four or more teeth per quadrant**

Note: D4341 is recorded two times, with noting the applicable area of the oral cavity code where the procedure was delivered.

D4321 **provisional splinting – extracoronal**

This is a temporary stabilization of teeth to reduce mobility during other treatment. Although only one code is submitted, the teeth numbers should be indicated on the claim.

D1330 **oral hygiene instructions**

Visit #3

Pocket depths were recorded, and homecare was again addressed as well as the patient's smoking habit. It was determined that osseous surgery would be necessary in both quadrants of the mandibular arch. No bone grafts would be needed, although the dentist decided that it would be advantageous to place a biologic material in between teeth #24 and #25 when the patient returns.

D0171 **re-evaluation – post-operative office visit**

D1330 **oral hygiene instructions**

D1320 **tobacco counseling for the control and prevention of oral disease**

Visit #4

The patient was sedated with oral medication and nitrous oxide. Using local anesthetic, flaps were elevated and the mandible was debrided, roots scaled and planed, with some osteoplasty where needed. Before replacing the flaps, Emdogain, a biologic material, was placed between the central incisors. Sutures and periodontal dressing were placed. Post-surgical instructions were given and the patient was dismissed to a relative.

D9248 **non-intravenous conscious sedation**

D9230 **inhalation of nitrous oxide/analgesia, anxiolysis**

D4260 **osseous surgery (including elevation of a full thickness flap and closure) – four or more contiguous teeth or tooth bounded spaces per quadrant**

Note: D4260 is reported twice along with the appropriate area of the oral cavity quadrant code.

D4265 **biologic materials to aid in soft and osseous tissue regeneration**

Visit #5

Two weeks later, sutures were removed, healing evaluated, and the patient was given oral hygiene instructions.

D0171 **re-evaluation – post-operative visit**

D1330 **oral hygiene instructions**

Clinical Coding Scenario #14:
Flap Surgery for Debridement and Evaluation

How could the following visits be coded?

Visit #1

A patient is evaluated for a problem on tooth #3. Symptoms include pain when biting, a pocket on the distobuccal of 8 millimeters, and edema with bleeding on probing but no suppuration. A root canal was completed on this first molar five years ago, but the patient did not have a crown placed, as recommended. A radiograph indicates minimal bone loss in the area with no pathology at the apex. The patient has a history of periodontal treatment including osseous surgery six years ago but has had quarterly maintenance appointments alternating between the general dentist and periodontist. It was decided to schedule the patient for osseous surgery to treat the continued deterioration.

D0140 limited oral evaluation – problem focused

D0220 intraoral – periapical first radiographic image

Visit #2

The patient was anesthetized using local anesthesia. A flap was elevated, and the area of concern debrided. Once exposed, it was found that a vertical fracture of the distobuccal root had occurred. After conferring with the patient, the best treatment option was determined to be extraction and a bone graft in anticipation of eventual placement of an implant. A resorbable membrane was placed in conjunction with the bone graft as well as a biologic materials to encourage regeneration.

D4241 gingival flap procedure, including root planing – one to three contiguous teeth or tooth bounded spaces per quadrant

D7140 extraction, erupted tooth or exposed root (elevation and/or forceps removal)

D7953 bone replacement graft for ridge preservation – per site

D4266 guided tissue regeneration – resorbable barrier, per site

D4265 biologic materials to aid in soft and osseous tissue regeneration

Visit #3

A post-operative visit was done, removing sutures and evaluating healing of the surgical site. The patient will be seen for follow-up over the next three months prior to implant placement.

D0171 re-evaluation – post-operative office visit

Clinical Coding Scenario #15:
Recession and Frenum Pull

How could the following visits be coded?

Visit #1

A 25-year-old presents with a strong frenum attachment facially between teeth #24 and #25. These central incisors also have 3–4 millimeters of recession on the facial, classified as Miller Class 2 recession. A periapical radiograph was taken to determine the prognosis of the teeth involved. A photo of the mandibular anterior was also taken. Orthodontic treatment is planned, and periodontal treatment should be completed prior to starting the orthodontic therapy. The patient is scheduled for a frenectomy and two connective tissue grafts.

D0140 limited evaluation – problem focused

D0220 intraoral – periapical first radiographic image

D0350 2D oral/facial photographic image obtained intra-orally or extra-orally

Visit #2

A frenectomy was done and connective tissue grafts were performed on teeth #24 and #25 using donor tissue from the patient's palate. After sutures were placed, the patient was given post-operative instructions and an appointment in two weeks for suture removal was scheduled.

D7961 buccal / labial frenectomy (frenulectomy)

D4273 autogenous connective tissue graft procedure (including donor and recipient surgical sites) first tooth, implant, or edentulous tooth position in graft

D4283 autogenous connective tissue graft (including donor and recipient surgical sites) – each additional contiguous tooth, implant, or edentulous tooth position in same graft site

Both the frenectomy and the soft tissue grafts are reported separately. Some carriers will benefit only the most inclusive procedures done at the same visit. In this case, those are the soft tissue grafts.

Visit #3

The sutures were removed. The patient was given oral hygiene instructions and appointed for follow-up three weeks later.

D0171 re-evaluation – post-operative visit

D1330 oral hygiene instructions

Clinical Coding Scenario #16:
Periodontal Pocketing and Subgingival Decay

<u>Visit #1</u>

A patient is seen with a chief complaint of pain in the mandibular left. An examination revealed decay on tooth #19 with periodontal disease present on adjacent teeth. A comprehensive periodontal evaluation is completed with full mouth radiographs. The diagnosis includes subgingival decay tooth #19 – Distal with localized moderate periodontitis on teeth #18 and #20. Pocket depths are 7 millimeters on tooth #18 – Distal and 5–6 millimeters on tooth #20 – Distal. The final treatment plan includes osseous surgery to address the pocketing present and crown lengthening for tooth #19.

D0180 **comprehensive periodontal evaluation – new or established patient**

or

D0150 **comprehensive oral evaluation – new or established patient**

D0210 **intraoral – complete series of radiographic images**

<u>Visit #2</u>

A full thickness flap is elevated from teeth #18–21, including a distal wedge on tooth #18. After debridement, osseous contouring is performed flattening the shallow crater on the distal of the second molar. The interproximal bone between teeth #18 and #19 is reduced to allow access for restorative in the area of decay. Some bone contouring is also completed on tooth #20 to eliminate pocketing. The flap is repositioned apically with sutures, and periodontal dressing is placed. Post-operative instructions are given.

D4261 **osseous surgery (including elevation of a full thickness flap and closure) – one to three contiguous teeth or tooth bounded spaces per quadrant**

D4249 **clinical crown lengthening – hard tissue**

As with other procedures, such as soft tissue grafts, carriers may reimburse based on the most inclusive procedure, in this case osseous surgery. Providers should always code for what is done, so both the osseous surgery and the clinical crown lengthening are documented in the patient record and reported on the claim.

<u>Visit #3</u>

The patient is evaluated, and the sutures removed. Oral hygiene instructions are given and the patient is appointed for a check in three weeks.

D0171 **re-evaluation – post-operative visit**

D1330 **oral hygiene instructions**

1. *Our patient has pocketing and an osseous defect on the distal of the last tooth in a quadrant. All other teeth in the quadrant have pockets that are three millimeters or less. We are not sure whether the treatment procedure to report is osseous surgery (D4261) or a distal wedge (D4274). Which is appropriate?*

   If there is an osseous defect evident radiographically on the distal of the last tooth in a quadrant, and treatment of the defect includes osseous contouring and possibly a bone graft, then the treatment should be coded as osseous surgery one to three teeth, D4261. If a bone graft is performed, use D4263 along with appropriate codes for membranes or biologics if they, too, apply.

   If the procedure involves only removal of soft tissue and debridement of the tooth surface, then the mesial/distal wedge procedure would apply. According to D4274, the descriptor states that "This procedure is performed in an edentulous area adjacent to a tooth, allowing removal of a tissue wedge to gain access for debridement, permit close flap adaptation, and reduce pocket depths." No osseous contouring or regeneration is done, but a flap is elevated and the area debrided including scaling and root planing.

2. *What is the code for reporting platelet rich plasma (PRP)?*

   Platelet rich plasma (PRP) is a concentrated suspension of the growth factors found in platelets. It is a procedure where a patient's blood is drawn and then centrifuged to obtain the PRP. This procedure should be coded using **D7921 collection and application of autogenous blood concentrate product**.

3. *We use the bone replacement graft codes D4263 and D4264 for periodontal defects around and adjacent to natural teeth. Do we use the same codes in periodontal defects around existing implants?*

   There are separate codes for bone grafts around natural teeth and for bone grafts around implants. If natural teeth are being treated, then D4263 and D4264 should be submitted. These codes apply "per site." If a bone graft is placed around an existing implant, then **D6103 bone graft for repair of peri-implant defect – does not include flap entry and closure** would be correct.

4. We use the bone replacement graft code D7953 when placing graft material in an extraction socket when removing a natural tooth. But if we place an immediate implant in the extraction site and place a bone graft around the implant, do we still use D7953 or do we use one of the periodontal bone graft codes D4263 or D4264?

The nomenclature for D7953 indicates that this procedure is appropriate to report when the service is for ridge preservation, and the code's descriptor also makes reference to "preservation of ridge integrity...clinically indicated in preparation for implant reconstruction." D4263 and D4264 specifically state that they apply to "natural" teeth.

The only appropriate code to use which would apply when placing an immediate implant and simultaneously placing bone graft material around the implant would be **D6104 bone graft at time of implant placement**. Note that the D6104 descriptor states that if a barrier membrane or biologic materials are used to aid in osseous regeneration they are reported separately. Codes D4265, D4266 or D4267 as applicable would then be reported.

5. If we remove an existing implant, and place a bone graft in the site, can we use the D7953 code?

Yes. You should be using two codes to describe what you are doing. The first would be D6100 ("implant removal, by report") and the second should be D7953 which states that the graft "is placed in an extraction or implant removal site at the time of extraction or removal." This descriptor statement means D7953 is appropriate in this situation.

6. What code should I use to report periodontal charting?

There is no separate code for periodontal charting. It is considered to be part of a comprehensive periodontal evaluation (D0180) or may be part of a comprehensive oral evaluation (D0150). It could also be considered part of a re-evaluation, post-operative office visit (D0171), such as that done after initial therapy.

7. Does **D4910 periodontal maintenance** include an evaluation?

The procedure does not include an evaluation. If one is performed, the type of diagnostic evaluation should be reported separately. In most cases, **D0120 periodic oral evaluation – established patient**. If a more comprehensive evaluation is done then **D0150 comprehensive oral evaluation – new or established patient** or **D0180 comprehensive periodontal evaluation – new or established patient** would be appropriate.

8. A patient needs multiple connective tissue grafts in the mandible. There are three to six millimeters of recession on the facial of teeth #23, #24, #25, #26, #27, and #28, with no attached gingiva. There is also no attached gingiva around the implant in the area of #29. The dentist plans on using Alloderm when performing connective tissue grafts on all involved teeth and the implant during one appointment.

    Should I just submit a code for the first tooth and then one code for the remaining teeth since they are contiguous? How do we submit for a soft tissue graft around an implant? And which connective graft code would apply, D4273 or D4275?

    In this case, the appropriate code would be **D4275 non-autogenous connective tissue graft procedure** for the first tooth involved. You would then use D4285 for grafts to each of the additional teeth or implants involved. In this specific case, D4275 would be submitted one time and D4285 would be submitted six times, regardless of the fact that the teeth are in two quadrants.

9. *I have many orthodontic patients who come in for a prophylaxis. Sometimes we find the tissue around brackets and wires is hyperplastic and bleeding with generalized pseudo-pocketing. There is no bone loss evident and homecare is poor. Although the hygienist spends more time on these patients than she would with a routine prophylaxis patient, we still have to code it as a D1110. Is this the only option for coding that we have?*

    The code for scaling in the presence of moderate to severe inflammation (D4346) would be appropriate in this case. Scaling and root planing is not necessary but the procedure is more involved than a routine prophylaxis. It does include full mouth. And remember that carriers may vary on the documentation required when submitting for reimbursement and limitations on the number of times this procedure is covered.

10. *My patient has had periodontal treatment in the past and is on periodic periodontal maintenance (D4910). The patient changed dental benefit plans and when we filed for our visit, the coverage was denied due to no history of periodontal treatment. What would best resolve this issue?*

    You should send in the current periodontal charting, radiographs and the patient's history of prior periodontal treatment. Ask for a review of the claim. Some insurers require periodontal treatment in the prior 24 months to be eligible.

11. *I plan anatomic crown exposure on teeth #27, #29, and #30. #28 is missing but this area will be involved in the procedure to achieve anatomically correct gingival relationships. Should I code this as D4230 or D4231?*

As four or more teeth or tooth bounded spaces (#28) are involved, you would code this as D4230. A tooth bounded space is a space created by one or more missing teeth that has a tooth on each side. In this case, the bounded space is counted the same as a tooth.

12. *I have a new patient that has so much plaque and calculus that it is difficult to determine a treatment plan. After doing a full mouth debridement and now being able to determine the patient's dental problems, can I do the exam on the same day?*

Typically not. The full CDT Code entry for **D4355 full mouth debridement to enable a comprehensive oral evaluation and diagnosis on a subsequent visit** makes it clear that a comprehensive oral evaluation procedure must be done on a separate day. This interval allows for healing of the inflamed tissues.

For a comprehensive guide on the D4355 procedure and its reporting visit the ADA's Coding Education resource at *ADA.org/~/media/ADA/Publications/Files/D4355_ADAGuidetoReportingFullMouthDebridement_v1_2018Jan.pdf?la=en.*

13. *A periodontal maintenance patient presents with a localized area of pocketing with 6 mm probing depths. If I treat this area today, is this included in the **D4910 periodontal maintenance**, whose descriptor indicates site specific scaling and root planing? Or can it be coded as **D4342 scaling and root planing – one to three teeth per quadrant**?*

The descriptor of D4910 includes site specific scaling and root planing. It is considered part of the periodontal maintenance appointment on the same day. If the change is significant, you may want to obtain a current periodontal chart and a radiographic image for the patient and then consider scaling and root planing (D4342) as a separate procedure. It is advantageous to have periodontal charting that demonstrates an increase in pocket depths that support the need for scaling and root planing. In these cases, it is best to obtain a pre-treatment estimate and complete the procedure at a separate appointment.

14. *I submitted a claim for a gingival flap and subgingival restoration on a tooth that was performed at one appointment for a patient. The dental benefits company denied benefits for not seeing the necessity of the flap. What should I do?*

There are two ways to code for this procedure. The first is to code for the flap that was elevated using D4241, followed by the code for the restoration, either **D2330 resin-based composite – one surface, anterior** or **D2391 resin-based composite – one surface, posterior**, depending on the tooth treated.

A second way to document this procedure would be to use one of the following codes first published in CDT 2021, with selection depending on whether the tooth is anterior, a premolar or a molar:

D3471   **surgical repair of root resorption – anterior**
For surgery on root of anterior tooth. Does not include placement of restoration.

D3472   **surgical repair of root resorption – premolar**
For surgery on root of premolar tooth. Does not include placement of restoration.

D3473   **surgical repair of root resorption – molar**
For surgery on root of molar tooth. Does not include placement of restoration.

In these cases, the restoration is also coded separately. The issue arises when, in many instances, the decay is not seen clearly or may not be seen at all on a radiograph. If there is minimal pocketing, periodontally, this creates another question from a carrier's perspective.

A good course of action would be to submit the routine attachments required, including periodontal charting and a periapical radiograph. Make sure the radiograph is of diagnostic quality showing the subgingival decay. Also include a short narrative, written on the claim form, explaining that there is subgingival decay that cannot be treated without elevating a flap. If the procedure has been performed, and you have the ability to take a photograph showing the flap elevated and the area of decay, send it as well, noting in the narrative that it is accompanying the claim. Many times insufficient supporting documentation results in denials and increases work as well as frustration for both the office and the carrier.

15. *What is the difference between the codes for osseous surgery in the Periodontics category and the codes for periradicular surgery in the Endodontics category?*

The periodontic osseous surgery codes (D4260 and D4261) document procedures that modify the boney support of teeth by reshaping the alveolar process. These procedures apply when treating teeth that have a diagnosis of periodontitis and must include removal of supporting (ostectomy) or non-supporting (osteoplasty) bone.

The endodontic periradicular surgery codes (D3471–D3473, added in CDT 2021 as replacements for the deleted D3427) document procedures that treat root surfaces. These procedures apply when the pathology is primarily due to an endodontic issue, normally at the apex of the tooth without periodontal involvement, and where an apicoectomy procedure (amputation of the apex of a tooth) is not required.

16. *I have a patient who has had periodontal surgery six years ago. Although we have encouraged him to alternate his maintenance appointments with the periodontist, he insists on remaining in our office for recall. How often should I schedule his appointments and how should I code these maintenance visits since he is not seeing a periodontist? His homecare is good and only minimal pocket depths are present in localized areas.*

Since the patient has had periodontal therapy in the past, he should be coded with D4910 for all his visits where the periodontal maintenance procedure is delivered, regardless of whether he is treated in a general dentist's office or a periodontist's office. The D4910 covers site-specific scaling and root planing, if needed. An evaluation code should accompany the D4910. This can be:

D0120   periodic oral evaluation – established patient

D0150   comprehensive oral evaluation – new or established patient

D0180   comprehensive periodontal evaluation – new or established patient

It is recommended that a comprehensive periodontal evaluation, D0180, be completed annually since patients who have had periodontal therapy in the past are at a higher risk for recurrence. The number of maintenance visits annually should be determined by the treating dentist, based on the patient's homecare, stability and risk factors such as smoking or diabetes. Most periodontal maintenance patients require a three-to four-month schedule.

17. *What is the difference between anatomical crown exposure and a gingivectomy?*

Anatomical crown exposure (D4230 and D4231) is performed on healthy gingival tissues in order to obtain the correct gingival relationship or contour. Both hard and soft tissue are normally removed. This is a procedure that sometimes is done after orthodontic treatment to provide improved esthetics, for example. A gingivectomy is performed when supragingival pocketing is present with or without inflammation. No bone is removed, only soft tissue.

18. *When is it necessary to take an intraoral photograph of a periodontal patient?*

When recession is present, a photograph of the area prior to treatment is recommended. A photograph is also helpful in cases where a fracture or subgingival decay is present and visible after a flap has been elevated. In cases where there is an unusual condition that can be seen more visually, photographs can be appropriate for multiple reasons. Not only will a photograph be helpful if an appeal is necessary when requesting benefits from a third-party carrier, but they are also a means to communicate with the patient the need for treatment. Last but by no means least, photographs are part of your legal documentation

Summary

Filing for benefits related to periodontal procedures can be frustrating. In order to reduce issues with carriers and patients, some things can be routinely done to avoid problems. Use this checklist as a reminder:

- Obtain proper documentation when evaluating a patient who requires periodontal treatment. Full periodontal charting should be present, which includes not only pocket depths, but also recession, amount of attached gingiva, furcation involvement, mobility, bleeding on probing, clinical attachment loss and any other periodontal condition found. The charting should be recent, usually less than six months old. Radiographic images should typically be less than one year old. Periapical images are preferred over bitewing or panoramic images. At times, especially for soft tissue grafts, photographic images may be helpful, but these are not normally submitted with the initial claim.

- A pre-treatment estimate is the best way to avoid problems with reimbursement. Although not a guarantee of benefits, it establishes guidelines for the patient related to payments. With some plans, pre-treatment estimates may be valid for a limited time and this should be taken into consideration.

- When submitting for periodontal reimbursement, attachments are essential. For scaling and root planing, as well as osseous surgery, periapical radiographs and charting are necessary. For soft tissue grafting, recession and the amount of attached gingiva must be evident on the charting. If initial therapy has been performed prior to any necessary osseous surgery, many carriers will require periodontal charting after the scaling and root planing has healed and prior to the osseous surgery for comparison pocket depths. This holds true for periodontal maintenance patients also. If it is determined that treatment such as scaling and root planing or osseous surgery is needed and a patient has been on a periodontal maintenance schedule, then previous, as well as recent charting, should be available to demonstrate changes, normally seen as increased pocket depths between appointments.

Chapter 5: D4000–D4999 Periodontics

Contributor Biography

Marie Schweinebraten, D.M.D. is a practicing periodontist in Duluth, GA. She has been active in the dental tripartite, including serving on the ADA Council on Dental Benefit Programs and as Fifth District Trustee. While appointed to the Council on Dental Benefit Programs she represented the ADA on the Code Maintenance Committees. Presently she serves as Insurance Consultant for the American Academy of Periodontology, representing the AAP on the Code Maintenance Committee the past five years. Dr. Schweinebraten has given code workshops and is a certified insurance consultant.

Chapter 6: D5000–D5899
Prosthodontics, removable

Betsy K. Davis, D.M.D., M.S.

Introduction

This Prosthodontics category of service describes procedures which replace missing dentition in partially or completely edentulous patients. Stability and retention of a removable prosthesis reported with a code in this category of service is dependent on both hard and soft tissue support. Materials used in prosthesis fabrication have particular characteristics that are reflected in the nomenclatures of several codes used to document prosthesis fabrication and placement.

Because most of the materials used for a well-fitting prosthesis can be modified or repaired there is a significant portion of codes in this category to describe various repair, reline, and adjustment procedures. Such procedures are delivered to maintain or modify a prosthesis when changes occur to the supporting structures. It is important to note that all procedure codes in this category are inherently based on either a partial or complete denture. Moreover, nomenclatures of most codes specifically designate the involved arch — maxillary or mandibular.

Key Definitions and Concepts

The Glossary of Prosthodontics Terms from the Academy of Prosthodontics contains descriptors for all removable prosthodontic procedures, and is an excellent resource for comprehensive definitions of prosthodontic procedures. It is available at *www.academyofprosthodontics.org*.

Complete Denture: A removable prosthesis that replaces an entire arch of dentition and associated structures.

Partial Denture: A removable prosthesis that replaces a portion of missing dentition and associated structures.

The ADA Glossary definition of partial denture is: "Usually refers to a prosthetic device that replaces missing teeth. See fixed partial denture or removable partial denture."

The ADA Glossary definition of removable partial denture is: "A removable partial denture is a prosthetic replacement of one or more missing teeth that can be removed by the patient."

Immediate Partial or Immediate Complete Denture: A removable prosthesis that is specifically designed to replace a portion or all of the missing dentition in an arch, which is inserted immediately following extraction of teeth. Adaptation of the prosthesis frequently involves placement of a soft lining material at insertion, which is included as part of the routine delivery of care for these procedure codes.

It is important to note that an immediate denture procedure code only applies to the initial insertion appointment. Post-insertion visits for purposes of adjustments, repairs, or relines are documented with the code applicable to the type of denture subject to the procedure.

> The ADA Glossary definition of **immediate denture** is: "Prosthesis constructed for placement immediately after removal of remaining natural teeth."

Overdenture: A removable prosthesis that covers and is partially supported by natural teeth, roots, and/or dental implants.

> The ADA Glossary definition of **overdenture** is: "A removable prosthetic device that overlies and may be supported by retained tooth roots or implants."

Prosthesis: An artificial replacement of an absent part of the human body; designed to restore form and function.

> The ADA Glossary definition of **prosthesis** is: "Artificial replacement of any part of the body."

Changes to This Category

There are no new codes for this category. However, there are 16 editorial changes – none of which affect the nature of or manner by which these procedures are delivered to a patient.

The following eight changes bring consistency to how the clasping mechanism for the various types of removable prostheses are described in current code nomenclatures:

D5225 **maxillary partial denture – flexible base (including ~~any clasps,~~ retentive/clasping materials, rests, and teeth)**

D5226 **mandibular partial denture – flexible base (including ~~any clasps,~~ retentive/clasping materials, rests, and teeth)**

D5282 **removable unilateral partial denture – one piece cast metal (including ~~clasps~~ retentive/clasping materials, rests, and teeth), maxillary**

D5283   removable unilateral partial denture – one piece cast metal (including ~~clasps~~ retentive/clasping materials, rests, and teeth), mandibular

D5284   removable unilateral partial denture – one piece flexible base (including ~~clasps~~ retentive/clasping materials, rests, and teeth) – per quadrant

D5286   removable unilateral partial denture – one piece resin (including ~~clasps~~ retentive/clasping materials, rests, and teeth) – per quadrant

D5820   interim partial denture ~~(maxillary)~~ (including retentive/clasping materials, rests, and teeth), maxillary ~~Includes any necessary clasps and rests.~~

D5821   interim partial denture ~~(mandibular)~~ (including retentive/clasping materials, rests, and teeth), mandibular ~~Includes any necessary clasps and rests.~~

The following eight changes revise nomenclature wording to reflect contemporary terminology used to identify where the reline procedure is performed – "direct" or within the oral cavity; "indirect" or outside the oral cavity, which includes both in-office laboratories and external dental laboratories:

D5730   reline complete maxillary denture (~~chairside~~ direct)

D5731   reline complete mandibular denture (~~chairside~~ direct)

D5740   reline maxillary partial denture (~~chairside~~ direct)

D5741   reline mandibular partial denture (~~chairside~~ direct)

D5750   reline complete maxillary denture (~~laboratory~~ indirect)

D5751   reline complete mandibular denture (~~laboratory~~ indirect)

D5760   reline maxillary partial denture (~~laboratory~~ indirect)

D5761   reline mandibular partial denture (~~laboratory~~ indirect)

Clinical Coding Scenario #1:
Modification of Mandibular Complete Denture to Enable Placement on Implants

A patient presents with an existing mandibular complete denture which needs to be modified prior to placement on two implant fixtures recently integrated into the anterior mandible. Following the implant placement surgery the denture is relieved in the areas of implant support and retention, and a soft liner or tissue conditioner is placed to re-adapt the denture base.

How would you code these procedures related to changes made to the denture base?

> **D5875** **modification of removable prosthesis following implant surgery**
>
> **D5851** **tissue conditioning, mandibular**

Notes:

- D5875 is used to describe the procedure which modifies an existing removable prosthesis following implant surgery.

- **But**, in the event that a completely new implant supported mandibular overdenture will be fabricated with an implant attachment such as a locator, then the following codes in the Implant Services category would apply:

> **D6111** **implant/abutment supported removable denture for edentulous arch – mandible**
>
> **D6192** **semi-precision attachment – placement**

(Report each attachment assembly separately.)

Chapter 6: D5000–D5899 Prosthodontics, removable

Clinical Coding Scenario #2:
Removable Denture and Bone Loss

A patient presents with an existing mandibular removable partial denture which is supported by remaining anterior dentition, teeth #22 through #27. On examination, multiple teeth exhibit greater than 50 percent bone loss as demonstrated radiographically. Both #22 and #27 have existing PFM crowns, which have defective margins and recurrent decay.

The treatment plan involves removal of the remaining dentition, #22 through #27, with placement of new denture on the now completely edentulous mandible. An immediate mandibular complete denture will be fabricated in advance of the scheduled surgery, and inserted with a soft reline on the day of surgery.

How would you code the removable prosthodontic procedures completed in advance of the scheduled surgery?

The correct coding for the removable prosthesis is:

D5140   immediate denture – mandibular

How would you code future reline procedures for the removable denture placed on the day of scheduled surgery?

In this case, a chairside reline at a future visit would be coded as:

D5731   reline complete mandibular denture (direct)

As the immediate denture placed at the time of surgery has not been replaced with another prosthesis (e.g., implant/abutment supported removable denture) it is considered, for maintenance purposes such as relines and rebases, to be the same as a permanent complete denture. There are no codes for reline (and rebase) procedures applicable to any interim prosthesis.

Clinical Coding Scenario #3:
Complete Denture Repair

A patient presents relating that they dropped their maxillary complete denture, resulting in fracture of the buccal flange along the right side including the area comprising the tuberosity. The denture is otherwise in good condition, and the flange is able to be accurately re-assembled and repaired with acrylic resin.

How would you code this procedure?

D5512   **repair broken complete denture base, maxillary**

Clinical Coding Scenario #4:
Reinforcement of the Denture Base for a Complete Denture

A patient with a history of fracture and repair of the denture base due to an opposing arch of natural dentition and a Class III jaw relationship presents for a new maxillary complete denture. In order to strengthen the denture base, a metal substructure is added to the palatal aspect of the new denture to enhance resistance to fracture during function.

How would code this procedure?

D5876   **add metal substructure to acrylic complete denture (per arch)**

Clinical Coding Scenario #5:
Fractured Tooth and an Interim Prosthesis

A patient comes in with a fractured #3. The tooth is extracted by the oral surgeon with bone grafting/socket preservation. The oral surgeon requests an interim prosthesis to replace #3 during the healing process until an implant can be placed and an implant crown can be fabricated. The dentist fabricates a unilateral removable partial denture of a resin base to replace tooth #3.

How would you code for this prosthesis?

D5286   **removable unilateral partial denture – one piece resin (including retentive/clasping materials, rests, and teeth) – per quadrant**

Clinical Coding Scenario #6:
Fractured Teeth and a Removable Partial Denture

An 87-year-old patient presents to the office upon referral from the oral surgeon. The patient fractured teeth #7, #8, #9, and #10 as a result of a fall. The surgeon extracted teeth #7 through #10. A removable partial denture replacing teeth #7–10 was fabricated by the restorative dentist and inserted immediately at the time of the extractions. After several months of healing, she is in need of a new prosthesis to be used as an interim measure until her remaining dental work can be completed.

How would you code the prosthesis inserted at the time of extraction?

D5221 **immediate maxillary partial denture – resin base (including retentive/clasping materials, rests and teeth)**
Includes limited follow-up care only; does not include future rebasing/relining procedure(s).

What code would be applicable to report the procedure for fabrication and placement of the prosthesis placed after several months of healing?

This interim prosthesis would be reported with **D5820 interim partial denture (including retentive/clasping materials, rests, and teeth), maxillary**.

Clinical Coding Scenario #7:
Second Stage Implant Surgery (a.k.a., Stage II Surgery) and Placement of the Modified Prosthesis

A patient, who has a removable complete denture modified to enable placement on implant bodies, presents for surgery to exposure the previously placed implants. During this visit the dentist will complete the denture modification with placement of locators followed by prosthesis insertion.

What CDT codes are used to document the several procedures involved in this implant case?

D5875 **modification of removable prosthesis following implant surgery**
Attachment assemblies are reported using separate codes.

D6011 **surgical access to an implant body (second stage implant surgery)**
This procedure, also known as second stage implant surgery, involves removal of tissue that covers the implant body so that a fixture of any type can be placed, or an existing fixture be replaced with another. Examples of fixtures include but are not limited to healing caps, abutments shaped to help contour the gingival margins or the final restorative prosthesis.

D6191 **semi-precision abutment – placement**
This procedure is the initial placement, or replacement, of a semi-precision abutment on the implant body.

D6192 **semi-precision attachment – placement**
This procedure involves the luting of the initial, or replacement, semi-precision attachment to the removable prosthesis.

Clinical Coding Scenario #8:
Locator Attachment Repair

A patient presents to the office and is upset that her maxillary denture is loose. She demands that all six locator attachments receive new plastic housings and the dentist evaluates the situation. Upon closer examination the dentist determines that three of the attachments can be repaired, but three of the locator abutments on the implants are worn due to bruxism and cannot be repaired. Hence, three new locator abutments were placed.

How would you code the procedures delivered during this encounter?

D0140 **limited oral evaluation – problem focused**

D6091 **replacement of replaceable part of semi-precision or precision attachment (male or female component) of implant/abutment supported prosthesis, per attachment**

Note: This service is reported three times as the nomenclature states it is a "per attachment" procedure.

D6191 **semi-precision abutment – placement**
This procedure is the initial placement, or replacement, of a semi-precision abutment on the implant body.

Note: This service is reported three times as the nomenclature and descriptor use the singular form to describe the appliance ("abutment") and procedure's nature and scope.

Coding Q&A

1. *For a patient whose maxillary arch is fully edentulous, when would I report an immediate denture procedure (D5130) and when would I report the complete denture procedure (D5110)?*

   An immediate denture is a prosthesis that may be placed for aesthetic or clinical reasons and is inserted immediately following extraction of teeth when the definitive prosthesis is not available. A complete denture is the definitive prosthesis. The dentist determines the longevity of an immediate denture.

   Note: The above also applies to immediate partial dentures.

2. *How do I properly code refitting the denture base of an existing removable partial denture when additional teeth are added to this prosthesis?*

   If the entire denture base needs to be updated in an existing removable partial denture, meaning the borders of the edentulous area are developed to re-establish proper extension and contour, then the correct code for this procedure would be either **D5720 rebase maxillary partial denture** or **D5721 rebase mandibular partial denture**.

   The code to add an additional tooth to this existing partial denture is **D5650 add tooth to existing partial denture**.

3. *How do I code for a partial denture that needs an adjustment and a repair?*

   A maxillary partial denture that has a broken clasp assembly typically requires both a repair and an adjustment once the new clasp assembly is joined to the framework. This should be coded as **D5630 repair or replace broken retentive/clasping materials – per tooth** and **D5421 adjust partial denture – maxillary**.

4. *Is the procedure documented with code "**D5876 add a metal substructure to an acrylic full denture (per arch)**" applicable to fabrication of a new denture, or to the repair of an existing denture?*

   This procedure may be reported in either situation. The clinical scenario contained in the CDT Code Action Request that led to this code's addition in CDT 2019 states that this procedure is delivered to:

   > Patients who present with a broken denture or who have a history of heavy bruxism may be candidates for a substructure to be added to their denture. Additionally, patients with certain disabilities including the lack of fine motor skills or manual dexterity may need a substructure to prevent breakage of a new denture.

Chapter 6: D5000–D5899 Prosthodontics, removable

5. *How do I properly code the placement of a locator abutment on an implant?*

   D6191 semi-precision abutment – placement is the proper code for the initial placement or replacement of a semi-precision attachment on an implant body. It is recorded for each individual abutment.

6. *A patient has lost tooth #5 and grinds their teeth. The dentist decides to fabricate a unilateral partial denture with a metal base to address these conditions. How would you code this denture procedure?*

   D5282 removable unilateral partial denture – one piece cast metal (including retentive/clasping materials, rests, and teeth), maxillary

7. *A patient recently had insertion of immediate maxillary and mandibular complete dentures. Due to shrinkage, change of anatomical contour, the dentures are worn out and lack retention, stability, support. However, the patient is not ready for her definitive implant prostheses. She is in need of a new maxillary and mandibular dentures until she can have her definitive implant supported prosthesis. How would you code the dentures?*

   D5810 interim complete denture (maxillary)

   D5811 interim complete denture (mandibular)

   Interim prosthesis are provisional prosthesis designed for a limited period of time until the definitive restoration is ready to be fabricated.

Summary

The procedure codes listed in this category describe services related to either a partial or complete denture that is natural tooth borne. These removable denture procedures are not the same as those that are implant borne and listed in the CDT Code's Implant Services category. Keeping this concept in mind when coding for a procedure will simplify the correct code decision-making process.

Note: The inclusion of select procedure codes from the Implant Services category illustrate the differences in appropriate code selection.

Contributor Biography

Betsy K. Davis, D.M.D., M.S. is Professor in the Department of Otolaryngology/ H&N Surgery and holds the Keith and Wendy Wellin Endowed Chair in Maxillofacial Prosthodontics and Dental Oncology at the Medical University of South Carolina.

She is an adjunct faculty member in the Department of Bioengineering at Clemson University. Dr. Davis' research focuses on rehabilitation of the maxillofacial patient. She is also the Past-President for the American Academy of Maxillofacial Prosthetics, past Treasurer for the International Society for Maxillofacial Rehabilitation, and a representative for the American College of Prosthodontists and American Academy of Maxillofacial Prosthetics to CMS (Centers for Medicare and Medicaid Services).

Chapter 7: D5900–D5999
Maxillofacial Prosthetics

By Terri Bradley, C.P.C.

Introduction

The CDT Code's Maxillofacial Prosthetics category of service is very unique as the majority of codes address procedures for devices often used for patients with cancer, trauma (such as gunshot wounds), cleft palate, etc. Due to the various medical conditions of these patients, the majority of the codes and services in this category would be submitted to medical carriers. There are, however, codes for procedures in this section such as medicament carrier fabrication or splints that would be covered by dental carriers and not necessarily by medical carriers.

Key Definitions and Concepts

Splint: A prosthetic device which uses existing teeth or the alveolar process as points of anchorage to aid in the stabilization of broken bones (i.e., mandible, alveolar ridge) during healing. Splints are used to reestablish normal occlusion after trauma or procedures such as orthognathic surgery. These devices are stabilized by hard tissue.

> The ADA Glossary definition of **splint** is "A device used to support, protect, or immobilize oral structures that have been loosened, replanted, fractured or traumatized. Also refers to devices used in the treatment of temporomandibular joint disorders."

Stent: A prosthetic device which is used to apply pressure to soft tissue to aid in healing and to prevent scarring during healing. It can be used after surgery to aid in tissue closure and healing. Stents are often utilized for procedures post periodontal surgery, such as skin grafting.

Obturator: A prosthetic device which artificially replaces part of or all of the maxilla and associated teeth lost due to cancer, trauma or congenital defects. Obturators can be classified as interim, surgical and definitive.

> The ADA Glossary definition of **obturator** is "A disc or plate which closes an opening; a prosthesis that closes an opening in the palate."

Oral Prosthesis: An oral prosthesis is an artificial replacement which is either fixed or removable and aids in restoring normal form and function.

 © American Dental Association

Changes to This Category

There are two new codes and one code deletion in this category – the new codes replace the deleted code:

D5995 **periodontal medicament carrier with peripheral seal – laboratory processed – maxillary**

A custom fabricated, laboratory processed carrier for the maxillary arch that covers the teeth and alveolar mucosa. Used as a vehicle to deliver prescribed medicaments for sustained contact with the gingiva, alveolar mucosa, and into the periodontal sulcus or pocket.

D5996 **periodontal medicament carrier with peripheral seal – laboratory processed – mandibular**

A custom fabricated, laboratory processed carrier for the mandibular arch that covers the teeth and alveolar mucosa. Used as a vehicle to deliver prescribed medicaments for sustained contact with the gingiva, alveolar mucosa, and into the periodontal sulcus or pocket.

~~**D5994**~~ ~~**periodontal medicament carrier with peripheral seal– laboratory processed**~~

~~A custom fabricated, laboratory processed carrier that covers the teeth and alveolar mucosa. Used as a vehicle to deliver prescribed medicaments for sustained contact with the gingiva, alveolar mucosa, and into the periodontal sulcus or pocket.~~

Clinical Coding Scenario #1:
Implant Placement Guide

Four months after an extraction and socket preservation, a patient returns for endosteal implant placement at site #30. You fabricate a guide for the implant placement surgery. In the past, you have used **D5982 surgical stent** and you were recently told this is wrong.

How would you code this encounter?

The correct code to report for this scenario is **D6190 radiographic/ surgical implant index, by report**, which is in another CDT Code category of service (Implant Services). Code D5982 in Maxillofacial Prosthetics is **not** the appropriate code to report in this case as it is applicable when reporting a surgical stent to apply pressure to soft tissues to facilitate healing and prevent cicatrization or collapse.

Clinical Coding Scenario #2:
Obturator for Cancer Patient

A patient was referred to you for fabrication of an obturator. The patient was recently diagnosed with mucoepidermoid carcinoma of the maxilla. He currently has a surgical obturator that was fabricated for him pre-operatively but no longer fits well. You plan on fabricating another obturator for him instead of modifying the ill-fitting prosthesis.

What other obturator(s) might you fabricate for your patient and how would you code for this prosthesis?

The provider can provide the patient with either an interim (D5936) or a definitive (D5932) obturator depending on the clinical condition. If the patient requires an interim obturator they will likely require the fabrication of a definitive prosthesis once healing is complete.

Clinical Coding Scenario #3:
Obturator for Palatal Perforation Due to Cocaine Use

A patient with a history of cocaine abuse presents with palatal perforation and nasal communication due to snorting cocaine. The patient states that they are having a hard time eating and drinking. You decide to make an obturator for your patient. The patient is not pursuing surgical treatment at this time.

How would you code for fabricating the appliance used in this treatment?

   D5932 obturator prosthesis, definitive

What other obturator(s) might you fabricate for your patient and how would you code for this?

If the patient decides to pursue surgical treatment, you can code **D5931 obturator prosthesis, surgical**. Any obturator adjustments (to the surgical or definitive obturator), can be coded with **D5933 obturator prosthesis, modification**.

Clinical Coding Scenario #4:
Appliance for Patient Undergoing Radiation Therapy

Your patient is diagnosed with squamous cell carcinoma and is scheduled to undergo radiation therapy. In order to best protect the unaffected tongue and oral mucosa, you decide to fabricate an oral appliance.

How would you code this appliance fabrication procedure?

You would use **D5984 radiation shield**.

Clinical Coding Scenario #5:
Protecting Dentition During Cancer Treatment

A patient was recently diagnosed with cancer of the tongue and will be undergoing radiation therapy in the very near future. The patient's oncologist suggested the patient see you to discuss ways to protect the dentition during cancer therapy. The doctor recommends fluoride trays for the patient.

How would you code for the fluoride tray fabrication?

D5986 fluoride gel carrier

Synonymous terminology: fluoride applicator.

A prosthesis, which covers the teeth in either dental arch and is used daily to apply topical fluoride in close proximity to tooth enamel and dentin for several minutes daily.

Clinical Coding Scenario #6:
Snoring and Treatment Appliances

A patient comes in stating that his wife complained his snoring is so loud at night that some nights she sleeps in the other room. He has seen his medical doctor and has been told that he does not have obstructive sleep apnea; he is just a loud snorer and his snoring seems to be worse after a high stress day.

The doctor fabricates a snore guard for the patient.

How would you code for this appliance fabrication?

Many people are unaware that the Maxillofacial Prosthetics category includes a number of non-orthodontic treatment appliances. However, there is not a specific code for the snore guard. Since such an appliance is similar to other appliances in the Maxillofacial Prosthetics category, it would be appropriate to use this code:

D5999 unspecified maxillofacial prosthesis, by report

Clinical Coding Scenario #7:
Mouth Lesions

A 50-year-old woman comes to the office stating that she has painful lesions in her mouth. Upon clinical inspection, it is noted that the tissue is erythematous and the lesions look erosive in nature, and there are some bullae present. You suspect that the patient has pemphigus vulgaris. The patient states that the lesions have been there for four days and that she has been self-treating with salt water rinses. You prescribe a topical steroid for the lesions and arrange for the lab to create a medicament carrier that will cover the affected areas.

How would you code for fabricating this type of medicament carrier?

D5991   vesiculobullous disease medicament carrier
A custom fabricated carrier that covers the teeth and alveolar mucosa, or alveolar mucosa alone, and is used to deliver prescription medicaments for treatment of immunologically mediated vesiculobullous diseases.

Clinical Coding Scenario #8:
Post-radiation Trismus

A 67-year-old female patient has recently completed her radiation treatment for pT4N2M0 squamous cell carcinoma. The patient reports that since completing radiation, she has had a difficult time opening her mouth more than 15 mm. The patients TMJs are asymptomatic bilaterally. She is worried that lack of mouth opening will harm her oral health and lead to increased weight loss. Her lip opening is within normal limits.

The doctor fabricates a trismus appliance.

How would you code for this fabrication procedure?

D5937   trismus appliance (not for TMD treatment)

This prosthesis can be used to aid in opening the bite of a patient with trismus for causes other than TMJ dysfunction (i.e., radiation treatment).

Clinical Coding Scenario #9:
Malignant Neoplasm of the Hard Palate

Your patient has been diagnosed with a malignant neoplasm of the hard palate, and the planned treatment includes surgical removal of the neoplasm and radiation therapy. Prior to delivery of these treatments you fabricate a surgical obturator to be placed after the removal of the neoplasm, and a radiation shield. After the surgery, the plan is to fabricate both interim and definitive obuturator prostheses.

After the surgery however, due to the fit of the surgical obturator, an interim prosthesis is not needed by the patient and only the definitive prosthesis is created.

How would you code these appliance procedures?

    D5984   **radiation shield**

    D5931   **obturator prosthesis, surgical**

Note: If the surgical obturator is to be modified prior to placement of a definitive obturator, the modification procedure would be reported with: **D5992 adjust maxillofacial prosthetic appliance, by report**.

    D5932   **obturator prosthesis, definitive**

Maintenance of the definitive obturator would be coded as:

    D5993   **maintenance and cleaning of a maxillofacial prosthesis (extra-or intra-oral) other than required by adjustments, by report**

Clinical Coding Scenario #10:
Gunshot Wound and Ocular Prosthesis

A 30-year-old male was involved in an altercation and sustained a gunshot wound to the left side of his head. Evaluation and imaging obtained in the emergency department revealed left side orbital blow out fracture and left side globe rupture. The patient was taken emergently to the operating room for enucleation of the left globe and repair of facial fractures. His left eye was removed during surgery. The patient is seen in your clinic post-operatively to be evaluated for prosthesis for his left eye to replace the eye that was removed.

How would you code for the post-operative encounter services?

D0999 unspecified diagnostic procedure, by report
This "999" code is applicable to the in-clinic evaluation that led to fabrication of the prosthesis for the patient's left eye.

D5916 ocular prosthesis
Synonymous terminology: artificial eye, glass eye.

A prosthesis, which artificially replaces an eye missing as a result of trauma, surgery or congenital absence. The prosthesis does not replace missing eyelids or adjacent skin, mucosa or muscle.

Ocular prostheses require semiannual or annual cleaning and polishing. Occasional revisions to re-adapt the prosthesis to the tissue bed may be necessary. Glass eyes are rarely made and cannot be re-adapted.

Clinical Coding Scenario #11:
Patient with Maxillary Hypoplasia

An 18-year-old female patient presents with maxillary hypoplasia. The treatment plan for her is a LeFort 1 (three pieces) for which a surgical splint needs to be fabricated.

How do you code for the surgical splint?

D5988 surgical splint

Synonymous terminology: Gunning splint, modified Gunning splint, labiolingual splint, fenestrated splint, Kingsley splint, cast metal splint.

Splints are designed to utilize existing teeth and/or alveolar processes as points of anchorage to assist in stabilization and immobilization of broken bones during healing. They are used to re-establish, as much as possible, normal occlusal relationships during the process of immobilization. Frequently, existing prostheses (e.g., a patient's complete dentures) can be modified to serve as surgical splints. Frequently, surgical splints have arch bars added to facilitate intermaxillary fixation. Rubber elastics may be used to assist in this process. Circummandibular eyelet hooks can be utilized for enhanced stabilization with wiring to adjacent bone.

Coding Q&A

1. *I am a maxillofacial prosthodontist working in a large academic setting. The patients I am treating have some pretty significant medical conditions. What are the codes I would use to bill to a dental carrier and a medical carrier for the surgical, interim and definitive obturator prosthesis?*

   CDT codes are used on claims filed with dental benefit plans; CPT codes are used on claims filed with medical benefit plans.

   Surgical obturator: CDT code is D5931; CPT code is 21076.

   Interim obturator prosthesis: CDT code is D5936; CPT code is 21079.

   Definitive obturator prosthesis: CDT code is D5932; CPT code is 21080.

   If the claim is being filed with the patient's medical benefit plan using the appropriate (i.e., not dental) claim format a diagnosis (ICD-10-CM) code is required. One example of an ICD-10-CM diagnosis code applicable in this scenario is: **C05.0 Malignant neoplasm of the hard palate**. Keep in mind the diagnosis code reported on the claim must be supported by the documentation in the patient's healthcare record.

2. *What is the difference between a surgical, interim and definitive obturator? The terms are so confusing!*

   A surgical obturator is created and used during surgery and immediately post-operatively. The interim prosthesis is used for the duration of the healing, which can be anywhere from two to six months. After about six months, the definitive prosthesis is given to the patient, and it may last for many years.

3. *A patient has an obturator fabricated pre-operatively for placement immediately after a tumor removal surgery. Due to the excellent fit and comfort of this obturator, the patient decides they do not want another until the final prosthesis is fabricated. Some time later that patient returns and states that the obturator does not fit as well as it had before. What code would you use to document the necessary adjustment?*

   You would use **D5993 obturator prosthesis, modification**.

4. *Are obturators used only for cancer patients?*

   No, obturators can be used for patients with a various medical conditions. Patients with palatal perforations due to infection, disease, recreational drug use, or cleft palate may require an obturator as part of their treatment. Not all patients will require a definitive obturator. Some may need a surgical or interim obturator while receiving treatment or in between reconstructive surgeries.

5. *I'm still a little confused about the different types of obturators and when they're used. Can you go into more detail?*

   Surgical obturators (D5931) are delivered to the patient on the date of surgery. It may not fit exactly and will likely require some adjustment. An interim obturator (D5936) is intended to be used prior to the fabrication of a definitive obturator during the healing period. The patient will likely have this for a number of months. Sometimes, if the fit is good, a patient will opt to have their surgical obturator modified rather than have an interim obturator fabricated. A definitive obturator (D5932) is fabricated after healing has occurred. It is designed to be the patient's "final" obturator, though if the patient has it for a number of years it will likely need to be replaced.

6. *I noticed there's a code for a feeding aid (D5951). When would I use this?*

   A feeding aid is used in infants with cleft palates prior to surgery. The prosthesis is placed in the infant's mouth during feeding to help aid in suckling and swallowing. After surgery, the device is not needed. Its use is meant to be intermittent and interim in nature.

7. *What is the difference between "**D5986 fluoride gel carrier**" and "**D5995 periodontal medicament carrier with peripheral seal – laboratory processed – maxillary**"?*

   A fluoride gel carrier is used for application of topic fluoride only and it only covers the teeth. The periodontal medicament carrier, however, covers both the teeth and the alveolar mucosa. It is used to deliver medications to tissues (gingiva), membranes (alveolar mucosa), and into periodontal pockets. Report D5995 for a maxillary medicament carrier and D5996 for a mandibular medicament carrier.

8. *In dental coding, is there a separate code for a snoring appliance versus an appliance for patients with sleep apnea?*

   There is not a specific CDT code for either appliance. The best choice of code is to use **D5999 unspecified maxillofacial prosthesis, by report**. For medical coding, it is important to remember that while many patients with sleep apnea do snore, not all patients who snore have sleep apnea and the medical codes for the various appliances are very different. Diagnosis of obstructive sleep apnea is required to bill for an oral sleep apnea (OSA) appliance to a medical benefit plan.

9. *Is a sleep study required before I can code for a sleep apnea appliance?*

    There is no specific code for a sleep apnea appliance, so you would use **D5999 unspecified maxillofacial prosthesis, by report**. The patient will need to have a formal diagnosis of obstructive sleep apnea. This usually includes a sleep study.

    If you file a claim with the patient's medical benefit plan the following codes are applicable:

    - HCPCS procedure – E0486 oral device/appliance used to reduce upper airway collapsibility, adjustable or non-adjustable, custom fabricated, includes fitting and adjustment.
    - ICD-10-CM diagnosis – G47.33 Obstructive Sleep Apnea

10. *What is the difference between a trismus appliance and a commissure splint?*

    Both a trismus appliance (D5937) and a commissure splint (D5987) aim to accomplish the same goal: increasing the mouth opening of the patient. Commissure splints are used to increase the opening of the lips specifically. Trismus appliances are used to increase the opening of the oral aperture, not the lips themselves.

11. *What are some examples of vesiculobullous diseases?*

    Examples of vesiculobullous diseases include:

    - Paraneoplastic pemphigus
    - Pemphigus vulgaris
    - Bullous pemphigoid
    - Erythema multiforme
    - Herpes Simplex

12. *A patient requires medication to be delivered to soft tissue areas in the oral cavity due to painful ulcerated lesions. Which prosthesis would be fabricated and how would it be coded?*

    The patient would require a disease medicament carrier, not a periodontal medicament carrier, as a seal is not required. The applicable procedure is documented with CDT code **D5991 vesiculobullous disease medicament carrier**.

Chapter 7: D5900–D5999 Maxillofacial Prosthetics

13. *Can I use the "periodontal medicament carrier" and "vesiculobullous disease medicament carrier" codes on the same patient? Are these codes somewhat interchangeable?*

These two codes are not interchangeable. While both are used to describe medicament carriers, the need for these two appliances are quite different. **D5991 vesiculobullous disease medicament carrier** can only be used for patients who have a vesiculobullous disease. The periodontal medicament carrier (D5995 or D5996 depending on the involved arch) is used primarily to treat periodontal disease and deliver medications targeted at the pathogens that cause various periodontal diseases. These appliances are treating two different disease processes. D5995 or D5996 is used to treat diseases that are periodontal in nature, while D5991 is used to treat mucocutaneous diseases involving mucous membranes and skin.

14. *I have a patient who is eight years old and who has a speech impediment due to a palatal defect. The patient is not yet ready for surgery and is having a difficult time with socialization. How can I code for the prosthesis I made?*

The correct code for this scenario would be **D5952 speech aid prosthesis, pediatric**. This prosthesis is used temporarily, or as an interim prosthesis to close a palatal defect. The defect may be developmental or surgical in nature. It is not intended to be used as a permanent prosthetic device.

15. *I have a patient that has a nasal prosthesis and now needs a new one fabricated. She has been wearing the prosthesis for several years after having extensive surgery on her nose to treat her diagnosis of skin cancer. We still have her original mold. How do I code for the new nasal prosthesis?*

The correct code to report would be **D5926 nasal prosthesis, replacement** as the patient's new artificial nose is produced from the previously made mold. A replacement prosthesis does not require fabrication of a new mold.

16. *A patient well known to your practice presents with an obturator that they have had for eight years stating that one of the clasps broke off last night. You offer to send the prosthesis to the lab for replacement of the clasp. How do I code for this repair procedure?*

In this case, the correct code is **D5993 maintenance and cleaning of a maxillofacial prosthesis (extra-or intra-oral) other than required adjustments, by report**.

Summary

Due to the severity of the medical condition of so many of the patients seen by maxillofacial prosthodontists (i.e., cancer, gunshot wound, cleft, ameloblastoma, etc.), the majority of the procedures will be billed to medical carriers. Thus, it is important to ensure that you are using the proper CPT code if there is one (there are not always individual CPT codes for all CDT codes) when coding. If there is no specific CPT code, you may bill the medical carrier using the CDT code.

The other pitfall to coding for these procedures for the coder (not necessarily the provider) is a clear understanding of what is actually happening and why is the prosthesis being fabricated in the first place. The definitions are very specific and it is necessary to understand the nuances and differences between them.

Contributor Biography

Terri Bradley, C.P.C., is the owner of Terri Bradley Consulting and OMS Billing Solutions. With a hands-on background spanning more than 30 years, Terri is a practice management expert devoted to her clients. She is highly sought after for speaking engagements offering medical/dental/OMS coding and billing workshops across the country. Her publications include the *Fonseca Oral and Maxillofacial Surgery* textbook chapter (Volume III, released fall 2017) and *Dictations and Coding in Oral and Maxillofacial Surgery.*

Chapter 7: D5900–D5999 Maxillofacial Prosthetics

Chapter 8: D6000–D6199
Implant Services

By Linda Vidone, D.M.D.

Introduction

The CDT Code's Implant Services category is somewhat unique and challenging compared to other categories of service because it includes separate entries for procedures that address:

- Surgical placement of the implant post (or body or fixture)
- Placement of connecting components when needed
- The final prosthetic restoration (single crowns, bridges or dentures)

Once these three basic concepts of implant procedures (addressed in greater detail below) are understood, it will become less challenging and even easy to select the appropriate CDT Code to document the procedures performed.

Note: When performing implant procedures, it's important to remember that not all codes are in the Implant Services category. For example, codes for membrane placement (D4266 and D4267) are in the Periodontics category (D4000–D4999) and codes for sinus augmentation (D7951 and D7952) are in the Oral Maxillofacial Surgery category (D7000–D7999).

Key Definitions and Concepts

Basic Implant

This image illustrates all components of a single implant. Please note that the connecting element (abutment) may not be present in all cases. The dentist's clinical decision-making determines whether the implant crown will be supported and retained by an intermediary abutment, or if it may be placed directly on the implant body.

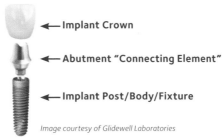

←— Implant Crown

←— Abutment "Connecting Element"

←— Implant Post/Body/Fixture

Image courtesy of Glidewell Laboratories

Implant Post/Body/Fixture

The two most common types of implant posts are endosteal and mini implants. The size and type of implant fixture determines the proper code to document the surgical implant placement procedure.

Surgical Placement of an Implant Body: Endosteal Implant (D6010): Placement of full-sized implant fixture into the jawbone.

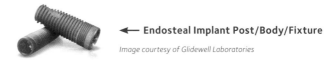

←— Endosteal Implant Post/Body/Fixture

Image courtesy of Glidewell Laboratories

Surgical Placement of Mini-Implant (D6013): Placement of mini implant fixture into the jawbone. These are smaller in diameter than full sized implants, yet are still considered permanent. They are typically used to support removable prostheses, but implant-supported crowns can be placed on the mini-implants as well.

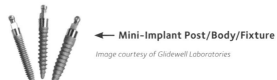

←— Mini-Implant Post/Body/Fixture

Image courtesy of Glidewell Laboratories

Connecting Elements for Implant Crowns, Implant Retainer Crowns and Implant Prostheses

Abutments, both prefabricated (D6056) and custom (D6057), are the "connecting elements" that are placed, when needed, between the implant post and the restorative crown (definitive prosthesis), retainer crown (for a fixed partial denture), or prosthesis such as a fixed hybrid denture. Abutments are not always needed, but when placed are reported separately from the from the crown restoration.

Prefabricated Abutment (D6056): A manufactured component. The procedure includes modification and placement.

←— **Prefabricated Abutment**

Image courtesy of Glidewell Laboratories

Custom Abutment (D6057): Created by a laboratory for a specific individual, usually if there are aesthetic concerns. The procedure includes placement. Custom abutments are custom cast by a laboratory or CAD/CAM milled.

←— **Custom Abutment**

Image courtesy of Glidewell Laboratories

Semi-precision Abutment – placement (D6191): One component part of the manufactured connection between a prosthesis and implant body. The procedure involves placement of this prefabricated abutment (a.k.a, "locator") onto the implant post.

←— **Semi-precision Abutment**

Image courtesy of Glidewell Laboratories

Note: Placement of the second component part of this connection (a.k.a, "keeper assembly") into the prosthesis is a separate procedure documented and reported with its own code **D6192 semi-precision attachment – placement**.

Connecting Bar – Implant Supported or Abutment Supported (D6055): A device to help stabilize prostheses. Attaches to abutments or directly to the implants themselves to make the prosthesis more secure. Hader® and Dolder® are two types of connecting bars that can be designed to use other types of retentive mechanisms, such as semi-precision attachments. The entire bar is reported as a single unit; however, an abutment would be documented for each implant that supports the connecting bar.

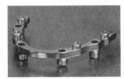

← **Connecting Bar – Implant Supported or Abutment Supported**

Image courtesy of Glidewell Laboratories

Implant Prostheses (Includes Single Crowns, Fixed Bridges and Dentures)

There are two types of single unit implant crowns – abutment supported, and implant supported. Selection of the appropriate crown procedure code is determined by the type of material used for the crown and the type of attachment.

Most of us are familiar with the type of material used (porcelain, metal, etc.). However, there is sometimes confusion over appropriate coding when there are ways to attach the restorative prosthesis to its supporting structure: via an intermediary abutment or directly by the implant.

Note: Both abutment supported and implant supported crowns are may be retained by either cemented or screw retaineds, but neither of these options is a determining factor in code selection.

Abutment Supported Single Unit Crowns (D6058–D6064, D6094, and D6097): These are crowns that are attached to an abutment (D6056 or D6057), not directly to the implant post. The applicable abutment procedure code is submitted with the applicable single unit crown procedure code. These crowns obtain stability from the abutment. This is the most common type of implant crown.

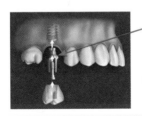

— **Abutment**

Image courtesy of Glidewell Laboratories

Implant Supported Single Unit Crowns (D6065–D6067 and D6082–D6088): Implant crowns are attached directly to the implant post (one-piece retained crown). *Even though a separate abutment may be used in the manufacturing process, it is delivered as an integral part of the one-piece crown.* Typically, single unit implant supported are screw retained and the access opening sealed with composite material. These crowns obtain stability directly from the implant.

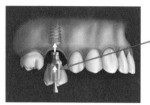

— No abutment

Image courtesy of Glidewell Laboratories

Implant Supported Fixed Partial Dentures (Implant Bridges)

There are two types of implant retainer crowns: abutment supported and implant supported. Retainer crowns will have one or more pontics attached, the total number of pontics being determined (and reported separately with their applicable code) by the edentulous space being bridged. Selection of the appropriate retainer crown procedure code is based on the same criteria used for single implant crowns: the type of material used and the method of attachment.

Note: Both abutment supported and implant supported retainer crowns may be retained by either cement or screws, but neither of these options is a determining factor in code selection.

Abutment Supported Retainer Crowns (D6068–D6074 and D6194–D6195): These are retainer crowns that are attached to an abutment (D6056 or D6057), not directly to the implant post. The applicable abutment procedure code is submitted with the applicable retainer crown procedure code.

Implant Supported Retainer Crowns (D6075–D6077, D6098–D6099, and D6120–D6123): Implant retainer crowns are attached directly to the implant post. *No abutment is used with this type of crown.*

Implant/Abutment Supported Dentures

There are two types of implant or abutment supported dentures: removable and fixed (also known as hybrid). Implant dentures, unlike single unit crowns and retainer crowns, are *not* determined by the type of attachment system.

Denture procedure code selection is determined by two factors:

- Is the denture replacing a full or partial complement of teeth?
- Will the patient be able to remove the denture by themselves, or is assistance needed from the dentist or dental staff?

If the patient is able to remove the denture by themselves, it is a removable implant denture. If the patient is unable to remove the denture and requires the assistance of dentist or dental staff, then the denture is a fixed implant denture.

Although a fixed implant bridge and fixed implant denture appear similar, the denture's supporting implant locations do not have a specific relationship to the missing natural teeth. This is why a fixed implant denture is referred to as a "hybrid" denture.

Implant/Abutment Supported Removable Dentures: Overdentures are supported by implants; the patient is able to remove them. These dentures typically have prefabricated abutments placed, a connecting bar, and a precision or semi-precision attachment. (Note these components are not included in the denture and should all be submitted as separate procedures.) Codes for removable complete dentures are D6110 and D6111; codes for removable partials are D6112 and D6113.

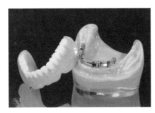

← **Implant/abutment supported removable dentures**

Image courtesy of Zest Dental Solutions

Implant/Abutment Supported Fixed (Hybrid) Dentures: Implant dentures that the patient cannot remove and are either screwed directly on the implant or connected via abutments. (Note abutments are not included in the denture and when used should be submitted as separate procedures.) The implant supported dentures are heavily advertised as an "All-on-4®." Yet there can be more implants. In addition to All-on-4, another common name for implant supported dentures is hybrid denture. Codes for fixed complete dentures (dentures that replace all missing teeth) are D6114 and D6115. Typically, four to eight implants are utilized and are not in absolute tooth positions. Codes for fixed partials are D6116 and D6117.

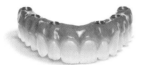

← **Hybrid dentures**

Image courtesy of Glidewell Laboratories

Changes to This Category

Implant techniques and materials continue to advance and improve, and these evolutionary changes prompt CDT Code changes as well. In the Implant Services category CDT 2021 contains two additions, one deletion, two revisions and one editorial change. Some of these changes are interrelated and others are stand-alone.

The following deletion and two additions are related to clarify and allow accurate documentation of semi-precision attachment placement procedures.

> ~~D6052~~ ~~semi-precision attachment abutment~~
> ~~Includes placement of keeper assembly.~~

This code was deleted as it neither adequately nor clearly described the procedure's scope or the component parts used when the service is delivered to a patient. The two new replacement codes, which fill the coding gap created by this deletion, are:

D6191 semi-precision abutment – placement
This procedure is the initial placement, or replacement, of a semi-precision abutment on the implant body.

D6192 semi-precision attachment – placement
This procedure involves the luting of the initial, or replacement, semi-precision attachment to the removable prosthesis.

These additions recognize that there are two attachment procedures during placement of a semi-precision assembly: one involves placement of the semi precision abutment on the underlying supporting structure (e.g., implant post); the other involves placement/luting of the semi-precision attachment to the removable prosthesis. These components may be placed, or replaced, independent of each other.

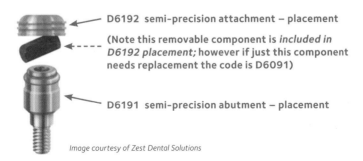

D6192 semi-precision attachment – placement

(Note this removable component is *included in D6192 placement;* however if just this component needs replacement the code is D6091)

D6191 semi-precision abutment – placement

Image courtesy of Zest Dental Solutions

In addition, there are two stand-alone (i.e., not related to any other change) CDT code revisions:

D6011 <u>**surgical access to an implant body (second stage implant surgery)**</u>
~~Surgical access to an implant body for placement of a healing cap or to enable placement of an abutment.~~ <u>This procedure, also known as second stage implant surgery, involves removal of tissue that covers the implant body so that a fixture of any type can be placed, or an existing fixture be replaced with another. Examples of fixtures include but are not limited to healing caps, abutments shaped to help contour the gingival margins or the final restorative prosthesis.</u>

The previous definition of D6011 did not clearly and fully describe the nature and scope of the procedure, nor did it acknowledge that clinical needs may prompt repeated removal of overgrown gingival tissue.

D6091 **replacement of** <u>**replaceable part of**</u> **semi-precision or precision attachment (male or female component) of implant/abutment supported prosthesis, per attachment**
~~This procedure applies to the replaceable male or female component of the attachment.~~

The D6091 revision clarifies the nomenclature's wording to specify that the procedure involves replacement of an attachment's replaceable part or parts. This allows consistency with the comparable procedure within the removable Prosthodontics category, **D5867 replacement of replaceable part of semi-precision or precision attachment (male or female component)**.

The stand-alone editorial change corrects the descriptor so that it is consistent with the nomenclature's wording:

D6098 **implant supported retainer – porcelain fused to predominantly base alloys**
A metal-ceramic retainer for a fixed partial denture that gains retention, support and stability from an ~~abutment on an~~ implant.

Note: When selecting the appropriate CDT code for a denture retainer the key determinants are the type of material used in fabrication and whether an abutment is placed between the retainer and the implant body. A retainer crown may be retained by either cement or a screw, but neither of these options is a determining factor in code selection.

Abutment vs. Retainer

When implant procedures were first introduced in CDT-1 (effective January 1, 1990), confusion arose over the term abutment, a word with different meanings within the Implants category of service and within the Prosthodontics category of service. For Implants, "abutment" was associated with the piece that connected the implant body with the restorative prosthesis. In Prosthodontics, the term was used to describe a supporting (anchor) tooth in a fixed bridge.

The current and continuing usage for the term "abutment" applies only to the piece that connects the implant body with the restorative prosthesis. "Retainer" is the term solely used to describe the anchor tooth (natural or prosthetic) for a fixed partial denture.

CPT Codes Applicable to Implant Procedures

Claims against a patient's medical benefit plan use the AMA's CPT (Current Procedural Terminology) procedure codes on the medical claim format. Keep in mind there are no CDT codes that exactly match CPT codes regarding implant restorations. Medical carriers may benefit for the implant placement and necessary bone grafting, but the final restorative prosthesis is typically never a benefit.

A sample of CPT codes for implant placement and bone grafting are in the following tables:

Surgical Placement and Removal of Dental Implants	
Code	Nomenclature
20670	Removal of implant, superficial
20680	Removal of implant, deep
21248	Reconstruction of maxilla/mandible endosteal implant, partial (1–3 per jaw)
21249	Reconstruction of maxilla/mandible endosteal implant, complete (4–6 per jaw)
21085	Diagnostic/surgical stent

Bone Grafts	
Code	Nomenclature
21210	Graft, bone, nasal, maxillary, or malar areas (includes obtaining graft)
21215	Graft, bone, mandibular areas (includ es obtaining graft)
0232T	Platelet rich plasma
41899	Nonspecific code (Used for guided tissue regeneration)

Clinical Coding Scenario #1:
Abutment Supported Porcelain Implant Crown Tooth #7

The patient has a long history of dental treatment on #7 that began when hit by a ball in her mouth when she was 14 years old. The affected tooth (#7) received a root canal, post and core, and crown at the time of the accident. At age 22 she received retreatment of the root canal, apicoectomy, a new post and core, and a new crown procedures.

The patient is now 30 years old and presents with tooth #7 re-infected. The dentist suspects a vertical fracture and determines through the oral evaluation that she has class 2 mobility with 7 mm pocket on the buccal, and the adjacent teeth are perfectly healthy with no restorations nor do they need restorations.

The mobility and pocket depth findings for #7 indicate a poor prognosis for retention and the dentist proposes a lengthy multi-part treatment plan that leads to a single tooth abutment supported implant crown as the final restorative prosthesis.

What codes would document the services for each part of the treatment plan?

Part 1: Extraction of #7 with Ridge Preservation and Insertion of a "Flipper"

D7210 extraction, erupted tooth requiring removal of bone and/or sectioning of tooth, and including elevation of mucoperiosteal flap if indicated

D7953 bone replacement graft for ridge preservation – per site

Notes:
- Bone in this area is thin, therefore it is imperative that the ridge be preserved.
- This procedure is also referred to as "socket preservation" with the placement in the extraction site at the time of the extraction to preserve the size and shape of the bone.

D4266 guided tissue regeneration – resorbable barrier, per site

Note: The D7953 procedure does not include placement of a barrier membrane to prevent tissue from invading the bone graft site and there is no separate code for a membrane with ridge preservation. D4266 is used to document placement of the barrier membrane.

D5820 interim partial denture (including retentive/clasping materials, rests, and teeth), maxillary

Note: D5820 is the "flipper" procedure.

Part 2: Implant Placement Surgery and Second Stage Surgery and Provisional Implant Crown

The patient was unhappy with the removable appliance and wanted a tooth as soon as possible. The dentist decided at second stage surgery to fabricate and insert a provisional implant crown.

Note: The implant post is surgically placed and followed by second stage surgery six months later.

    D6010   **surgical placement of implant body: endosteal implant**

    D6011   **surgical access to an implant body (second stage surgery)**

    D6085   **provisional implant crown**

Part 3: Final Restoration – Custom Abutment and Abutment Supported Porcelain Crown

Note: In this case, esthetics were a concern. A custom abutment was placed due to angulation concerns and final material chosen was porcelain since the patient has a high smile line.

    D6057   **custom fabricated abutment – includes placement**

    D6058   **abutment supported porcelain/ceramic crown**

Chapter 8: D6000–D6199 Implant Services

Clinical Coding Scenario #2:
Implant Supported Mandibular Denture for an Edentulous Patient

The patient has worn a complete mandibular denture for over 10 years with an occasional reline. The most recent reline was two years ago. Before this there were no problems with fit or retention, but since the last reline the patient has been using an adhesive to glue in the denture with limited success. The patient is also edentulous on the maxillary but is happy with her denture. The patient had previously declined a recommendation to replace the denture with implants and fabricate an overdenture that would be placed on the implants. Now the patient has agreed to implant treatment.

What codes would be used to document services delivered as the treatment progressed?

Initial Services

Since the patient has been edentulous for over ten years, a cone beam CT scan was necessary to evaluate the mandibular jaw bone dimensions. This enables an assessment to determine whether bone augmentation is needed prior to implant placement. A surgical guide was made and used during radiographic exposure for treatment planning and will be used again during implant placement.

> **D0365** cone beam CT capture and interpretation with field of view of one full dental arch – mandible
>
> **D6190** radiographic/surgical implant index, by report

Implant Post Placement

The cone beam image revealed there was enough bone to place two implants in positions of teeth #22 and #27. However, after placing the implant bodies a few threads were exposed, so a bone graft and membrane were also necessary.

> **D6010** surgical placement of implant body: endosteal implant

Note: Report D6010 twice as two implant bodies were placed, one for #22 and the second for #27.

> **D6104** bone graft at the time of implant placement

Note: The bone graft procedure (D6104) does not include placement of a barrier membrane and there is no separate code for membranes with implant bone grafts. Use one of the following codes, as applicable, to report barrier membrane placement.

D4266 **guided tissue regeneration – resorbable barrier, per site**

D4267 **guided tissue regeneration – non-resorbable barrier, per site (includes membrane removal)**

Second Stage Surgery and Placement of the Restorative Prosthesis

The patient will continue to wear her existing denture as the implants heal. After the implants have successfully integrated, the next step is to begin the restorative treatment. Second stage surgery is followed by placement of semi-precision abutments. A newly fabricated mandibular complete overdenture is inserted with the semi-precision attachments in the denture.

These procedures are documented as follows:

D6011 **surgical access to an implant body (second stage surgery)**

Note: Report D6011 twice as the procedure is required for each of the two implant bodies placed.

D6191 **semi-precision abutment – placement**

Note: Report D6191 twice as the procedure is required for each of the two implant bodies placed.

D6111 **implant/abutment supported removable denture for edentulous arch – mandibular**

Note: This code is used for removable complete dentures that are either directly supported by the implant body, or by the abutments placed on the implant body.

D6192 **semi-precision attachment – placement**

Note: Report D6192 twice since this procedure involves the luting of the initial semi-precision attachment to the removable denture.

Replacement of Semi-Precision Attachment Replaceable Component

The patient is made aware that it is normal for the attachment's replaceable components to wear over time and will periodically need replacement. This future procedure is documented with the following CDT Code:

D6091 **replacement of replaceable part of semi-precision or precision attachment (male or female component) of implant/abutment supported prosthesis, per attachment**

Clinical Coding Scenario #3:
Implant Supported Maxillary Fixed Complete Denture

The patient in scenario two was so happy with the results of her lower denture she would now like implants on her maxilla. The final prostheses for this arch will be an abutment supported fixed complete denture.

What codes would be used to document services delivered as the treatment progressed?

Initial Services

Since the patient has low sinuses a cone beam scan was necessary to evaluate their exact location as well as the jaw bone dimensions. This enables an assessment to determine whether sinus elevation and bone augmentation is needed prior to implant placement. A surgical guide was made and used during radiographic exposure for treatment planning and will be used again during implant placement.

> **D0366** **cone beam CT capture and interpretation with field of view of one full dental arch – maxilla, with or without cranium**

> **D6190** **radiographic/surgical implant index, by report**

Implant Post Placement and Sinus Elevation

The restorative dentist would like six implants placed since the final restoration will be a fixed denture. The cone beam image revealed there was enough bone in areas of teeth #7 and #10 however in areas of #3, #5, #12, and #14 sinus elevation will be needed. Note the patients existing denture will be utilized after implant placement and sinus elevation.

> **D6010** **surgical placement of implant body: endosteal implant**

Note: Report D6010 six times since six implant bodies were placed, one for #3, #5, #7, #10, #12 and #14.

> **D7951** **sinus augmentation with bone or bone substitutes via a lateral open approach**

or

> **D7952** **sinus augmentation via a vertical approach**

Note: The appropriate sinus augmentation procedure is determined by the dentist's clinical judgment. Report the appropriate sinus elevation twice – once on the right side and once on the left and both these procedures include obtaining the bone or bone substitutes.

Second Stage Surgery and Placement Interim Prosthesis and Final Prosthetic

After three to six months of osseointegration, implants are uncovered, and an interim prosthesis is fabricated. An interim prosthesis was fabricated to evaluate the patient's esthetic and functional needs as well as soft tissue healing and assist with design of the definitive prosthesis. After healing is complete a newly fabricated implant supported fixed complete denture is inserted.

These procedures are documented as follows:

D6011   surgical access to an implant body (second stage surgery)

Note: Report D6011 six times as the procedure is required for each of the six implant bodies placed.

D6119   implant/abutment supported interim fixed denture for edentulous arch – maxillary

Note: D6119 is used during the healing prior to fabrication and placement of permanent prosthetic.

D6114   implant/abutment supported fixed denture for edentulous arch – maxillary

Note: This code is used for fixed complete dentures that are either directly supported by the implant body, or by the abutments placed on the implant body.

Clinical Coding Scenario #4:
Implant-borne Prosthesis

A patient with a fully edentulous mandible is ready to receive an implant/abutment supported overdenture. The oral surgeon performs the first stage surgery to place the implant fixtures. After osseointegration, the surgeon performs a second stage surgery and places prefabricated abutments before referring for completion of the prosthesis.

D6010 **surgical placement of implant body: endosteal implant**

D6011 **surgical access to an implant body (second stage implant surgery)**

D6056 **prefabricated abutment – includes modification and placement**

Modification of a prefabricated abutment may be necessary.

Note: The patient's record and claim submissions must report the number of implant bodies placed (D6010 procedure) and the number of prefabricated abutments placed (D6056 procedure).

The same patient presents with fully osseointegrated implant fixtures and is ready to receive the removable mandibular denture supported by the abutments on the implants. This denture will be retained with semi-precision attachments. The applicable CDT codes for placing the prosthesis in this case are:

D6111 **implant/abutment supported removable denture for edentulous arch – mandibular**

Note: D6111 applies if the prosthesis placed is newly fabricated. However, if the patient has an existing denture that will be modified to be supported by the new attachments, the procedure to report is **D5875 modification of removable prosthesis following implant surgery**.

D6191 **semi-precision abutment – placement**
This procedure is the initial placement, or replacement, of a semi-precision abutment on the implant body.

D6192 **semi-precision attachment – placement**
This procedure involves the luting of the initial, or replacement, semi-precision attachment to the removable prosthesis.

Notes:

- D6191 is reported for each semi-precision abutment and D6192 is reported for each semi-precision attachment that is placed within the overdenture and required to retain the prosthesis.

- For procedure D6192, the terms housing and keeper are synonyms for the term attachment.

A few years later, the patient states that the overdenture feels loose, and the dentist determines that the appropriate course of action is to replace worn components of the attachments as well as reline the prosthesis for patient comfort – all done in-office. The applicable CDT codes for this later encounter are:

D6091   **replacement of replaceable part of semi-precision or precision attachment (male or female component) of implant/abutment supported prosthesis, per attachment**

D5731   **reline complete mandibular denture (direct)**

Clinical Coding Scenario #5:
Removal of a Broken Implant Retaining Screw

Five years ago, a dentist replaced tooth #19 with an implant post that successfully osseointegrated and an implant supported crown. The patient came in for an emergency since he felt "something was loose." The radiograph image shows the post is still osseointegrated with no bone loss. However, the implant retaining screw is broken in the apical third of the implant chamber. The dentist was not able to retrieve the screw with a cavitron. In order to successfully retrieve the broken screw, the dentist had to purchase a screw retrieval kit.

How do you code for this visit?

D0140 **limited oral evaluation – problem focused**

D0220 **intraoral – periapical first radiographic image**

D6096 **remove broken implant retaining screw**

This procedure assumes the implant retaining screw is broken and the fragments are remaining in the body of the implant as well as the implant retained crown. This code is only submitted when removing the screw cannot be performed using standard and conventional techniques for removal. It does not report tightening of an intact screw or routine removal. When submitting to a dental plan, always submit a narrative with any supporting documentation.

Clinical Coding Scenario #6:
Tightening of an Implant Screw

Two years ago, a dentist placed a screw retained porcelain fused to metal implant crown on tooth #12. Today the patient was returning for a cleaning, exam and four bitewings. The patient had no concerns in her mouth, but the hygienist noticed that the implant screw was loose and needed to be tightened. After the prophy was completed, four bitewing radiographs were taken. The dentist performed a periodic exam, which showed that the screw was slightly loose, and proceeded to tighten the implant screw.

How would you code for this visit?

D1110 **prophylaxis – adult**

D0274 **bitewings – four radiographic images**

D0120 **periodic oral evaluation – established patient**

There is no separate code for tightening an implant retaining screw. This service may be reported with the unspecified implant services code D6199 accompanied by a detailed narrative.

Note: The Code Maintenance Committee considers tightening loose screws as inclusive to the implant maintenance procedure (D6080), which was not performed in this scenario. D6080 can be used to tighten an implant screw only if the fixed prosthesis was removed, inspected, cleansed and reinserted.

Clinical Coding Scenario #7:
Cantilever Implant

The patient desperately wants implants. Upon review of the cone beam image the proposed treatment is one surgical implant on tooth #5 with implant crown on #5 and a pontic on #4 cantilevering tooth #4 off tooth #5.

What code reports this structure that will be placed to replace teeth #4 and #5?

D6010 **surgical placement of implant body: endosteal implant**

(tooth #5)

D6076 **implant supported retainer for FPD – porcelain fused to high noble alloys**

(tooth #5)

D6240 **pontic – porcelain fused to high noble metal**

(tooth #4)

A porcelain fused to high noble metal cantilever (fixed) bridge on a natural tooth would be submitted with the same pontic code, D6240, plus **D6750 retainer crown – porcelain fused to high noble metal**.

Remember that the pontic codes, found in the Fixed Prosthodontic category of the CDT Code, can be used with all bridges whether the bridge is on natural teeth or implants. All pontic codes (D6205–D6253) can be used with either an abutment or implant supported bridge. Be sure the implant crown retainer material is consistent with the pontic material.

Clinical Coding Scenario #8:
Implant/Abutment Supported Interim Fixed Denture for Edentulous Arch – Maxilla

A patient is completely edentulous on his upper jaw and he chooses implants as an option. The implants will not be in relative tooth positions since the surgeon will place the implants where the ridge is sufficient. The final prosthesis will be a complete abutment supported fixed denture (a hybrid prosthesis) placed on pre-fabricated abutments. The dentist will be placing abutments and an interim fixed denture for this patient on the day of surgery so the patient doesn't have to go without teeth.

How do you code for the different prostheses in this scenario?

D6010   surgical placement of implant body: endosteal implant

(Repeat for the number of implants placed)

D6056   prefabricated abutment – includes modification and placement

(Repeat for the number of abutments placed)

D6119   implant/abutment supported interim fixed denture for edentulous arch – maxillary

D6114   implant/abutment supported fixed denture for edentulous arch – maxillary

Clinical Coding Scenario #9:

Implant Overdenture – Mandibular

A 45-year-old patient has worn a complete mandibular denture for five years since she lost her teeth due to periodontal disease. She would like a more stable denture. Since her finances are limited, she opted for an overdenture which will be supported by two mini-implants in location of teeth #22 and #27. She will utilize her current denture as a temporary denture while the implants heal, but ultimately wants a new overdenture.

What codes should the dentist submit for the mini implants and the overdenture?

D6013   surgical placement of mini implant

(teeth #22 and #27)

D6111   implant/abutment supported removable denture for edentulous arch – mandibular

(mandibular implant overdenture)

D6192   semi-precision attachment – placement

(teeth #22 and #27)

Note: D6192 is the correct code for luting of the semi-precision attachment keeper assembly in the denture.

Clinical Coding Scenario #10:

Cervitec Gel Application around an Implant to Treat Gingivitis

A dentist placed an implant and implant supported crown on tooth #6 five years ago. The implant is stable and radiographs show no bone loss around the implant fixture. The patient has very good oral hygiene. However, every time the patient presents for periodontal maintenance the tissue around the implant is inflamed. The dentist recently took a course and learned about a product she can apply to the tissue to treat this type of tissue inflammation around the implant. She purchased the material and will apply the gel on the gingival tissue and the implant restoration.

How would you code this procedure?

D6199   unspecified implant procedure, by report.

Currently, there is no CDT code to support application of the material that reduces tissue inflammation.

Clinical Coding Scenario #11:
Implant Removal

Two years ago, a dentist in another state placed an implant post and implant supported crown on tooth #14. Unfortunately, the patient admitted she began smoking again and has since developed diabetes. The implants have developed peri-implantitis and are extremely loose. The dentist needs to remove the implant crowns, the implant posts, as well as place a bone graft material and membrane.

How would you code these procedures?

This procedure involves the surgical removal of a failed implant. A narrative describing the procedure must be submitted with the claim. The narrative should include the location of the removed implant and the description of the procedure performed. It is also helpful to the carrier to say when the implant was initially placed, as well as to provide a radiographic image.

D6100   **implant removal, by report**

D7953   **bone replacement graft for ridge preservation – per site**

Use one of the following codes to report barrier membrane placement:

D4266   **guided tissue regeneration – resorbable barrier, per site**

or

D4267   **guided tissue regeneration – non-resorbable barrier, per site (includes membrane removal)**

Currently there is no CDT code to remove the implant crown and would be considered inclusive to D6100. However, if there are complex issues, use **D6199 unspecified implant procedure, by report**.

Clinical Coding Scenario #12:
Submerging a Fractured Implant

A new patient comes to your office with a fractured implant #23. The implant post was placed three years ago and restored with an implant supported crown. The dentist gives the patient all her options and they come to a mutual decision to bury the implant rather than remove it with a trephine since the jaw bone is so thin. Then a fixed partial denture will be fabricated. The dentist opens the area, grinds down the head of the implant, decontaminates the remaining screw channel with Peridex and places a connective tissue graft to reduce the height of the pontic on the proposed fixed partial denture.

How would you code these procedures?

Currently there is no CDT code to report "burial" of the implant. Describe the procedure with a clear and concise narrative. The narrative should include the location of the implant and the description of the procedure performed. If submitting a claim to a dental carrier, it is also helpful to include when the implant was initially placed, as well as a radiographic image, so you would use the following:

D6199   **unspecified implant procedure, by report**

D4273   **autogenous connective tissue graft procedure (including donor and recipient surgical sites) first tooth, implant, or edentulous tooth position in graft**

or

D4275   **non-autogenous connective tissue graft (including donor and recipient surgical sites) first tooth, implant, or edentulous tooth position in graft**

Clinical Coding Scenario #13:
Cement Removal around the Implant Crown

A patient presents with pain around her #10 implant. The pain has persisted since the crown was put on. After the original dentist (the one that placed the crown on the implant) couldn't help her, the surgeon that placed the implant referred her to your practice. The patient brings her treatment records with all her radiographs, so the dentist knows which implant system was used. The dentists observes cement around the implant crown causing bone loss.

Since it is an anterior tooth in an esthetic area, the dentist does not want to cut any gingival tissue. So she chooses to remove the crown and abutment. The dentist drills through the crown. She then locates the screw holding the crown onto the implant, removes the crown, cleans the cement and screws it all back together. This eliminates the patient's pain and most likely stops the bone loss.

How would you code this procedure?

D6080   **implant maintenance procedures when prostheses are removed and reinserted, including cleansing of the prostheses and abutments**

Note: You cannot submit D6092 re-cement or re-bond implant/abutment supported crown since this procedure is an inherent part of the D6080 procedure.

Note: Third-party payer reimbursement for this or any other procedure reported with a CDT code depends upon a dental benefit plan's coverage provisions, and the provisions of any participating provider contract in effect.

Additional procedures that may be performed to remove excess cement include:

D6081   **scaling and debridement in the presence of inflammation or mucositis of a single implant, including cleaning of the implant surfaces, without flap entry and closure**

The following code is utilized when a bony defect has occurred, and the implant surface is debrided and cleaned. It includes flap entry and closure.

D6101   **debridement of a peri-implant defect or defects surrounding a single implant, and surface cleaning of the exposed implant surfaces, including flap entry and closure**

This next code is utilized when a bony defect has occurred, and the implant surface is debrided, cleaned and the dentist performs osseous contouring of the peri-implant defect. It includes flap entry and closure.

D6102   **debridement and osseous contouring of a peri-implant defect or defects surrounding a single implant and includes surface cleaning of the exposed implant surfaces, including flap entry and closure**

Clinical Coding Scenario #14:
Changing Healing Abutments

A dentist placed full sized implants on teeth #8 and #9 one month ago and the implants are successfully integrating. A week ago the dentist performed second stage surgery and placed two healing caps (gingival contours) with a cuff height of 2 mm. However, when the patient returned for suture removal, it was clear the collar of the healing caps that had been placed were too short. The gingival tissue has already overgrown. The dentist had misjudged the tissue depth and therefore needed to place healing caps with an increased cuff height. The dentist had already performed second stage surgery and was not sure of the code.

How would you code this procedure?

D6011 **surgical access to an implant body (second stage implant surgery)**
This procedure, also known as second stage implant surgery, involves removal of tissue that covers the implant body so that a fixture of any type can be placed, or an existing fixture be replaced with another.

Per its descriptor, this procedure includes replacement of an existing fixture so D6011 is used again to report the service delivered to both implants. Even though this code should be used to document and report replacing the healing caps there are dental benefit plans with coverage provisions that only reimburse once per implant.

Clinical Coding Scenario #15:
Essix Retainer as a Temporary

A 74-year-old patient has existing crowns on all her maxillary teeth, many of which have been treated endodontically. Unfortunately, tooth #9 has a fracture and the dentist needs to remove it and place an implant. Since esthetics are a concern, the dentist would like to use an Essix retainer as a temporary while the implant is healing. Even though an Essix retainer is traditionally used for orthodontic retention, the dentist is not using it as a retainer so she doubts it would be appropriate to use the orthodontic code.

How would you code this temporary procedure?

There is no existing code that specifically describes an Essix retainer but there are codes that might describe this situation.

D5899 unspecified removable prosthodontic procedure, by report
Used for a procedure that is not adequately described by a codes. Describe the procedure

D5820 interim partial denture (including retentive/clasping materials, rests, and teeth), maxillary

Note: D5820 is often used to report a "flipper", which includes an Essix retainer.

Clinical Coding Scenario #16:
Implant Crown Repair

A patient presented to a dental office for a periodic cleaning and exam visit. The patient's chief complaint was that they felt like they may have a crack in one of their molars that they would like the dentist to look at. Oral evaluation revealed the implant crown on #30 had a chip in the porcelain on the distal occlusal and had become a food trap. Treatment options presented to the patient were to repair the chip on the existing crown with a bonded resin or to have a whole new crown and custom abutment fabricated. The patient chose to have it repaired for now. The repair was made with Porcelain Etch, Clearfil SE, Flowable (SureFill SDR), light-cured resin (Quixx).

How would you code this procedure?

> **D6090 repair implant supported prosthesis, by report**
> This procedure involves the repair or replacement of any part of the implant supported prosthesis.

Be sure to include brief narrative, including the original date of placement and a description of the repair, when reporting D6090 on a claim.

Clinical Coding Scenario #17:
Replacement of Clips on Hader Bar

A patient currently wears a lower implant supported overdenture. Implants are in positions #22 and #27 with a Hader bar connecting them. After many years of wear, it is now evident that the plastic clips in the metal housings require replacement.

What is the proper code for replacement of plastic clips on a Hader Bar?

> **D6091 replacement of replaceable part of semi-precision or precision attachment (male or female component) of implant/abutment supported prosthesis, per attachment**

Note: A clip is a replaceable part and therefore the code D6091 describes the procedure. Note submit this code per clip (per attachment) not per visit.

Coding Q&A

1. *My patient does not have implant coverage but does have crown coverage. Would I be able to use the code D2740 instead of D6065 to report an implant supported porcelain/ceramic crown?*

   No. If implants are not a covered benefit under the patient's benefits, reporting D2740 is misrepresenting a service to gain insurance reimbursement. You must report the procedure performed (D6065) regardless of insurance reimbursement. This statement also applies for retainer crowns. Reporting implant retainer crowns (D6075) as retainer crowns on natural teeth (D6740) to gain insurance reimbursement is also misrepresenting a service.

   Note: Even though you may be submitting the implant crowns appropriately, occasionally benefit plans may reimburse the implant crown as an alternate benefit of a natural tooth crown.

2. *I submitted the following codes on a claim to my patient's dental insurance carrier for two implant procedures for tooth #12:*

   D6066   implant supported crown – porcelain fused to high noble alloys

   D6056   prefabricated abutment – includes modification and placement

   The carrier has not reimbursed the procedures, stating, "Implant abutments must be submitted with an abutment supported prosthetics. Please resubmit with the appropriate codes." What do I do?

   The insurance carrier is correct. When using an abutment (either D6056 or D6057), it must be followed by an abutment-supported prosthesis. In this case, since an abutment was used, the correct code is **D6059 abutment supported porcelain fused to metal crown crown (high noble metal)**. The code D6066 is an implant supported crown that does not require an abutment.

3. *What is the difference between a temporary anchorage device (TAD) (D7292, D7293 or D7294) and a mini implant (D6013)?*

   Although both TADs and mini implants look similar, a TAD is typically smaller, has an area for orthodontic wire, is used for orthodontic anchorage or as part of orthodontic treatment, and is removed after a period of time. A mini implant (D6013) is not typically removed and usually supports a removable denture.

4. *A patient is having endosteal implants placed for a complete implant supported denture. The dentist will fabricate a stent-like appliance for the surgeon to be sure the implants are placed exactly where the dentist needs them. Would the appliance be documented as **D5982 surgical stent, D5988 surgical splint** or **D6190 radiographic/surgical implant index, by report**?*

The correct code for this appliance, which is a guide and not a stent, is:

D6190 radiographic/surgical implant index, by report
An appliance, designed to relate osteotomy or fixture position to existing anatomic structures, to be utilized during radiographic exposure for treatment planning and/or during osteotomy creation for fixture installation.

D5982 surgical stent is not correct because a stent is an appliance that applies pressure to soft tissues to facilitate healing and prevent collapse of soft tissue.

D5988 surgical splint is not correct as it uses existing teeth and/or alveolar processes as points of anchorage to assist in stabilization and immobilization of broken bones during healing.

5. *I noticed there are no pontic codes in the CDT Code's Implant Services category. When reporting a fixed partial denture placed on implants, how do I report the pontic?*

Pontic codes, found in the Fixed Prosthodontic category of the CDT Code, can be used with all bridges whether the bridge is on natural teeth or implants. All pontic codes (D6205–D6253) can be used with either an abutment or implant supported bridge. Be sure the implant crown retainer material is consistent with the pontic material.

6. *I placed an implant on tooth #30 two years ago. The patient has since developed peri-implantitis. There is radiographic evidence of bone loss only on the mesial aspect, so I am confident this can successfully be treated with bone grafting. Would the osseous surgery procedure be documented with D4261, and the bone graft documented with D4263?*

No, the D426x procedure codes are not appropriate for documenting surgical repairs and bone grafting in conjunction with implants. The correct codes in this situation are:

D6102 debridement and osseous contouring of a peri-implant defect or defects surrounding a single implant and includes surface cleaning of exposed implant surfaces, including flap entry and closure

D6103 bone graft for repair of peri-implant defect – does not include flap entry and closure
Placement of a barrier membrane or biologic materials to aid in osseous regeneration are reported separately.

7. *The current CDT manual does not include **D6020 abutment placement or substitution: endosteal implant**. What code should I use now to document this procedure?*

There were concurrent changes in CDT 2005 that included deletion of D6020 and revision to the implant abutment codes (D6056–D6057). These revisions clarified that the abutment procedures included placement. The current codes and their nomenclatures follow:

D6056   prefabricated abutment – includes modification and placement

D6057   custom fabricated abutment – includes placement

8. *We have several patients that have implant supported mandibular complete dentures. However, they have natural teeth in their maxillary arch. What procedure code would be used to report cleaning of the implants and can this code be submitted with a prophy (D1110) and a periodic oral evaluation (D0120)?*

The answer depends on whether or not the prosthesis placed on the implants is removed.

If the prosthesis is not removed cleaning both the natural teeth and implant bodies may be reported with the applicable prophylaxis code. The CDT code descriptors for both D1110 and D1120 were revised in CDT 2021 to indicate that these procedures apply to both natural dentition and implants placed within that dentition:

D1110   prophylaxis – adult
Removal of plaque, calculus and stains from tooth structures and implants in the permanent and transitional dentition. It is intended to control local irritational factors.

D1120   prophylaxis – child
Removal of plaque, calculus and stains from tooth structures and implants in the primary and transitional dentition. It is intended to control local irritational factors.

However, if the prosthesis is removed the following code is reported:

D6080   implant maintenance procedures when prostheses are removed and reinserted, including cleansing of prostheses and abutments
This procedure includes active debriding of the implant(s) and examination of all aspects of the implant system(s), including the occlusion and stability of the superstructure. The patient is also instructed in thorough daily cleansing of the implant(s). This is not a per implant code, and is indicated for implant supported fixed prostheses.

Implant maintenance (D6080) can be submitted for the same date of service that the patient receives a prophylaxis (D1110) or periodontal maintenance (D4910), because the implant maintenance procedure does not include services rendered to natural teeth in the patient's mouth. A periodic oral evaluation D0120 can also be submitted on this date of service.

However, when both the D6080 and D1110 are performed on the same date of service some dental benefit plan limitations and exclusions provisions may, for claim adjudication, consider D6080 to be inclusive in the D1110 (or D4910) and D0120 procedure and not provide additional reimbursement.

9. *I placed provisional crowns on three implants to allow time for healing which should take about six months. There are provisional crowns in the Restorative category of service, but what about reporting the provisional implant crown procedure?*

CDT 2017 filled this procedure reporting gap by addition of **D6085 provisional implant crown** (a provisional implant crown can either be abutment or implant supported). This procedure is similar to other provisional codes (e.g., **D2799 provisional crown**) in that there is neither a requirement that the provisional implant crown be used for a specific time period, nor prohibition on use if the final impression for the permanent implant crown has been taken. Keep in mind, a benefits plan may not cover this procedure or make the code inclusive of the final prosthesis. Report D6085 for each provisional crown placed.

10. *A patient presents with a complete lower denture made 11 months ago at another dental office. She is unhappy with the fit and now realizes she should have had the implants her dentist recommended. The treatment plan consists of two mini implants and two Zest locators on an overdenture. Is there any way to still use her existing denture after we place the implants and locator attachments?*

Yes, the existing denture can be used. This is a retrofitting procedure where the internal surface of the existing denture is modified to accommodate the retentive elements. The code is:

D5875   modification of removable prostheses following implant surgery

Surgical implants are coded as **D6013 surgical placement of mini implant** and the two locators on the overdenture are coded as **D5862 precision attachment, by report**. A Zest locator is just one example of a precision attachment.

Any relines are reported separately.

11. *I placed a prefabricated abutment (D6056) and an abutment supported porcelain fused to metal crown (D6059). Six months later the patient presented with the implant crown in his hand. I took a radiographic image which showed no problems with the implant fixture or abutment, so I cemented the implant crown back in his mouth. Is there a code for this procedure?*

Yes, the code you would use is:

D6092 re-cement or re-bond implant/abutment supported crown

12. *My patient comes in every three months for periodontal maintenance (D4910). She has all her teeth with the exception of implants on teeth #2 and #4 which I placed one year ago. A restorative dentist has since placed the abutments and abutment supported crowns. She noticed bleeding around the implants after the implant crowns were placed so she came to my office to have them evaluated. I took a radiographic image and noticed that around both of her implants, the gingival tissue was inflamed due to excess cement from the implant crown placement. However, there were no threads exposed and no bone loss present.*

I need to scale and debride around the implants; should I use the code D4346?

No. For scaling and debridement of the implants, use D6081. You would submit it twice – once for #2 and also for #4 since this is a per implant code.

D6081 scaling and debridement in the presence of inflammation or mucositis of a single implant, including cleaning of the implant surfaces, without flap entry and closure
This procedure is not performed in conjunction with D1110, D4910 or D4346.

13. *My patient has an implant on tooth #7 which was placed four years ago. The implant is well integrated with the bone and the patient is happy with the esthetics of the crown. However, there is now slight recession present on the buccal and I plan on performing a connective tissue graft. But I can't find a code in the implant section. What code would I use?*

The correct soft tissue graft codes are located in the Periodontics section and the code you choose depends on if you are performing an autogenous or non-autogenous connective tissue graft:

D4273 autogenous connective tissue graft procedure (including donor and recipient surgical sites) first tooth, implant or edentulous tooth position in graft

D4275 **non-autogenous connective tissue graft (including recipient site and donor material) first tooth, implant, or edentulous tooth position in graft**

14. ***D6010 surgical placement of an implant body*** *does not include placement of a healing cap. The implant has osseointegrated and is ready to be uncovered. What code would be used for placement of a healing cap?*

    Surgical exposure of the implant is called "uncovering" or "second stage surgery," and is reported separately as D6011. The descriptor of **D6011 surgical access to an implant body (second stage implant surgery)** states:

    > "This procedure, also known as second stage implant surgery, involves removal of tissue that covers the implant body so that a fixture of any type can be placed, or an existing fixture be replaced with another. Examples of fixtures include but are not limited to healing caps, abutments shaped to help contour the gingival margins or the final restorative prosthesis."

    Note that some benefit plans consider this procedure to be inclusive under D6010.

15. *Is an interim abutment the same as a healing cap?*

    No. An interim abutment (D6051) is used while awaiting definitive treatment during a healing phase and is ultimately replaced by either **D6056 prefabricated abutment – includes modification and placement** or **D6057 custom fabricated abutment – includes placement**. A healing cap is placed at the time of second stage surgery and just maintains an access opening to the implant body prior to the restorative phase of implant treatment.

16. *What code reports blocking out an implant restorative access hole?*

    There was a request to add a code for this procedure in CDT 2018. However, the Code Maintenance Committee (CMC) did not accept the request for a separate CDT code as the committee considers blocking out an implant restorative access hole to be a component of the implant crown procedure.

    However, if you block out an implant restorative access hole beyond the normal practice or if the patient loses the composite in the access hole of his implant crown, then submit as **D6199 unspecified implant procedure, by report** along with a detailed narrative.

17. *Is there a code for an immediate implant placement?*

    There is no distinction in the surgical implant placement codes. They can be submitted whether the implant is placed at the time of tooth extraction or post extraction.

18. *I just placed a UCLA-type single crown which is screw retained and I am using a composite to seal the access opening. What are the codes for the crown and the composite material placed?*

There is no separate code for a UCLA-type crown. These are implant supported crowns (D6065-D6067). There is no separate code for closure of the access opening with composite material at insertion.

19. *My patient is edentulous on the mandibular arch and would like a definitive prosthesis as soon as possible, so I am going to use the Trefoil system. What is the code for the Trefoil bar?*

The Trefoil bar is a pre-manufactured titanium bar with a unique retention mechanism that can be adjusted to compensate for inherent deviations from the ideal implant position and enable the passive fit of the definitive prosthesis. This is a type of a connecting bar and therefore the code is D6055.

20. *My patient is missing tooth #10 and the orthodontist moved #11 into the position of #10. I removed tooth H and placed an implant in the position of #11. What tooth number do I use for implant placement and fixture? I tried to use #11, but the dental carrier is telling me that the tooth is present.*

Per the instructions on the ADA claim form in box 27, teeth are based on morphology and not anatomical position. Therefore, the correct tooth number for the implant placement and crown is for tooth #10.

21. *When coding a screw retained full contour implant supported zirconia crown, what is the proper CDT code?*

Zirconia is a ceramic and therefore the appropriate code is:

D6065 implant supported porcelain/ceramic crown

22. *I placed an implant and screw retained crown on #14. The patient has all remaining teeth except for #15. The implant is osseointegrated but has an open contact between the dental implant crown and #13, which is a natural tooth. My concern is that food is beginning to get impacted and this can lead to peri-implantitis. I easily removed the crown, placed a healing abutment and sent the crown back to the lab to add porcelain. How do I code for this procedure?*

D6090 repair implant supported prosthesis, by report
This procedure involves the repair or replacement of any part of the implant supported prosthesis.

Be sure to include brief narrative, including the original date of placement and a description of the repair, when reporting D6090 on a claim.

23. *I took a course and I am about to restore my first case of an "All-on-4®" lower arch. What is the correct code?*

An "All-on-4®" denture is a trademark name given to a denture permanently attached to a jaw by four implants, hence the "four" in "All-on-4®." Note that this has changed over the years and the number of implants is not necessarily four, but the name is catchy, so it stuck. In this case the correct code is **D6115 implant/ abutment supported fixed denture for edentulous arch – mandibular**.

If you are performing an "All-on-4" in the maxilla the CDT would be:

> **D6114 implant/abutment supported fixed denture for edentulous arch – maxillary**

24. *I will be restoring my patient's upper arch with an "All-on 4" denture. I will be extracting remaining teeth, performing alveoloplasty, taking a cone beam image, placing full body implants and prefabricated abutments, modifying her existing denture as well as many other procedures. Since the patient does not have implant coverage with her current dental plan how should I code these procedures on a claim for reimbursement?*

You must utilize the proper CDT codes for the procedures you perform whether or not the dental benefit plan provides coverage. Keep in mind even if a patient doesn't have implant coverage, they still have coverage for extractions and some carriers may pay an alternate benefit (e.g., reimburse for a natural tooth borne denture in place of the implant denture).

25. *If a patient needs a prefabricated abutment does the implant surgeon or the restorative dentist submit the D6056?*

The practitioner who actually places the abutment submits the claim for this procedure (D6056). This person could be either the oral surgeon or the restorative dentist, depending on the circumstances.

26. *What code to I use for a prophy on a patient who has all her natural permanent teeth except for one that has been replaced with a healthy implant?*

The D1110 descriptor was revised in CDT 2021 to indicate the procedure is applicable to removal of plaque, calculus and stains from natural tooth structures and implants.

> **D1110 prophylaxis – adult**
> Removal of plaque, calculus and stains from tooth structures and implants in the permanent and transitional dentition. It is intended to control local irritational factors.

27. *If a dentist uses technology to mill an abutment with an implant crown or cements a prefabricated abutment into the implant crown outside the mouth, can he charge the patient for D6056 prefabricated abutment as well as the implant crown prior to delivery?*

    If the crown and abutment is attached directly to the implant body as one piece (that is, the abutment is an integral part of the crown), the abutment is not reported separately and the appropriate crown code would be an implant supported crown.

28. *What is the CDT code for replacement of O-rings?*

    The correct code is **D6091 replacement of replaceable part of semi-precision or precision attachment (male or female component) of implant/abutment supported prosthesis, per attachment.**

    Note: This code is reported per attachment replaced, meaning it is reported for each O-ring that is replaced and not per denture.

Summary

Coding for implants may appear challenging, but accurate coding helps ensure proper claim adjudication and reimbursement in accordance with dental benefit plan coverage provisions. However, it can be straightforward once you learn the basics. It's important to document the material used to fabricate the prosthesis and it must match the lab prescription. Some coding rules of thumb are in the following charts:

When the Final Prosthesis Is an Implant Crown or a Fixed Bridge

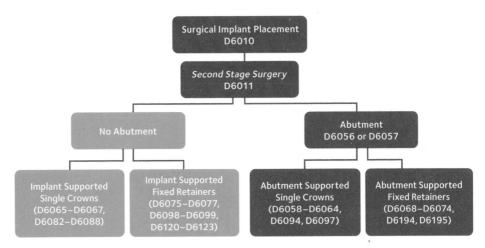

Chapter 8: D6000–D6199 Implant Services

When the Final Prosthesis is a Removable or Fixed Implant Denture

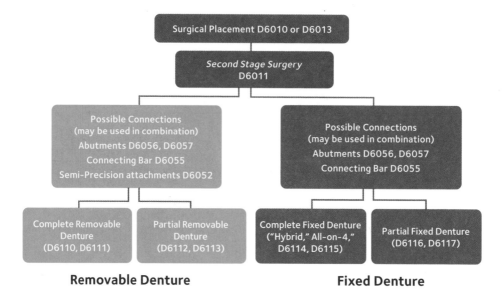

Reimbursement for surgical implant placement and restorations varies among dental benefit plans. Often when the surgical implant is not a benefit, the implant restorations are reimbursed as an alternative benefit. Even if a dental benefit plan does have implant coverage or has an implant rider, there still may be limitations and may not mean the plan includes benefits for implant maintenance related procedures. Pre-authorizing implants is highly recommended and may be a requirement of some patients' plans. A written estimate for the total cost of treatment – regardless of insurance coverage – should be presented, signed by the patient, and retained in the patient's file.

Contributor Biography

Linda Vidone, D.M.D., is the Chief Clinical Officer/V.P. Clinical Management at Delta Dental of Massachusetts. She has 20 years of dental experience in clinical private practice, as dental school faculty, and in the dental benefits industry. Dr. Vidone, a board-certified dental consultant, is a hands-on leader in the dental insurance industry, setting clinical policies and performing routine claim review while staying abreast of innovations in oral health care. She shares her unique knowledge of being on both sides of the claim form while lecturing nationwide on all aspects of dental benefits, dental coding, claim accuracy, utilization management and utilization review.

A graduate of Boston University School of Dental Medicine, Dr. Vidone holds a D.M.D. and C.A.G.S. in General Dentistry and Periodontology. She is currently a member of the Delta Dental Plan Association Policy Committee. She is President of the American Association of Dental Consultants and also serves as Chair of the Certification Committee. She is on National Association of Dental Plans Code workgroup and is a voting member of the American Dental Association's Code Maintenance Committee, where she represents American Health Insurance Plans She also maintains a private practice in periodontology in Brookline, Massachusetts.

Chapter 9: D6200–D6999
Prosthodontics, fixed

By Teresa Duncan, M.S.

Introduction

Fixed prosthodontics replace missing teeth using fabricated materials that are cemented onto existing natural teeth or roots. It is important to remember that the codes for pontics listed in this category of service are used when documenting both tooth borne fixed denture procedures and for pontics that are part of an implant borne denture.

Clinicians must take into account the patient's oral health habits along with existing restorations in order to determine if a fixed prosthetic is the best choice. When treatment planning for fixed prosthodontics, it is important to remember that multiple appointments and procedures are usually required, and it is advisable to inform the patient of the number of visits required.

Patients are often confused by the terminology used when discussing fixed prosthodontics. A treatment coordinator may be referring to a fixed partial denture between teeth #13 and #15, but the patient may not understand that this is the same as fixed bridgework. It is helpful to have visual aids and even tangible examples on hand. Consider adding models, videos and images to your case presentation tools. Often the only time the patient has even seen a bridge or fixed partial denture is right before it is cemented into his or her mouth.

From the beginning, your team should use the same language when discussing the components of fixed prosthodontics. They should also keep in mind that although most fixed prosthodontics are cemented permanently there can be situations in which the practitioner will choose to do so temporarily.

Key Definitions and Concepts

Retainer: As defined by the American College of Prosthodontics, a retainer is "any type of device used for the stabilization or retention of a prosthesis." The "Prosthodontics, fixed" category of service has codes for retainer inlays, onlays and crowns. A fixed partial denture would be comprised of two retainers and one or more pontics as needed for the prosthesis.

Abutment: When discussing fixed prosthodontics, the term used to describe the part of a tooth upon which the retainer will seat. There may be times when additional buildup material is needed in order to properly seat a retainer. Such build-up procedures are reported with CDT codes from the Restorative category.

Pontic: An artificial tooth created to take the place of a missing tooth. It will be attached to retainers. There is no supporting tooth or root below it. It may rest against but is not meant to be supported by the soft tissue. As bone resorbs, the soft tissue may pull away from the pontic.

Connector: The part that unifies the pontic and the retainer.

Fixed Partial Denture: A laboratory fabricated prosthetic that replaces missing teeth or empty tooth spaces. It is meant to stabilize the bite and maintain arch integrity. This means that it prevents teeth from shifting and changing the patient's bite which can lead to future required treatment. Also referred to as fixed bridgework or a bridge.

Cantilever Bridge: A fixed partial denture (bridge) in which a stabilizing retainer is not present on one end.

Changes to This Category

CDT 2021 contains no additions, revisions, deletions or editorial changes.

The fixed Prosthodontics category of service's most recent changes occurred when CDT 2020 was published. These were editorial changes and additions that enabled reporting of prostheses whose fabrication included titanium and titanium alloys – as well as high noble, noble and base alloys. These materials, described in the Classification of Metals table within the CDT Manual's Classification of Materials, are parsed on the basis of biocompatibility, not cost.

Clinical Coding Scenario #1:
Cantilever Bridge

A patient presents with tooth #27 missing and the dentist learned that this tooth has been missing for under a year. The dentist also observed that teeth #26 and #28 appeared to be in good condition. Upon further evaluation, the dentist determined that tooth #26 would not provide enough retention for a Maryland bridge and was reluctant to incorporate a virgin tooth in the prosthetic.

The patient was presented the information regarding Maryland bridge replacement and cantilever bridge replacement, with the doctor recommending a cantilever bridge off tooth #28 to preserve #26's tooth structure. Porcelain fused to high noble metal was the recommended material for this fixed prosthesis. The patient reviewed the treatment plan and opted for the cantilever bridge procedure.

What codes are used to document and report this procedure?

Tooth #28 is a retainer and the applicable code is:

D6750   retainer crown – porcelain fused to high noble metal

Note: Retainers, for coding purposes, are differentiated by their material.

(Refer to CDT 2021 for the full list of applicable codes based on the prosthetic's material.)

The pontic code for a "cantilever" bridge are the same as a conventional bridge, which for tooth #27 would be:

D6240   pontic – porcelain fused to high noble metal

As with the retainers, pontics may be made of different material.

Always refer to CDT 2021 to use the appropriate code.

Clinical Coding Scenario #2:
Maryland Bridge

A patient suffered an accident that damaged the dentition as follows:

- Two teeth were lost – #23 and #24

- One tooth was broken – #26

The doctor determined that #26 could not be restored and required extraction.

The initial treatment plan involved implants, which the patient declined due to cost. An alternative treatment plan was accepted. This alternative involved a Maryland bridge as this would preserve the remaining teeth and retain the option of implant in the future. The Maryland bridge consisted of a resin bonded porcelain-fused-to-metal (noble) bridge from teeth #22 to #27 with #25 acting as a pier.

What codes are used to document and report this procedure?

Teeth #22, #25 and #27 become retainers and the applicable code for each is:

D6545   retainer – cast metal for resin bonded fixed prosthesis

The pontic codes for a Maryland bridge are the same as a conventional bridge, which for teeth #23, #24, and #26 is (reported for each):

D6242   pontic – porcelain fused to noble metal

Note: Resin bonded bridge retainers (often referred to as wings) are differentiated by their material:

- All cast metal or porcelain fused to metal bridges would utilize the D6545 code noted above.

- The porcelain/ceramic retainer code (D6548) could only be used with a porcelain/ceramic pontic.

- Should the retainer be fabricated out of resin/composite, the applicable CDT code is **D6549 resin retainer – for resin bonded fixed prosthesis**.

Clinical Coding Scenario #3:
Three-Unit Fixed Partial Denture (Bridge) for Teeth #28–30

The patient presented with missing tooth #29 due to extraction at an oral surgery office and wished to replace this tooth. A treatment plan that offered the following options – fixed prosthetic; removable prosthetic; or implant placement and restoration – was presented and the patient chose a fixed prosthetic incorporating teeth #28 and #30 for retainers.

Informed consent was obtained and the patient returned for a tooth preparation appointment and a cementation appointment.

How would you code this scenario's treatment plan?

Tooth #28   **D6752   retainer crown – porcelain fused to noble metal**

Tooth #29   **D6242   pontic – porcelain fused to noble metal**

Tooth #30   **D6752   retainer crown – porcelain fused to noble metal**

Clinical Coding Scenario #4:

Three-Unit Fixed Partial Denture (Bridge) for Teeth #12–14 with Buildup on Molar Tooth

The patient presented with an existing fixed partial denture that needed to be replaced, and the dentist also determined that a gingivectomy would be necessary. The patient was presented the treatment plan and gave informed consent. Upon removal of the existing prosthetic the treating dentist decided that a buildup was needed to properly restore the molar tooth.

How would you code this scenario's initial treatment plan?

The initial treatment plan was for a replacement fixed partial denture involving teeth #12–14 and the doctor decided to use porcelain fused to noble metal based on soft tissue and material selection criteria. This plan was documented with the following codes:

Tooth #12 **D4212** **gingivectomy or gingivoplasty to allow access for restorative procedure, per tooth**

Tooth #12 **D6752** **retainer crown – porcelain fused to noble metal**

Tooth #13 **D6242** **pontic – porcelain fused to noble metal**

Tooth #14 **D6752** **retainer crown – porcelain fused to noble metal**

A flap of gingiva was prohibiting proper preparation of the tooth for the retainer crown so D4212 was appropriate in this situation.

Removal of existing decay during delivery of the D4212 procedure necessitated the addition of buildup material, and the dentist informed the patient of the change in treatment.

When the treatment plan changed to include the buildup the code for this additional procedure (below) was added:

Tooth #14 **D2950** **core buildup, including any pins when required**

It is important to note that this code is located in the Restorative section of the CDT manual.

Clinical Coding Scenario #5:
Fractured Tooth and Infection

A patient presents with painful and fractured tooth #5. The doctor took a radiograph that imaged the entire tooth as part of the focused oral evaluation. A two-phase treatment plan was presented and accepted. Descriptions of each phase, and applicable coding, follow.

How would you code each phase in this scenario?

First Phase

- Evaluation and diagnosis
- Extraction of #5 – no need to remove bone
- Impression of the extraction area and adjacent hard and soft tissues
- Creation and placement of a temporary fixed partial denture for healing and space maintenance

Codes for first phase procedures:

	D0140	**limited oral evaluation – problem focused**
	D0220	**intraoral – periapical first radiographic image**
Tooth #4:	**D6793**	**provisional retainer crown – further treatment or completion of diagnosis necessary prior to final impression**
Tooth #5:	**D7140**	**extraction, erupted tooth or exposed root (elevation and/or forceps removal)**
Tooth #5:	**D6253**	**provisional pontic – further treatment or completion of diagnosis necessary prior to final impression**
Tooth #6:	**D6793**	**provisional retainer crown – further treatment or completion of diagnosis necessary prior to final impression**

Second Phase

- Place permanent, porcelain/ceramic, fixed partial denture

Codes for second phase procedures:

Tooth #4:	**D6740**	**retainer crown – porcelain/ceramic**
Tooth #5:	**D6245**	**pontic – porcelain/ceramic**
Tooth #6:	**D6740**	**retainer crown – porcelain/ceramic**

Clinical Coding Scenario #6:
The Replacement of the Missing Tooth

During a comprehensive evaluation, which included an intraoral radiographic survey of the whole mouth, the patient stated that she would like to replace tooth #14 which had been "missing for years." The dentist recommended the following three treatment plan options:

- a fixed partial denture (recommended by the dentist)
- an implant placement and restoration
- the option to do nothing

The patient elected to proceed with the fixed partial denture. The patient and doctor both agreed to a titanium alloy as the patient complained of extreme sensitivity in previous restorations. Costs were presented to the patient who signed and agreed to the fact that the full cost would be the responsibility of the patient due to a "missing tooth clause" in the patient's dental benefit plan. After informed consent was obtained second and third appointments for the denture procedures were scheduled.

How would you code this scenario?

Visit #1: Initial Appointment

The patient presented for a comprehensive evaluation and had radiographs taken and reviewed.

> **D0150   comprehensive oral evaluation – new or established patient**
>
> **D0210   intraoral – complete series of radiographic images**

Visit #2: Restoration

Tooth #13: **D6753   retainer crown – porcelain fused to titanium and titanium alloys**

Tooth #14: **D6243   pontic – porcelain fused to titanium and titanium alloys**

Tooth #15: **D6753   retainer crown – porcelain fused to titanium and titanium alloys**

Visit #3: Cementation of Fixed Partial Denture

The patient presented for cementation of the fixed partial denture. After the new margins were verified and the patient stated they were happy, the doctor took a final bitewing radiograph to verify the margins were accurate.

> **D0270   bitewing – single radiographic image**

Clinical Coding Scenario #7:
Re-cementation of Fixed Partial Denture

A patient presented with his bridge for teeth #29–31 in his hand. He stated it had come out over the weekend. He also complained of sensitivity in the area.

A limited evaluation was completed, and the provider prescribed two periapical radiographs before re-cementation to assess health and stability of the teeth. The radiographs showed no periapical infections and confirmed the visual determination that no active caries was present. After removing cement from the bridgework, it was re-cemented with no incident. The patient was told to return in two weeks for assessment of bridge health and the sensitivity complaint.

How would you code this scenario?

Visit #1: Initial Appointment

D0140 **limited oral evaluation – problem focused**

D0220 **intraoral – periapical first radiographic image**

D0230 **intraoral – periapical each additional radiographic image**

D6930 **re-cement or re-bond fixed partial denture**

It is appropriate to document D0140 as the provider had to assess the situation before prescribing radiographs and treatment. However, some carriers may have benefit clauses that will preclude payment of the evaluation due to frequency limitations.

Visit #2: Post-operative Appointment

D0171 **re-evaluation – post-operative office visit**

Clinical Coding Scenario #8:
Fixed Partial Denture for a Child

During a periodic evaluation and prophylaxis visit, it was determined that a child could benefit from a space maintainer for primary tooth C. The primary tooth had been shed earlier than anticipated. A panoramic radiograph revealed that eruption would not occur for some time. The parent was given the option of a removable or fixed space maintainer. The parent's concern was function and aesthetics.

It was decided that a more permanent space maintainer was necessary. The patient presented for treatment with no issues. The final appointment included cementation and oral instructions. The parent was advised to call the provider with any issues.

How would you code this scenario?

Visit #1: Initial Appointment

D0120   periodic oral evaluation – established patient

D1120   prophylaxis – child

D0330   panoramic radiographic image

Visit #2: Operative Appointment

D6985 pediatric partial denture, fixed

Visit #3: Post-operative Appointment

There is no separate procedure code for the cementation as it is an integral part of the denture procedure.

D1330   oral hygiene instructions

1. *Should I present a treatment plan for an implant if my recommendation is to place a fixed partial denture?*

   Yes, you should always present all available options to the patient. The patient must be aware of all the options available to restore their oral condition. However, you can present a recommended treatment.

2. *We placed a pediatric partial denture on a child but it has come loose. Is there a re-cementation code for this prosthetic?*

   The code **D6930 re-cement or re-bond fixed partial denture** is appropriate. The age of the patient is not a determining factor when using this code.

3. *We have had to temporarily cement fixed bridgework. Is there a separate code for that?*

   Sometimes a fixed partial denture is temporarily cemented so that the clinician can observe the oral condition for a time period. If the fixed partial denture is intended to be the permanent restoration, then there is not a separate code. You are simply delaying the permanent delivery. You may want to use code **D6999 unspecified fixed prosthodontic procedure, by report** to request reimbursement. This will require a narrative and supporting images.

4. *Our patient presented with a multi-unit bridge that had come out. It is a large bridge with five pontics in addition to the retainers. Can we charge the re-cement fee for multiple teeth?*

   Existing code **D6930 re-cement or re-bond fixed partial denture** is per prosthetic. The number of units is not a factor.

5. *I'd like to place a post and core buildup in a tooth that previously had endodontic therapy as this tooth will serve as the abutment for a fixed bridge retainer. Are the post and build-up codes found in this category or in Endodontics?*

   Neither. The post and core procedure codes are actually found in the CDT Code's Restorative category of service.

   D2952   post and core in addition to crown, indirectly fabricated

   D2954   prefabricated post and core in addition to crown

   There is no post and core buildup code that is specific to only crowns or only fixed partial dentures.

6. *I would like to place a temporary bridge while a site is healing. We are planning to treat adjacent teeth but would like to preserve the tooth space in the meantime. What code should I use?*

    You are referring to a provisional fixed partial denture which means the provisional retainer crowns are documented with code D6793 and the provisional pontic(s) with code D6253 (for each provisional pontic in the temporary bridge).

7. *I plan to use a precision attachment. Do I bill for the male and female component separately?*

    The precision attachment code D6950 includes both the male and female part and should be recorded per tooth.

8. *We are placing a fixed partial denture made from a porcelain fused to a titanium alloy. Should I use the high noble code for the retainer crowns and the pontic?*

    There is no reason to use a procedure code that does not correctly reflect the material used. Since both the retainer crowns and pontics are porcelain fused to a titanium alloy the applicable codes are:

    D6753 retainer crown – porcelain fused to titanium and titanium alloys and **D6243 pontic – porcelain fused to titanium and titanium alloys.**

9. *Should I pass the laboratory costs through to the patient?*

    The codes for fixed restorations include laboratory charges and milling expenses and any minor occlusal adjustments made at the seat appointment. Many third-party contracts also exclude such services as they consider them to be part of the procedure. Always review the full code definition and your third-party contract if you are unsure.

10. *I was told by a carrier that the patient has a missing tooth clause. What does that mean and why does it matter in this category?*

    A missing tooth clause means that benefits are not available to replace a tooth that was missing prior to the date of service. If your patient agrees to replace a missing tooth with a fixed partial denture then the full cost will be the patient's responsibility. Always advise the patient if this is the case so that they can plan their financial obligations.

11. *We took impressions for a fixed partial denture and provided the patient with a temporary bridge. The patient has not replied to any of our requests for a cementation appointment. Can we collect on the full amount of the prosthetic? We have already paid the laboratory bill.*

You may seek compensation for costs incurred although there is no specific CDT code for an incomplete procedure. When there is no specific CDT code consider a "999 unspecified procedure" code such as **D6999 unspecified fixed prosthodontic procedure, by report**.

This will require a narrative and supporting images. In addition you will need to evaluate your materials and labor costs and decide on an appropriate fee. Documentation of your attempts to reach the patient should be entered into the clinical record to represent the treatment timeline. The patient's record should document the preparation of teeth to receive the prosthesis and any temporary or provisional restoration provided to the patient.

12. *Are there general guidelines for third-party-requested documentation for this category?*

Every plan will have its own set of requirements but in general the radiographs and intra-oral images should be of clear diagnostic quality and labeled for orientation. A common requirement is a full set of radiographs or panoramic image that shows both arches. Radiographs and intra-oral images should be current (within 12–24 months according to the carrier guidelines). Other requirements could include the date of extraction (for tooth to be replaced) and the reason for extraction. Replacement of an existing fixed prosthetic may also require radiographs showing any open margins, breakages or missing tooth structure (upon removal of structure).

Summary

The selection of a fixed prosthodontics code should be made with the following items in mind:

1. Material used in restoration

2. Is it to replace a missing tooth or tooth space?

3. Is the end result meant to be part of a permanent placement?

4. Diagnostic procedures are separate from fixed prosthodontic codes

5. Any soft tissue preparation is separate from the fixed prosthodontic code

In some situations, a fixed prosthetic is part of an implant case. Specifically, the pontic codes for a fixed partial denture that is supported by implants are found in the Prosthodontics, fixed category. There are no pontic codes that are specific to implant restoration cases.

If you cannot find an appropriate code for your procedure, then use:

D6999 unspecified fixed prosthodontic procedure, by report

When using a "by report" code remember to include a diagnosis, description of procedure and prognosis. Include any supporting documentation such as radiographs and intraoral images. Clear and current documentation will always be needed for communications with carriers.

Contributor Biography

Teresa Duncan, M.S. is the president of Odyssey Management, Inc. She lectures nationally on the topics of insurance administration; case and financial presentations; and practice manager skill improvement. These topics are also tackled on her podcast and in her book. She may be reached via her website at *www.OdysseyMgmt.com*. Her website contains many management and insurance articles, as well as complimentary webinars.

Chapter 9: D6200–D6999 Prosthodontics, fixed

Chapter 10: D7000–D7999
Oral & Maxillofacial Surgery

By James Mercer, D.D.S.

Introduction

Oral and maxillofacial surgery is a broad area. It encompasses not only the discipline of oral surgery, but also that of implant services, radiologic imaging, trauma, facial cosmetic procedures and anesthesia services. Some of the procedures are medical in nature and need to be submitted to medical carriers along with ICD-10-CM codes. However, there are still many procedures which are purely dental in nature.

Key Definitions and Concepts

Autogenous Graft: A graft that is taken from one part of a patient's body and transferred to another.

Anesthesia Definitions: A patient's level of consciousness is determined by the anesthesia provider's documentation of a patient's level of consciousness and is not dependent upon the route of administration of anesthesia.

> **Deep Sedation**: A drug-induced depression of consciousness during which patients cannot be easily aroused but respond purposefully following repeated or painful stimulation. The ability to independently maintain ventilator function may be impaired. Patients may require assistance in maintaining a patent airway. Cardiovascular function is usually maintained.

> **General Anesthesia**: A drug-induced loss of consciousness during which patients are not arousable. The ability to maintain ventilator function is often impaired. Cardiovascular function may be impaired.

> **Minimal Sedation**: A minimally depressed level of consciousness that retains the patient's ability to independently and continuously maintain an airway and respond normally to tactile stimulation and verbal command. Ventilatory and cardiovascular functions are unaffected.

> **Moderate Sedation**: A drug-induced depression of consciousness during which patients respond purposefully to verbal commands either alone or accompanied by light tactile stimulation. Spontaneous ventilation is adequate. Cardiovascular function is usually maintained.

> **Anxiolysis**: The diminution or elimination of anxiety.

Provisional: Formed or preformed for temporary purposes or used over a limited period.

Soft Tissue Impacted Tooth: Occlusal surface of the tooth is covered by soft tissue.

Partial Bone Impacted Tooth: Part of the crown is covered by bone.

Full Bone Impacted Tooth: Most or all of the crown is covered by bone.

Changes to This Category

There are five changes to this category in CDT 2021. The first two are additions for documenting discrete procedures, and fill gaps in the code set:

D7993 surgical placement of craniofacial implant – extra oral
Surgical placement of a craniofacial implant to aid in retention of an auricular, nasal, or orbital prosthesis.

D7994 surgical placement: zygomatic implant
An implant placed in the zygomatic bone and exiting though the maxillary mucosal tissue providing support and attachment of a maxillary dental prosthesis.

The other three changes are related. Two codes were added to enable more accurate documentation of procedures that have been reported with a single code until CDT 2021 became effective. These new codes replace one deleted code.

The two new codes are:

D7961 buccal / labial frenectomy (frenulectomy)
and
D7962 lingual frenectomy (frenulectomy)

These codes clarify the location(s) in the oral cavity where the procedure is performed. This added clarity will enable more robust patient recordkeeping, help claim adjudication processing, and reduce the request for additional information when multiple sites require this procedure.

The deleted code is;

~~**D7960 frenulectomy – also known as frenectomy or frenotomy – separate procedure not incidental to another procedure**~~
~~Removal or release of mucosal and muscle elements of a buccal, labial or lingual frenum that is associated with a pathological condition, or interferes with proper oral development or treatment.~~

Clinical Coding Scenario #1:
Connective Tissue Grafts – Autogenous and Non-autogenous

A 55-year-old male who is a patient of record presented to an oral surgeon's office six years after placement of two separate implants for teeth #12 and #13. The exam revealed loss of 3 mm of attached gingiva on the buccal aspect of the implants. X-rays revealed minimal bone loss on the implants. There was one thread on each implant exposed. Along with debridement of the area, the treatment plan consisted of placing a connective tissue graft on the buccal of both implants.

How would you code for the autogenous grafts?

D4273 **autogenous connective tissue graft procedure (including donor and recipient surgical sites) first tooth, implant or edentulous tooth position in graft**

D4283 **autogenous connective tissue graft procedure (including donor and recipient surgical sites) – each additional contiguous implant in same graft site**

Note: D4273 is the code used when the procedure involves two surgical sites, donor and recipient. The recipient site has a split thickness incision and the connective tissue is from a separate donor site leaving an epithelized flap for closure. D4283 is used to code for additional sites adjacent to the first site.

If using a non-autogenous connective graft, the procedures are coded as follows:

D4275 **non-autogenous connective tissue graft (including recipient site and donor material) first tooth, implant or edentulous tooth position in graft**

D4285 **non-autogenous connective tissue graft procedure (including recipient surgical site and donor material) – each additional contiguous tooth, implant and edentulous tooth position in the same graft site**

Clinical Coding Scenario #2:
Harvesting Bone and Hard Tissue Grafting

Two years following an ATV accident, the patient was still dealing with the after effects of the comminuted fracture of his anterior maxilla. A traumatic defect and oro-nasal fistula, not much different from a congenital alveolar cleft, still existed.

The patient's oral surgeon recommended closure of the fistula and reconstruction of the bony deficit prior to prosthetic reconstruction. The doctor planned to do this as an in office procedure utilizing an autogenous bone graft from the tibia.

What codes would be used to document these procedures?

Two codes would be used to document the planned services to be delivered in the doctor's office:

D7955 **repair of maxillofacial soft tissue and/or hard tissue defect**
Reconstruction of surgical, traumatic, or congenital defects of the facial bones, including the mandible, may utilize graft materials in conjunction with soft tissue procedures to repair and restore the facial bones to form and function. This does not include obtaining the graft and these procedures may require multiple surgical approaches. This procedure does not include edentulous maxilla and mandibular reconstructions for prosthetic considerations.

D7295 **harvest of bone for use in autogenous grafting procedure**
Reported in addition to those autogenous graft placement procedures that do not include harvesting of bone.

Note: The harvesting code D7295 was added in CDT 2011. This addition provides a means to report the separate procedure of obtaining osseous material for the purpose of grafting to a distant site. It enables documentation of the harvesting procedure when the grafting procedure (e.g., D4263; D7953; D7955) does not include obtaining bone to be grafted.

Clinical Coding Scenario #3:
Implant Placement with Inadequate Bone Volume

A 36-year-old female patient presents for placement of an implant in the mandibular right posterior. Tooth #30 had been extracted two years ago. There is inadequate bone volume in the site where the implant will be placed and ridge augmentation is required.

How do you code for the graft?

D7950 **osseous, periosteal, or cartilage graft of the mandible or maxilla – autogenous or nonautogenous, by report**

This procedure is for ridge augmentation or reconstruction to increase height, width and/or volume of residual alveolar ridge. It includes obtaining graft material. Placement of a barrier membrane, if used, should be reported separately.

How do you code for the barrier membrane if used?

D4266 **guided tissue regeneration – resorbable barrier, per site**

or

D4267 **guided tissue regeneration – non-resorbable barrier, per site (includes membrane removal)**

Clinical Coding Scenario #4:
Zygomatic Implants

A 65-year-old female is referred for evaluation for maxillary implants. The patient has a severely atrophic maxilla posteriorly and a history of failed bilateral maxillary sinus augmentation. After obtaining a cone beam CT of the maxilla and comprehensive evaluation, the treatment plan is to place four implants in the anterior region and one zygomatic implant on each side of the maxilla to support a maxillary fixed complete denture.

How do you code for the implants?

D6010   surgical placement of implant body: endosteal implant

Report D6010 four times – once for each of the anterior implants.

D7994   surgical placement: zygomatic implant
An implant placed in the zygomatic bone and exiting though the maxillary mucosal tissue providing support and attachment of a maxillary dental prosthesis.

Report D7994 two times – once for each of the zygomatic implants.

Previously, the code **D6199 unspecified implant procedure, by report** would have been used for documenting the two zygomatic implant procedures.

Clinical Coding Scenario #5:
Autogenous Bone Graft

A 45-year-old male presents for extraction of non-restorable tooth #5 and placement of an implant at a later date. An autogenous bone graft is placed with a membrane at the time of extraction to increase the bone volume and preserve ridge integrity at the future implant site.

After coding for the extraction, how do you code for the graft and membrane portion of the procedure?

D7953 **bone replacement graft for ridge preservation – per site**
Graft is placed in an extraction site or implant removal site at the time of the extraction or removal to preserve ridge integrity (e.g., clinically indicated in preparation for implant reconstruction or where alveolar contour is critical to planned prosthetic reconstruction). Does not include obtaining graft material. Membrane, if used should be reported separately.

D7295 **harvest of bone for use in autogenous grafting procedure**
Reported in addition to those autogenous graft placement procedures that do not include harvesting of bone.

D4266 **guided tissue regeneration – resorbable barrier, per site**

or

D4267 **guided tissue regeneration – non-resorbable barrier, per site (includes membrane removal)**

How would you code for this procedure if the implant is placed at the same time of the extraction and the graft?

D6010 **surgical placement of implant body: endosteal implant**

D6104 **bone graft at time of implant placement**

Placement of a barrier membrane, or biologic materials to aid in osseous regeneration are reported separately.

What code would also be reported if a barrier membrane were placed?

D4266 **guided tissue regeneration – resorbable barrier, per site**

or

D4267 **guided tissue regeneration – non-resorbable barrier, per site (includes membrane removal)**

Clinical Coding Scenario #6:
Possible Orbital Fracture

A 23-year-old male presents to the office after being punched in the face the night before. He has severe periorbital swelling of the left eye. The surgeon is unable to perform an adequate clinical exam and does not have a CBCT in the office. But she does have a cephalometric x-ray machine capable of taking a flat plate extra-oral film. She takes a Waters view film to rule out an orbital fracture.

How do you code for this diagnostic imaging procedure?

D0250   extra-oral – 2D projection radiographic image created using a stationary radiation source, and detector

D0250 covers a class of images which can be obtained utilizing a flat plate radiographic image to view aspects of the skull and facial bones when a CBCT scan is not available.

Clinical Coding Scenario #7:
Extraction of Full Bony Impacted Teeth

A 20-year-old male presents to the oral surgeon's office for extraction of full bony impacted teeth #1, #16, #17 and #32. The procedure was performed utilizing deep IV sedation. The procedure lasted 53 minutes.

How would you code for the deep sedation anesthesia procedure?

> **D9222   deep sedation/general anesthesia – first 15 minutes**

(Report D9222 once for minutes one through 15.)

> **D9223   deep sedation/general anesthesia – each subsequent 15 minute increment**

(Report D9223 three times for the additional 38 minutes (16 through 53). D9223 documents each additional full or partial 15-minute increment.)

What code would be reported if 53 minutes of moderate IV sedation were appropriate?

> **D9239   intravenous moderate (conscious) sedation/analgesia – first 15 minutes**

(Report D9239 once for minutes one through 15.)

> **D9243   intravenous moderate (conscious) sedation/analgesia – each subsequent 15 minute increment**

(Report D9243 for the additional 38 minutes (16 through 53). D9223 documents each additional full or partial 15-minute increment.)

What code would be reported if the extraction procedure could be performed with non-IV conscious sedation?

> **D9248   non-intravenous conscious sedation**

This procedure would be reported once as it is not time-based.

Clinical Coding Scenario #8:
Extraction of Full Bony Impacted Tooth and Periodontal Defect

A 32-year-old male presents for extraction of a full bony impacted horizontal tooth #17. On exam the patient has an increased probing depth and osseous defect on the distal of tooth #18 with bone loss to the mid root of tooth #18. The treatment plan is to extract tooth #17 and perform a bone graft at the time of extraction to regenerate the bone on distal aspect of tooth #18.

How do you code for the procedure?

D7240 removal of impacted tooth – completely bony
Most or all of crown is covered by bone; requires mucoperiosteal flap elevation and bone removal.

D4263 bone replacement graft – retained natural tooth – first site in quadrant

Use of D7953 for the graft would be the incorrect code since the purpose of the graft is not ridge preservation of the extraction socket of tooth #17. The purpose of the delivered procedure (D4263) is to stimulate periodontal regeneration on the distal of tooth #18.

If additional biologic materials are used the following code would also be appropriate:

D4265 biologic materials to aid in soft and osseous tissue regeneration

If a barrier membrane was used the following codes may be used depending on the type of membrane.

D4266 guided tissue regeneration – resorbable barrier, per site

D4267 guided tissue regeneration – non-resorbable barrier, per site (includes membrane removal)

Clinical Coding Scenario #9:
Removal of Non-vital Bone (Two Different Cases)

Patient A

Patient A, a 55-year-old male, is referred for evaluation of pain in the area of a previously extracted tooth #31. Examination reveals exposed loose bone lingual to where tooth #31 had been extracted. There is no swelling or signs of acute infection at the time of presentation. The patient tells you tooth #31 was extracted five weeks prior to your exam due to infection and non-restorability. The initial plan is to provide local would care and removal of the loose bone.

How would you code for this the removal of the loose bone?

D7550 **partial ostectomy/sequestrectomy for removal of non-vital bone**
Removal of loose or sloughed-off dead bone caused by infection or reduced blood supply.

Patient B

Patient B, a 65-year-old female complaining of jaw pain, is referred for evaluation of a large area of mandibular exposed bone 9 weeks after extraction of tooth #31. She has a history of treatment with oral bisphosphonates for osteoporosis. There is no history of radiation therapy to the area. On examination of the mandible, there is obvious loose exposed bone. Part of the treatment plan is to remove the loose bony sequestra to eliminate the source of soft tissue irritation.

How would you code for the removal of the loose bone?

D7550 **partial ostectomy/sequestrectomy for removal of non-vital bone**
Removal of loose or sloughed-off dead bone caused by infection or reduced blood supply.

Since the treatment may be more extensive than the first case described above and not completely described by D7550 you may consider using the following code.

D7999 **unspecified oral surgery procedure, by report**
Used for a procedure that is not adequately described by a code. Describe the procedure.

This is a "by report" code that may be used when no other code adequately describes the procedure you performed. You should include a narrative describing the procedure with the claim form.

Clinical Coding Scenario #10:
Orthognathic Surgery Planning

An oral and maxillofacial surgery office recently installed a cone beam radiography machine. It was used to treatment plan some anticipated orthognathic surgery for a patient. Following image capture, several axial and lateral views were constructed to plan the surgery. A panoramic view was also produced to send to the patient's orthodontist.

After consultation with the orthodontist, the surgeon constructed a 3D virtual model, which they viewed together on the computer, to properly locate a temporary implant to anchor the orthodontic appliance. The virtual model could be manipulated on the screen to allow them to visualize other anatomical structures in the area and their relationship to the teeth to determine the ideal location to place the implant.

A transmucosal endosseous implant was placed as a temporary fixation device for the patient's braces. The temporary implant will be removed when orthodontic treatment is completed.

How could you code for procedures delivered during the initial treatment planning visit (includes initial scan, coronal and sagittal views, and panoramic view)?

D0367   cone beam CT capture and interpretation with field of view of both jaws; with or without cranium

This code was added effective January 1, 2013 specifically to report procedures related to cone beam imaging technology. It replaces the separate cone beam data capture (D0360) and two-dimension reconstruction (D0362) codes. The image capture includes two-dimensional sectional (tomographic) views from the axial (coronal or frontal) and lateral (sagittal) planes, as well as the panoramic view.

How could you code the subsequent consultation procedure (3D virtual model)?

D0393   treatment simulation using 3D image volume

The 3D virtual model is a three-dimensional image reconstructed from data acquired during the treatment planning visit.

How could you code the temporary implant placement procedure that required a surgical flap?

D7293 **placement of temporary anchorage device requiring flap; includes device removal**

Temporary implants also represent a new kind of technology for which codes were added effective January 1, 2007. The correct code to use for this type of implant depends upon whether it will be used for fixation or an interim restoration. In this case, the implant is being used as a fixation device for orthodontics, so the correct code comes from the CDT Code's Oral & Maxillofacial Surgery category.

Note: If the temporary implant does not require a surgical flap, the correct code would be **D7294 placement of temporary anchorage device without flap; includes device removal**.

Clinical Coding Scenario #11:
Treating a Traumatic Wound a Mouthguard Could Have Prevented

An eight-year-old patient arrived at the oral and maxillofacial surgeon's office literally screaming. The doctor understood why when he saw the patient who was injured during a baseball game. A headfirst slide had resulted in a lower lip full of gravel and a chin raspberry in the making.

An intramuscular injection of 40 mg of ketamine provided a reasonable amount of sedation and allowed sufficient time to completely debride the wound, followed by placing sutures in the cut in the patient's lip. No teeth were broken. The doctor recommended a mouthguard for protection.

What codes would be used to document and report procedures delivered during this visit?

The CDT Code for a parenteral sedative is:

D9248   non-intravenous conscious sedation

Note: Effective January 1, 2007, **D9610 therapeutic drug injection, by report** was revised to exclude the reporting of sedative agents.

There is not a code for traumatic wound debridement, but **D7999 unspecified oral surgery procedure, by report** could be used for that procedure.

Suture placement is reported with a code based on the size of the wound:

D7910   suture of recent small wounds up to 5 cm

The code to use when making a mouthguard:

D9941   fabrication of athletic mouthguard

Clinical Coding Scenario #12:
Coronectomy (Two Different Cases)

An oral and maxillofacial surgeon completed consultations with two patients, both of whom faced similar complications.

Patient A

Patient A, a 38-year-old male, presents with chronic pericoronitis associated with a deep mesio-angular impaction of tooth #32. There is gingival inflammation and substantial bone loss surrounding the crown. The root of the tooth extends well past the inferior alveolar nerve canal and it is the dentist's opinion that removal of the entire tooth is a substantial risk to the nerve.

Patient B

Patient B, a 19-year-old female, presents for evaluation and treatment of a dentigerous cyst, associated with an impacted supernumerary tooth in the area of #20, displaced inferiorly and is encroaching on the left mental foramen. After evaluation and examination, the dentist determines that total removal of the supernumerary tooth risks injury to the inferior alveolar nerve.

What procedure codes would be used to document the services delivered today, and planned for a future date?

Each patient's record would have the same procedure codes.

For today's consultation:

> **D9310   consultation – diagnostic service provided by dentist or physician other than requesting dentist or physician**

For the planned procedure:

> **D7251   coronectomy – intentional partial tooth removal**

Note: D7251 was added to the CDT Code effective January 1, 2011. Its addition enables documentation of intentional partial tooth removal that is performed when a neurovascular complication is likely if the entire impacted tooth is removed. The procedure avoids complications involving the inferior alveolar nerve and the lingual nerve.

Clinical Coding Scenario #13:
Oroantral Fistula

A 23-year-old male is referred to the oral surgeon for evaluation of a partial boney impacted tooth #1. A clinical exam reveals pain on palpation. A panoramic image shows that the roots are in close proximity to the sinus and that there is no cystic lesion present. The procedure for the extraction of #1 is reviewed including risks and alternate treatments. The patient elects to have the tooth removed utilizing general anesthesia.

The patient returns for the surgery. After extracting the tooth, a large oroantral opening is noted and a mucoperiosteal flap is elevated with a buccal releasing incision to obtain primary closure. The procedure takes 20 minutes and the patient heals without incident.

How do you code for procedures related to the surgery encounter?

D7230   removal of impacted tooth – partially bony
Part of crown covered by bone; requires mucoperiosteal flap elevation and bone removal.

D7261   primary closure of a sinus perforation
Subsequent to surgical removal of tooth, exposure of sinus requiring repair, or immediate closure of oroantral or oronasal communication in absence of fistulous tract.

D9222   deep sedation/general anesthesia – first 15 minutes

D9223   deep sedation/general anesthesia – each subsequent 15 minute increment

Note: D9223 is reported once since the entire anesthesia time is 20 minutes.

If during the extraction there was no oroantral opening but the patient returned a few weeks later with an oroantral opening with a fistulous tract but no signs of infection, and the oroantral opening was closed at this subsequent visit with a primary closure, what would be the correct code for the closure procedure?

D7260   oroantral fistula closure
Excision of fistulous tract between maxillary sinus and oral cavity and closure by advancement flap.

Clinical Coding Scenario #14:
TMD Therapy

You have been treating a 32-year-old female who previously presented with complaints of several years of headaches, facial pain and "popping" in her left TM joint with occasional locking. Her treatment plan includes but is not limited to a splint for her temporomandibular joint dysfunction and in-office physical therapy.

How do you code for the device and physical therapy?

D7880 occlusal orthotic device, by report
Presently includes splints provided for the treatment of temporomandibular joint dysfunction.

D9130 temporomandibular joint dysfunction – non-invasive physical therapies
Therapy including but not limited to massage, diathermy, ultrasound, or cold application to provide relief from muscle spasms, inflammation or pain, intending to improve freedom of motion and joint function. This should be reported on a per session basis.

You feel an MRI is needed to further evaluate the soft tissue of the joint. The mandible needs to be in a specific position at the time of the MRI and a device is used to position the mandible for the MRI.

How do you code for the device?

If the occlusal orthotic device is used that is also being used in her ongoing treatment, then no additional code is needed. If you construct an additional device to position the jaw for the MRI, then you may use:

D7899 unspecified TMD therapy, by report
Used for procedure that is not adequately described by a code. Describe procedure.

Clinical Coding Scenario #15:
Hyperplastic Tissue Excision

A 77-year-old male presents with ill-fitting dentures and requests new dentures. You determine that prior to constructing new dentures, he will require excision of some excess tissue in the maxilla related to irritation from his current dentures.

How would you code for the excision in the maxilla using a laser vs. excision using a scalpel?

The codes are procedure based rather than instrument based. Therefore the same code is used for either instrumentation.

D7970   excision of hyperplastic tissue – per arch

Clinical Coding Scenario #16:
Non-opioid Post-operative Pain Management

A 17-year-old female is referred for extraction of painful impacted teeth #1, #16, #17, and #32. During the consultation, the patient's mother expresses concern about her daughter receiving opioids as part of the post-operative pain management protocol. To address this concern, following the manufacturer's instructions, the surgeon plans to infiltrate bupivacaine liposome injectable suspension at the surgical sites at the end of the procedure.

How would you code for the bupivacaine liposome injectable suspension?

D9613   infiltration of sustained release therapeutic drug – single or multiple sites
Infiltration of a sustained release pharmacologic agent for long acting surgical site pain control. Not for local anesthesia purposes.

Chapter 10: D7000–D7999 Oral & Maxillofacial Surgery

Clinical Coding Scenario #17:
Using a 3D Printer as Part of a Patient's Restoration Process

A 32-year-old female is referred for restoration of missing teeth #7, #8, #9, and #10 with implants. The dentist incorporates a 3D printer into his digital workflow for fabrication of his surgical guides. How do I code for this new step leading up to the implant placement?

One of the following codes may be used for documenting the referred patient's clinical oral evaluation. The code reported must be supported by your documentation in the patient's chart.

D0140 **limited oral evaluation – problem focused**

An evaluation limited to a specific oral health problem or complaint

This may require interpretation of information acquired through additional diagnostic procedures. Report additional diagnostic procedures separately. Definitive procedures may be required on the same date as evaluation.

Typically, patients receiving this type of evaluation present with a specific problem or dental emergencies, trauma, acute infections, etc.

D0160 **detailed and extensive oral evaluation – problem focused, by report**

A detailed and extensive problem focused evaluation entails extensive diagnostic and cognitive modalities based on the findings of a comprehensive oral evaluation. Integration of more extensive diagnostic modalities to develop a treatment plan for a specific problem is required. The condition requiring this type of evaluation should be described and documented.

Examples of conditions requiring this type of evaluation may include dentofacial anomalies, complicated perio-prosthetic conditions, complex temporomandibular dysfunction, facial pain of unknown origin, conditions requiring multi-disciplinary consultation, etc.

The following code may be reported for the digital or analog diagnostic cast:

D0470 **diagnostic cast**

Also known as diagnostic models or study models.

The following codes may be used to report the CBCT. The selection of the code depends on the field of view and if the procedure includes image capture and interpretation (D0366–D0367) or image capture is separate from interpretation (D0382–D0383):

D0366 **cone beam CT capture and interpretation with field of view of one full dental arch – maxilla, with or without cranium**

D0367 **cone beam CT capture and interpretation with field of view of both jaws; with or without cranium**

D0382 **cone beam CT image capture with field of view of one full dental arch – maxilla, with or without cranium**

D0383 **cone beam CT image capture with field of view of both jaws, with or without cranium**

The following code may be used to report the merging of the CBCT data and the digital cast information. It also includes the virtual planning of the surgical guide and implant positions:

D0393 **treatment simulation using 3D image volume**
The use of 3D image volumes for simulation of treatment including, but not limited to, dental implant placement, orthognathic surgery and orthodontic tooth movement.

The following code may be used when the surgeon fabricates the guide. The code is "by report" so it may be used to report different types of guides. It is important to include a detailed description of the guide when submitting the code.

D6190 **radiographic/surgical implant index, by report**
An appliance, designed to relate osteotomy or fixture position to existing anatomic structures, to be utilized during radiographic exposure for treatment planning and/or during osteotomy creation for fixture installation.

Clinical Coding Scenario #18:
Extraction for a Patient with Cardiovascular Disease Who Takes Anti-platelet Agents

A 72-year-old man presents for extraction of non-restorable teeth #29, #30, and #31. Review of his medical history reveals a history of cardiovascular disease. He is currently taking two anti-platelet agents. In consultation with the patient's physician, the surgery will be performed while continuing the antiplatelet agents. Bleeding will be controlled with local hemostatic measures including intra-socket wound dressing.

Is there a code available to describe the use of the intra-socket dressing?

> **D7922** **placement of intra-socket biological dressing to aid in hemostasis or clot stabilization, per site**
>
> This procedure can be performed at time and/or after extraction to aid in hemostasis. The socket is packed with a hemostatic agent to aid in hemostasis and or clot stabilization.

Coding Q&A

1. A patient presents to the office for a follow up treatment for bruxing and an adjustment was made to his occlusal guard. What is the correct code?

   D9943   occlusal guard adjustment

2. An immediate implant and a provisional crown was placed in the #8 position. What is the proper code for the crown?

   D6085   provisional implant crown

3. A 75-year-old male with severe cardiac disease, including a history of aortic valve replacement, presents to the office for evaluation of his remaining dentition for extraction. The surgeon gives the patient antibiotics to be taken at home one hour prior to the scheduled appointment for his extractions. Due to the severity of his cardiac condition, the surgeon contacted the patient's cardiologist to discuss the planned procedure.

   How do you code for the medication and the phone consultation with the cardiologist?

   D9630   drugs or medicaments dispensed in the office for home use

   D9311   consultation with a medical health care professional

4. A 19-year-old patient presents for their initial visit. After reviewing their past medical history, it is noted that the patient admits to vaping. During the visit, you have a detailed conversation with the patient about the risks and adverse effects this may have on oral and systemic health. The patient indicates they would like to stop vaping and methods of cessation are discussed in detail. Is there a code for this counseling?

   The proper code to use is:

   D1321   counseling for the control and prevention of adverse oral, behavioral, and systemic health effects associated with high-risk substance use
   Counseling services may include patient education about adverse oral, behavioral, and systemic effects associated with high-risk substance use and administration routes. This includes ingesting, injecting, inhaling and vaping. Substances used in a high-risk manner may include but are not limited to alcohol, opioids, nicotine, cannabis, methamphetamine and other pharmaceuticals or chemicals.

5. *I was forwarded a panoramic radiographic image for interpretation and a report that I did not capture. How do I code for my interpretation of the image?*

    D0391   interpretation of diagnostic image by a practitioner not associated with the capture of the image, including report

6. *A patient needed an extraction, and it turned into a very difficult procedure. The doctor removed most of the tooth, but was unable to remove the entire root and the patient was referred to an oral surgeon immediately. Is there a code for a partial extraction?*

    There are no partial extraction codes available. To report this procedure, use code **D7999 unspecified oral surgery procedure, by report**.

7. *I was not able to complete the extraction of an erupted tooth as the crown separated from its roots, and my attempts to remove them were unsuccessful. How should I document this incomplete extraction?*

    There is a no code for an incomplete extraction of an erupted tooth, therefore CDT code **D7999 unspecified oral surgery procedure, by report**" would be used to document what was completed. Details of what occurred would be in the report's narrative.

8. *When an erupted tooth extraction is incomplete what procedure is reported when another dentist is extracting only the residual roots?*

    D7140 if the separated root is exposed and can be extracted with forceps or elevation. If removal requires cutting soft or bony tissue it is the D7250 procedure.

9. *The patient has been to another dentist who attempted to extract a tooth, but did not successfully remove all structure and roots remain. What is the applicable procedure and its code to for me to document only removal of the residual roots?*

    It depends. If the residual root can be extracted using an elevator and forceps the applicable procedure is D7140 as this code's nomenclature states the procedure is applicable to extraction of the entire tooth or only the root, or both. However, if removal of the residual root requires cutting tissue (soft and bone), the applicable procedure and its code is D7250.

10. *I removed a portion of the patient's fractured tooth, but not the entire tooth, to provide immediate relief of pain. How should I report this procedure?*

There is no code that specifically refers to removal of a portion of a fractured tooth to relieve pain. When there is no procedure code whose nomenclature and descriptor reflect the service provided, an "unspecified...procedure, by report" code may be considered (e.g., **D7999 unspecified oral surgery procedure, by report**).

11. *I am an oral surgeon and extracted a fully erupted tooth. My extractions are usually documented with CDT code D7210. For this patient, however, there was no need for any of the surgical actions listed in this code's nomenclature and descriptor. Is D7210 appropriate to document the service, or should I consider D7140?*

Selection of the appropriate code comes through consideration of the full code entries, as follows:

D7140 **extraction, erupted tooth or exposed root (elevation and/or forceps removal)**
Includes routine removal of tooth structure, minor smoothing of socket bone, and closure, as necessary.

D7210 **extraction of erupted tooth requiring removal of bone and/or sectioning of tooth, and including elevation of mucoperiosteal flap if indicated**
Includes related cutting of gingiva and bone, removal of tooth structure, minor smoothing of socket bone and closure.

As you did not perform any of the actions listed in the D7210 entry, D7140 is the only applicable CDT code to document and report the service.

12. *When extracting an erupted tooth, what procedure is reported when: a) the crown and root are extracted in one piece; or b) during the course of the procedure the crown and root separate and are extracted individually?*

There are separate codes for each scenario –

a. D7140 is reported when a dentist completes the erupted tooth extraction procedure and the crown and root are extracted in one piece.

b. D7210 is reported when the crown and root separated during the extraction procedure (for any reason) and both were removed, with the removal of the root tip requiring bone removal.

13. *According to its descriptor code, **D7241 removal of impacted tooth – completely bony with unusual surgical complications** can be used for a completely impacted tooth with an "aberrant tooth position." Would a completely impacted wisdom tooth that is radiographically very close to the mandibular nerve justify use of this procedure code?*

Perhaps. The dentist serving the patient is in the best position to determine whether the observed clinical condition of the patient's dentition and the procedure provided matches a dental procedure code (e.g., D7241). Radiographic images may not provide enough visual information to determine the extent of bony coverage, aberrant tooth position or other unusual circumstances.

Should a dentist determine that a specific code does not adequately apply to the service rendered, we recommend that the service be reported using an "unspecified procedure, by report" code (e.g., D7999 unspecified oral surgery procedure, by report).

14. *I have used D3427 in the past for exploration and repair of root resorption. I see that D3427 has been deleted. What code do I use now?*

There are now six new codes. Three for surgical repair and three for exploration without repair or apicoectomy:

Repair codes:

D3471 surgical repair of root resorption – anterior
For surgery on root of anterior tooth. Does not include placement of restoration.

D3472 surgical repair of root resorption – premolar
For surgery on root of premolar tooth. Does not include placement of restoration.

D3473 surgical repair of root resorption – molar
For surgery on root of molar tooth. Does not include placement of restoration.

Exploration without repair:

D3501 surgical exposure of root surface without apicoectomy or repair of root resorption – anterior
Exposure of root surface followed by observation and surgical closure of the exposed area. Not to be used for or in conjunction with apicoectomy or repair of root resorption.

D3502 surgical exposure of root surface without apicoectomy or repair of root resorption – premolar

Exposure of root surface followed by observation and surgical closure of the exposed area. Not to be used for or in conjunction with apicoectomy or repair of root resorption.

D3503 surgical exposure of root surface without apicoectomy or repair of root resorption – molar

Exposure of root surface followed by observation and surgical closure of the exposed area. Not to be used for or in conjunction with apicoectomy or repair of root resorption.

15. *Which soft tissue biopsy code should I use?*

There are three codes for soft tissue biopsies, differentiated by the depth and structural integrity of the tissue sample.

D7286 incisional biopsy of oral tissue – soft tissue
For partial removal of an architecturally intact specimen only. This procedure is not used at the same time as codes for apicoectomy/periradicular curettage. This procedure does not entail an excision.

D7287 exfoliative cytological sample collection
For collection of non-transepithelial cytology sample via mild scraping of the oral mucosa.

D7288 brush biopsy – transepithelial sample collection
For collection of oral disaggregated transepithelial cells via rotational brushing of the oral mucosa.

Code D7286 would be used for incisional tissue samples that maintain the original structure. Codes D7287 and D7288 are used for cell sampling biopsies that do not maintain tissue architecture.

16. *What is the appropriate code for reporting a supra-crestal fiberotomy?*

The available procedure code for reporting a supra-crestal fiberotomy is **D7291 transseptal fiberotomy, by report**.

17. *What is a fibroma and how would removal be reported?*

A fibroma is a benign tumor composed of fibrous or connective tissue, and the available procedure codes are:

D7410 excision of benign lesion up to 1.25 cm

D7411 excision of benign lesion greater than 1.25 cm

18. *How do I code removal of mandibular tori?*

If the bony elevations are located lingually **D7473 removal of torus mandibularis** may be reported by quadrant.

19. *What is a torus/exostosis and how would removal be reported?*

A torus/exostosis is a benign overgrowth of bone forming an elevation or protuberance of bone. They can form in the patient's palate, lingual or lateral aspect of the maxilla or mandible.

Available procedure codes may include:

D7471 removal of lateral exostosis (maxilla or mandible)

D7472 removal of torus palatinus

D7473 removal of torus mandibularis

20. *What is the difference between the procedures reported with the following three CDT codes?*

D4263 bone replacement graft – retained natural tooth first site in quadrant

Report when the bone graft is performed to stimulate periodontal regeneration when the disease process has led to a deformity of the bone around an existing tooth.

D7950 osseous, periosteal, or cartilage graft of the mandible or maxilla – autogenous or nonautogenous, by report

Report when the graft is used for augmentation or reconstruction of an edentulous area of a ridge.

D7953 bone replacement graft for ridge preservation – per site

Report when the bone graft is placed in an extraction site at the time of the extraction to preserve ridge integrity.

21. *How can I report a sinus lift procedure?*

There are two codes available for different approaches:

D7951 sinus augmentation with bone or bone substitutes via a lateral open approach

D7952 sinus augmentation via a vertical approach

22. *What is an operculectomy, and how would it be coded?*

In dentistry, an operculum is a small flap of tissue surrounding or partially covering the back molars and "ectomy" is a suffix referring to the removal of something. Therefore, an operculectomy is the surgical removal of a flap of tissue surrounding a partially erupted or impacted tooth.

The available procedure code is:

D7971   excision of pericoronal gingiva
Removal of inflammatory or hypertrophied tissues surrounding partially erupted/impacted teeth.

23. *The dentist performed a frenectomy on a child that had been diagnosed with ankyloglossia. What is ankyloglossia and how would treatment be documented?*

Ankyloglossia, more commonly referred to as "tongue tied," is a condition in which the lingual frenum is short and attached to the tip of the tongue, making normal speech difficult.

The available procedure code is:

D7962   lingual frenectomy (frenulectomy)

24. *A patient presents with a small sialolith in his right Wartons duct. Utilizing non-surgical manipulation which included dilatation and manual manipulation the stone was removed. How would you code for the removal of the stone?*

The correct procedure code is:

D7979   non-surgical sialolithotomy

25. *A restorative dentist refers a patient to your office for evaluation and removal of a broken retaining screw in an implant that you placed two years prior. You are able to remove the screw without damaging the implant. What would the proper code for this procedure be?*

Use the following code to correctly document this procedure:

D6096   remove broken implant retaining screw

26. *I am working with a maxillofacial prosthodontist and I have been using **D6199 unspecified implant procedure, by report** when placing craniofacial implants. Is that the correct code to use?*

The proper code to use is:

D7993   surgical placement of craniofacial implant – extra oral
Surgical placement of a craniofacial implant to aid in retention of an auricular, nasal, or orbital prosthesis.

27. *An orthodontist refers a patient to the oral surgeon because he would like to accelerate orthodontic movement, and by modifying the alveolus enable teeth to move into areas with limited bone. You determine that a corticotomy would be the appropriate treatment to enable the desired orthodontic movement. How would you code for this procedure?*

The proper code(s) for this procedure depends on the number and location of teeth involved and would be either:

D7296   corticotomy – one to three teeth or tooth spaces, per quadrant

or

D7297   corticotomy – four or more teeth or tooth spaces, per quadrant

Note: When the involved teeth cross the mid-line two quadrant codes must be reported.

28. *I am treating a patient for xerostomia. Is there a way to code for my assessment of the salivary flow?*

D0419   assessment of salivary flow by measurement
This procedure is for identification of low salivary flow in patients at risk for hyposalivation and xerostomia, as well as effectiveness of pharmacological agents used to stimulate saliva production.

29. *Can I use D7283 in conjunction with surgical exposure code D7280 even if no orthodontics is involved?*

D7283   placement of device to facilitate eruption of impacted tooth
Placement of an attachment on an unerupted tooth, after its exposure, to aid in its eruption. Report the surgical exposure separately using D7280.

In CDT 2019, the phrase "orthodontic bracket, band or other device" was deleted from the D7283 descriptor and the word "attachment" was substituted to demonstrate that this procedure can be done for purposes other than orthodontics. On many occasions, dental benefits companies see "orthodontic" in the descriptor (or even in the nomenclature) and deduct the claim payment from the orthodontic coverage although no orthodontic treatment was performed.

An example where this code would apply is an attachment which is placed after surgical exposure of a mesially impacted permanent first molar that is trapped by the deciduous second molar. The attachment is designed to "unlock" the permanent first molar and allow normal eruption. No orthodontics are being done and may never be done to achieve eruption.

Summary

Oral and maxillofacial surgery cases use codes from many different categories of service, as well as from the CPT medical codes, and requires a step-by-step approach to coding. With time, practice and patience, it will get easier to code for what you do.

Contributor Biography

James E. Mercer, D.D.S. is a board certified oral and maxillofacial surgeon practicing in Columbia, SC since 1988. He is a graduate of Vanderbilt University and The Ohio State University College of Dentistry. He completed a one-year general practice residency, a two-year research fellowship and his four-year specialty training in Oral and Maxillofacial Surgery at the Medical College of Georgia at Augusta University.

Dr. Mercer is a past chairman of the ADA's Council on Dental Benefit Programs and has been active in code maintenance nationally since 2003. He continues to be active in the tripartite and is currently a member of the American Association of Oral and Maxillofacial Surgeon's Committee on Health Care Policy, Coding, and Reimbursement representing them on the Code Maintenance Committee, the Dental Quality Alliance, and the SNODENT Maintenance Committee.

Chapter 11: D8000–D8999 Orthodontics

By Randall C. Markarian, D.M.D., M.S.

Introduction

Orthodontics is a unique CDT Code category of service when compared with others published in the CDT manual. This is due to the lower number of procedure codes and because a single code is used describe a procedure that involves a multi-visit and possibly multi-year treatment. It is advantageous for the dentist to understand the codes, even though there are only a few, so that they may choose the appropriate code to describe the service that they are providing. It is also important to note that even though the orthodontic treatment can be defined with a single code, codes from outside the orthodontic category are necessary to document what services were performed, especially diagnostic codes such as a comprehensive exam (D0150), panoramic radiograph (D0330), and diagnostic models (D0470).

Orthodontic treatment is a complex, dentist guided process which alters the structure of the dentofacial complex requiring a comprehensive clinical examination including: pre-treatment diagnostic records such as radiographs, photos, and models; diagnosis and treatment planning; informed consent; supervision of the treatment; remediation and re-assessment of the therapy; retention; and retrospective evaluation by the treating dentist.

Terminology used in the orthodontic codes can be somewhat different than what is used in other areas of dentistry. For example, understanding the definition of terms like adolescent dentition, limited treatment, interceptive treatment and comprehensive treatment influences the selection of the code used to document the procedure. A review of relevant terminology is the appropriate place to start.

Key Definitions and Concepts

Primary Dentition: The stage during which the deciduous (or "baby") teeth erupt and are present. Typically, orthodontic treatment does not begin prior to complete eruption of the primary dentition and the permanent first molars are usually in the process of erupting or have fully erupted. The age of a patient can vary based on development, but usually ranges from ages five to eight.

Transitional Dentition: This stage, also referred to as the mixed dentition, begins with the eruption of the first molars and is while the patient has both primary teeth remaining and the permanent teeth are erupting. The transitional dentition ends with the exfoliation of the final remaining primary tooth. The age of a patient in the transitional dentition will vary, but typically age ranges are from six to twelve years old.

Adolescent Dentition: The stage where primary teeth are exfoliated and permanent teeth are in the process of erupting or have fully erupted, with the exception of the third molars. The patient is still in a growing phase, and dramatic changes to the oral–maxillofacial complex typically occur during this time. Adolescent dentition typically occurs during ages eleven to eighteen depending upon the sex of the patient as males and females mature at different rates.

Adult Dentition: This final stage is the full permanent dentition with little or no patient growth remaining. Third molars, if present, are usually erupted unless there is lack of space for eruption or the teeth are malposed.

Limited Orthodontic Treatment: The category of orthodontic treatment that involves a specific, defined, and limited scope. Examples would be a single tooth in crossbite or a tooth that needs guidance during eruption. Limited treatment does not involve the entire dentition and can be done at any of the stages of dental development.

Codes exist for each stage of development:
- D8010 for the primary dentition
- D8020 for the transitional dentition
- D8030 for the adolescent dentition
- D8040 for the permanent dentition

Limited orthodontic treatment could involve palatal expansion or be a simple singular tooth movement with a retainer. Typically, limited coding can be used to report treatment using simple appliances and simple movements that are directed at improving a specific problem for the patient.

Interceptive Orthodontic Treatment: Treatments performed under this category should only be coded for treatment done during the primary dentition (D8050) or transitional dentition (D8060) stages of dental development. The rationale behind using an interceptive code rather than a limited treatment code is that the treatment provided will tend to correct a developmental issue that could lead to less or no treatment in the future when the patient reaches the adolescent or adult dentition.

The three main considerations for this type of treatment are as follows:

- Are there space concerns for eruption of the permanent dentition?
- Are there concerns about the patient's occlusion?
- Are there social or self-esteem issues?
- Can these concerns be improved or corrected with early intervention?

Diagnostic procedures, which become part of the patient's record, are important to accurately diagnose the case. Treatment modalities are likely to vary depending on the situation and severity, and may involve a partial set of braces or other orthodontic appliances (or a combination of braces and appliances). Treatment may be localized to one area of an arch, the entire arch or both arches.

Comprehensive Orthodontic Treatment: These treatments are the most complicated that the orthodontist can provide to a patient, and they must include careful diagnosis and treatment planning with complete and detailed orthodontic records. It involves correction of all of the patient's dentofacial issues including any skeletal, muscular, and dental alignment and occlusion issues. Comprehensive treatment can be provided during the transitional (D8070), adolescent (D8080), or permanent (D8090) dentition stage of dental development. These treatments may include a multi-disciplinary approach and involve treatment or consultation with other dental or medical providers such as oral surgeons and periodontists.

Clinical Coding Scenario #1:
Class II Malocclusion and Severe Crowding

A 12-year-old patient presents with a Class II malocclusion and severe crowding. The patient just lost her last deciduous tooth. Parents want the teeth straightened and bite corrected. The case has been diagnosed and treatment planned for full upper and lower braces and extraction of all four first bicuspids.

How would you code this treatment?

This case would be coded as **D8080 comprehensive orthodontic treatment of the adolescent dentition** because the patient is still experiencing erupting teeth and growth.

Clinical Coding Scenario #2:
Class I Crowding and Clear Aligners

A 35-year-old patient presents with a Class I crowding situation. The patient does not want fixed appliances (i.e., braces), but will agree to wearing a series of clear, plastic trays to straighten the teeth and improve the esthetics of the case.

How would you code this treatment?

Even though this treatment involves a specific appliance, the case should be coded as **D8090 comprehensive treatment of the adult dentition**.

Clinical Coding Scenario #3:
Crossbite with Lower Anterior Teeth

A nine-year-old patient's #8 tooth has erupted into crossbite with the lower anterior teeth. The parents are simply interested in getting the central incisor out of crossbite. Different treatment options were offered to the parents for correction of the problem. After the decision was made, treatment on the central incisor was initiated.

How would you code this treatment?

Since this is treating one particular issue or problem with no serious thought to further treatment later on in the patient's development, this case is best reported using **D8020 limited orthodontic treatment of the transitional dentition**.

Clinical Coding Scenario #4:
Thumb Sucking and Appliances

An eight-year-old patient has a thumb sucking habit that the parents are anxious to stop. An appliance was recommended and placed to aid in halting the habit.

How would you code this procedure?

Coding for appliances to stop harmful habits depends upon the design. For removable appliances the code is **D8210 removable appliance therapy**; for a fixed appliance, **D8220 fixed appliance therapy**.

Clinical Coding Scenario #5:
Removable Retainers to Stabilize Teeth

A patient has completed active treatment and is wearing removable retainers to stabilize the teeth. The retainers are becoming loose and require an appointment for the orthodontist to make adjustments to the appliances.

How would you code this visit?

This visit would be coded using **D8681 removable orthodontic retainer adjustment**.

Clinical Coding Scenario #6:
Claim for Diagnostic Services

A dentist wishes to submit a claim for diagnostic procedures needed to prepare the orthodontic treatment plan for reimbursement by a patient's dental benefits plan.

How would you code this claim?

The claim you submit would list each diagnostic procedure performed, which usually includes:

- A comprehensive patient examination
- Panoramic, cephalometric and photographic images
- Diagnostic study models

The case would then be submitted by selecting the codes for each of the procedures your office renders, none of which are from the CDT Code's Orthodontics category. Applicable codes in this scenario are from Diagnostics:

D0150 **comprehensive oral evaluation – new or established patient**

D0330 **panoramic radiographic image**

D0340 **2D radiographic (cephalometric) image – acquisition, measurement and analysis**

D0350 **2D oral/facial photographic images obtained intra-orally or extra-orally**

D0470 **diagnostic casts**

If your office provides a consultation, don't forget to submit for that component as well by using **D9450 case presentation, detailed and extensive treatment planning**. Many offices overlook this very important part of reporting treatment planning.

Clinical Coding Scenario #7:
Monitoring Growth and Development

After the initial orthodontic evaluation, many times orthodontists will not feel that orthodontic treatment should begin at that time. They will set an appointment for the patient to return in a few months in order to monitor their growth and development. They will then determine if treatment should begin at that point.

What code should be used to report these future visits?

D8660 **pre-orthodontic treatment examination to monitor growth and development**

Clinical Coding Scenario #8:
Discontinued Treatment and Removal of Braces

A 10-year-old patient's parents have decided that they would like to discontinue orthodontic treatment. As such, they also wish to have their child's braces removed.

How would you code for this scenario?

D8695 **removal of fixed orthodontic appliances for reasons other than completion of treatment**

Although it may not be needed, please consider requesting the parents sign a waiver of release for premature removal of braces.

The practice should make a decision about whether to provide retention based on the treatment progress made, and in conjunction with the patient's or parent's treatment wishes. In addition, the practice should ensure that the patient's results to-date are held should the decision be reversed and treatment continues.

Clinical Coding Scenario #9:
Removal of Orthodontic Braces and Appliances by General Dentist in an Emergency Situation

A patient with braces has been struck in the face. Since it's an emergency, the patient is rushed to his general dentist. In order to assess and repair the damage, the dentist must remove the patient's braces and appliances.

How would you code for the removal of the patient's braces and appliances?

> **D8695** removal of fixed orthodontic appliances for reasons other than the completion of treatment

Clinical Coding Scenario #10:
Re-cementing a Loose Fixed Appliance

A patient presents with a palatal expander that has a band loose on one side. The only way to take care of the problem is to remove the expander, clean and repair the appliance, polish the teeth involved and then re-cement the expander on the teeth.

How would you code for this treatment?

Since the loose appliance must be repaired before re-cementation, and that a palatal expander is placed in the maxillary arch, you would use:

> **D8696** repair of orthodontic appliance – maxillary

Clinical Coding Scenario #11:
Repair and Complete Reattachment of a Mandibular Fixed Retainer

The patient presents with a mandibular bonded lingual retainer with one side of the retainer having come un-bonded. Due to a distortion of the retainer wire, the retainer must be removed, all adhesive cleaned off and teeth polished. Once the retainer's proper form is restored, the retainer is re-bonded.

How would you code for this procedure?

This procedure is coded **D8699 re-cement or re-bond fixed retainer – mandibular**.

Clinical Coding Scenario #12:
Remote Patient Encounter Utilizing Teledentistry

A patient with adolescent dentition is unable to come to the office to have their aligners checked, and would like more aligners shipped to them. A videoconference examination and subsequent review of digital photos sent by the patient, are utilized to determine whether the patient should advance to further aligner trays.

How would you code for this encounter?

D8670 **periodic orthodontic treatment visit**

D9996 **teledentistry – asynchronous; information stored and forwarded to dentist for subsequent review**
Reported in addition to other procedures (e.g., diagnostic) delivered to the patient on the date of service.

In a teledentistry encounter both the applicable orthodontic procedure code and teledentistry code are documented in the patient record and recorded on a claim submission. In this case the applicable teledentistry code is D9996 as the photographs were forwarded to the orthodontist for review after the videoconference ended. If the images were transmitted in real-time the applicable teledentistry code reported would be "D9995 teledentistry – synchronous; real-time encounter" along with the periodic orthodontic treatment visit code (D8670).

The criterion for selection of the applicable teledentistry code is CDT code's nomenclature and descriptor, regardless of the type of treatment modality or appliance that is being used to treat the patient. As noted above the applicable teledentistry code is reported with the appropriate orthodontic treatment code.

There are limitations in use of teledentistry in orthodontics for reasons that include the difficulty in obtaining adequate quality photographs from patients to document their current condition, as well as being unable to double check the patient's occlusion remotely. Further, diagnostic information (e.g., images) captured remotely by a patient or person without professional training or licensure, are unlikely to be of the same diagnostic quality as those captured in-office.

Periodic orthodontic treatment visits utilzing teledentistry can, however, be useful for established patients that are away at college or for other extended period and when the dentist has a familiarity with the patient's malocclusion and treatment.

Clinical Coding Scenario #13:
Coding All Aspects of an Orthodontic Case

A 14-year-old patient with adolescent dentition is now undergoing comprehensive orthodontic treatment that will last approximately two years. The appropriate code for comprehensive treatment is **D8080 comprehensive orthodontic treatment of the adolescent dentition**, but that cannot be the only CDT code applicable to this case.

Which CDT codes must be included in the patient's record and on claim submissions so that all necessary services are documented?

Procedures and Codes for Diagnosing the Patient's Condition

An oral evaluation and diagnosis is necessary in order to develop an appropriate treatment plan, and the applicable CDT codes for these services are found in the Diagnostic category of service. Although they are not listed in the Orthodontics category, diagnostic procedures and their codes may be delivered and reported by any licensed dentist.

Codes that are typical for an orthodontist to deliver and report are:

D0150 comprehensive oral evaluation – new or established patient

D0330 panoramic radiographic image

D0340 2D cephalometric radiographic image – acquisition, measurement, and analysis

D0350 2D oral/facial photographic image obtained intra-orally or extra-orally

D0470 diagnostic casts

Note: The findings from these procedures will lead to development of the appropriate orthodontic treatment plan. It is possible that the orthodontist may determine that treatment should not start immediately. In that case, there is a monitoring procedure that may also be performed and reported with its own unique code in the Orthodontics category:

D8660 pre-orthodontic treatment examination to monitor growth and development

Codes During Active Treatment

Even though orthodontic treatments are coded under an "umbrella code," such as D8080 in this case, there are other codes that should be used in conjunction to fully describe the services provided to the patient.

The overarching "umbrella" code for the type of orthodontic treatment for the patient in this scenario is:

D8080 **comprehensive orthodontic treatment of the adolescent dentition**

During the active orthodontic treatment, each visit would be coded using:

D8670 **periodic orthodontic treatment visit**

When the orthodontic treatment is complete and patient will receive retainers. This procedure is coded with:

D8680 **orthodontic retention (removal of appliances, construction, and placement of retainer(s))**

All subsequent orthodontic retainer adjustments should be coded as:

D8681 **removable orthodontic retainer adjustment**

Many orthodontists will be confused by this coding since most third-party payers only pay a set amount for an orthodontic treatment and therefore the additional coding does not affect the reimbursement received. Utilization of the CDT codes is not directly about billing and insurance as much as it is about documenting in the patient record the treatment that was provided to the patient.

Coding Q&A

1. *Many offices now produce digital versus plaster study models for their cases. What code should be used to report digital study models (e.g., iTero scans)?*

   Code **D0470 diagnostic casts** is used to report fabricating any type of orthodontic study models. CDT coding is intended to be procedure specific, not modality or technique specific.

2. *What code or codes should be used to report multiple stages of orthodontic treatment?*

   It is best to use limited coding for the initial phase of orthodontic treatment when you are treating only a portion of the dentition (e.g., treatment of crossbite with an expansion appliance). Interceptive treatment is often the coding for initial orthodontic care that typically is followed later in the patient's development with comprehensive (full) treatment.

3. *What are the differences between limited, interceptive, and comprehensive codes and how should they be used?*

   Limited (D8010–D8040) and Interceptive (D8050–D8060) codes are generally used to report less complex cases or initial stages of treatment. Comprehensive (D8070–D8090) codes are generally reserved for more complex cases.

4. *What code should be used to report treatment using clear aligners?*

   Coding for treatments using clear aligner therapy would be the same code that would be used for a treatment utilizing orthodontic brackets. Choice of code is dependent on the nature of the treatment (limited or comprehensive) and the stage of dental development.

5. *When should an orthodontic practice use D8999 unspecified orthodontic procedure, by report?*

   This code should be used sparingly and only when there is no other coding strategy available. In most cases another code can be found that will adequately and appropriately report the procedure performed. If the code is used, make certain that the claim is accompanied by a narrative report to describe the patient's condition, the need for treatment and the treatment provided.

6. *Often times when orthodontic cases are completed, the orthodontist may wish to put final touches on the case to perfect the end result by slightly altering the shape of a tooth or teeth. What code should be used?*

   The code most often used to report slight revisions to tooth shape is **D9971 odontoplasty – per tooth**.

7. *What code should be used to report space maintainers – space maintenance codes or interceptive coding? How should holding arches be reported?*

   The appropriate space maintenance code (D1510; D1516–D1517; D1520; D1526–D1527; or D1575) should be used if only a single space is being held. Treatment with holding arches is best reported using limited treatment procedure codes (D8010–D8040) if several spaces are being held and the treatment is part of a larger plan to gain space for the eruption of the permanent dentition.

8. *A patient has been placed on recall appointments every four months to monitor growth and development and to determine the best time to start orthodontic treatment. How should these appointments be recorded?*

   These appointments should be reported using **D8660 pre-orthodontic treatment examination to monitor growth and development**.

9. *A patient is being seen for routine orthodontic treatment. How are these appointments coded?*

   These appointments are coded using D8670 periodic orthodontic treatment visit.

10. *A patient has lost her retainer and it must be replaced. What code would you use?*

    Replacement of lost or broken retainers is coded using either **D8703 replacement of lost or broken retainer – maxillary** or **D8704 replacement of lost or broken retainer – mandibular** depending on the arch involved.

11. *I have a new patient who began orthodontic treatment in a different city who now resides in my practice area and wishes to continue treatment locally. Does the fee structure of the orthodontist who initiated treatment apply to the services I deliver, and how would I correctly document these services?*

    You are responsible for determining your own fee schedule and it would be applicable to the ongoing treatment provided. Services you provide are documented with the appropriate CDT code from the Orthodontic (or other) category of service as applicable.

 © American Dental Association

12. *When should adolescent coding be used versus adult coding?*

   Adolescent coding should be used when the patient involved is approximately 11 to 13 years of age, presents with adult dentition and is expected to undergo further growth. Adult coding should be considered when the patient has full adult dentition (may or may not have third molars present), is approximately 17 years of age or older and is not expected to experience additional growth.

13. *How does a dentist bill for a tongue presser appliance?*

   D8210   removable appliance therapy

   D8220   fixed appliance therapy

14. *My patient successfully responded to the orthodontic treatment plan in less time than originally anticipated. What effect, if any, does this have on the case fee and procedure coding?*

   There is no effect. Your full fee for services delivered is applicable and these procedures are documented with the appropriate procedure code or codes.

15. *A patient comes in with three mandibular brackets off. Can I use code D8697 for that appointment to re-bond them?*

   No. That code is only for repairs to appliances on the mandibular arch, and these appliances do not include standard orthodontic brackets such as a palatal expander, a lip bumper, or other functional appliances. There is no specific CDT code for re-bonding brackets. The visit during which the rebonding occurs would be documented with the following codes:

   D8670   periodic orthodontic treatment visit

   D8999   unspecified orthodontic procedure, by report

16. *A patient presents with a lower lingual bonded retainer that developed a sharp edge, irritating the tongue. How would I code a procedure of smoothing and burnishing that sharp edge?*

   Any repair of a fixed mandibular retainer without having to remove the retainer is coded **D8702 repair of fixed retainer, includes reattachment – mandibular**.

17. *A patient comes in with a maxillary removable retainer that is broken in two pieces. A new retainer needs to be made. How should this be coded?*

   Since the maxillary removable retainer must be remade completely, the proper code for this is **D8703 replacement of lost or broken retainer – maxillary**.

18. *I am using a rapid palatal expander in conjunction with a complete set of braces, how do I code for the use of a fixed appliance like an RPE?*

The RPE is part of a comprehensive treatment and should be coded utilizing the appropriate comprehensive orthodontic treatment code for the patient's dentition.

19. *A patient has completed orthodontic treatment and is in retainers and have maxed their orthodontic benefit. When I adjust their retainer, how should I code for that?*

You could code for the adjustment **D8681 removable orthodontic retainer adjustment** regardless of the patient's dental benefit status.

Summary

To properly code for the orthodontic procedures that are performed, the dentist must correctly identify the scope of the treatment and the appropriate stage of dental development while understanding that codes outside of the orthodontic section are necessary to fully describe procedures provided. This is especially true of the pretreatment diagnostic workup. While, the smaller number of codes in the orthodontic section may appear to simplify the coding process, it is easy to be confused and overlook all of the codes needed to properly document the full treatment.

Contributor Biography

Randall C Markarian, D.M.D., M.S. has been practicing orthodontics in Swansea, Illinois since 1994. Dr. Markarian is a member of the Council on Dental Benefit Programs and is serving as the current chair. He is also a member of the American Association of Orthodontists Council on Orthodontic Healthcare. Dr. Markarian served on the ADA's Code Maintenance Committee and was the 2020 chair.

Chapter 12: D9000–D9999
Adjunctive General Services

By Charles D. Stewart, D.M.D.

Introduction

Dentistry and medicine concur that the word "adjunctive" refers to any treatment or service delivered with a primary treatment that increases the primary treatment's efficacy, or to assist with completion or reporting of the primary treatment. In other words, adjunctive treatment or therapy is generally a secondary treatment or activity in addition to the primary therapy. The word "general" in the dental or medical context means not specialized or limited in range of subject, application, activity, etc. Differentiation between primary and secondary treatment as noted above is consist with the ADA Glossary definition of adjunctive: "A secondary treatment in addition to the primary therapy." The CDT Code's Adjunctive General Services category is needed to properly identify and document procedures or treatments that are performed on patients or used to satisfy requirements of reporting not directly related to the procedure actually being performed.

The Adjunctive General Services category often contains the answer when an appropriate CDT code can't be found in any of the other 11 CDT Code categories. This twelfth category is unique, with CDT codes for clinical services and non-clinical services that include case management, and other administrative services. This uniqueness has led many to describe the Adjunctive category as a catchall for procedures and services that don't quite fit in the other CDT Code categories. Many of the CDT codes in this section are for care or administrative activities that happen outside of the mouth, but can, and usually do, occur in the practice administrative office or location setting.

The relevance and use of codes in the Adjunctive category has been recently demonstrated. In early 2020 there was a global health emergency developing, which evolved into the COVID-19 pandemic. Response to the pandemic led to emergency regulations and publication of guidelines that directly affected the practice of dentistry and how services can be provided to patients in need. The ADA, along with dental benefit plans, provided guidance to dental providers on reporting services performed remotely during this emergency, including the use of the two very important teledentistry codes contained in the Adjunctive category. Teledentistry encounters, also referred to as virtual encounters, will be discussed further in this chapter.

Key Definitions and Concepts

Anesthesia: A patient's level of consciousness is determined by the patient's response to the drugs or medications administered, not the route of the anesthetic agent administration. State dental licensing boards regulate the use of anesthesia techniques and license those who render this service. The ADA House of Delegates adopted and published anesthesia policy and guidelines, which are available at *ADA.org/en/member-center/oral-health-topics/anesthesia-and-sedation*. There are several anesthesia procedure codes such as local, regional, deep sedation, general anesthesia, etc.

Consultation: In a dental setting, a service or meeting provided by a dentist or other licensed dental professional where the dentist, patient, or other parties (e.g., another dentist, physician, or legal guardian) discuss the patient's dental needs, conditions and proposed treatment modalities. A consultation could be performed via a teledentistry model.

Medicament: Substance or combination of substances intended to be pharmacologically active, specially prepared to be prescribed, dispensed or administered by authorized personnel to prevent or treat diseases in humans or animals. This can be an agent that promotes recovery from an injury or ailment. It can also be referred to as a medicine. It can be a substance used for medical treatment. In dentistry, medicaments can be placed in the mouth or dispensed by a licensed dental professional, and may also be purchased as an over-the-counter treatment. Medicaments may be indicated based on results of clinical examination performed both in person and via a teledentistry model.

Microabrasion: Mechanical and chemical removal of a small amount of tooth structure to eliminate superficial enamel discoloration defects. This process uses chemical solutions and or pumice to remove thin layers of tooth enamel in order to eliminate yellow, white and brown spots, or stains and discolorations on the teeth. Microabrasion may be used as a step or process in a conservative restorative treatment. It also may be a definitive stand-alone procedure and as such should be reported using the appropriate CDT code.

Palliative: Action that relieves pain and symptoms without dealing with the underlying disease or cause of the condition.

The ADA Glossary definition of **palliative** is more concise: "Action that relieves pain but is not curative."

Parenteral: A technique of administration in which the drug bypasses the gastrointestinal (GI) tract. Examples of parenteral administration may include intramuscular (IM), intravenous (IV), intranasal (IN), submucosal (SM), subcutaneous (SC) or intraosseous (IO). Simply put, bypassing the gastrointestinal tract means the drug is not administered through the mouth or alimentary canal.

Special Health Care Needs: Include any physical, developmental, mental, sensory, behavioral, cognitive, or emotional impairment or limiting condition that requires medical management, health care intervention, and/or use of specialized services or programs. The condition may be congenital, developmental, or acquired through disease, trauma, or environmental cause and may impose limitations in performing daily self-maintenance activities or substantial limitations in a major life activity. Health care for individuals with special needs requires specialized knowledge, as well as increased awareness and attention, adaptation, and accommodative measures beyond what are considered routine. (This definition was developed by the American Academy of Pediatric Dentistry (AAPD) Council on Clinical Affairs.)

Teledentistry, Asynchronous: Also known as "store-and-forward," involves transmission of recorded health information to a dentist, who uses the information to evaluate a patient's condition or render a service outside of a real-time or live interaction. Such transmitted information can include radiographs, photographs, video, digital impressions, digital models and photomicrographs of patients. Transmission is through a secure electronic communications system. CAD-CAM technology can be considered an asynchronous encounter with appliance fabrication, design and treatment applications. This technology is currently used within Dentistry in several practice areas such as: diagnostic, preventive, restorative, prosthetics and orthodontics.

Teledentistry, Synchronous: Also referred to as live video or real-time, synchronous teledentistry involves live, two-way interaction between a person or persons (e.g., patient; dental, medical or health caregiver) at one physical location, and an overseeing supervising or consulting dentist or dental provider at another location. This type of interaction saw increased utilization during the 2020 COVID-19 pandemic.

Chapter 12: D9000–D9999 Adjunctive General Services

Changes to This Category

CDT 2021 contains only one change, a revision to the following code's nomenclature and descriptor that is in Adjunctive's "Miscellaneous Services" subcategory.

D9971 **odontoplasty** ~~1-2 teeth; includes removal of enamel projections~~ <u>– per tooth</u>
<u>Removal/reshaping of enamel surfaces or projections.</u>

As seen in the marked revisions D9971 is now a single tooth procedure, with a descriptor added that describes the procedure's purpose and scope. Code Maintenance Committee discussion in support of this change recognized the importance of being able to accurately and precisely report the service performed. This discussion acknowledged confusion with the existing code where many dentists thinking that it should only be used to report the removal of enamel projections such as mamelons on incisors.

However, odontoplasty is often used in orthodontics where the interproximal surfaces of teeth are adjusted to assist in proper alignment and positioning of the teeth being moved. The odontoplasty procedure may also be used in conjunction with the fabrication of a prosthetic, to establish guide planes, develop rest seats and to create other different retentive aspects. By the approval of the per tooth reporting the dental industry is now able to strengthen the ability of tracking individual tooth outcomes and add to the data vitally needed for future evidence based dentistry models.

Review of Notable Past CDT Changes

CDT 2020 was the first version that included a code for dental case management that recognized a patient's unique physical condition or needs:

D9997 **dental case management – patients with special health care needs**
Special treatment considerations for patients/individuals with physical, medical, developmental or cognitive conditions resulting in substantial functional limitations, which require that modifications be made to delivery of treatment to provide comprehensive oral health care services.

A review of the incidence of claim submission of D9997 shows a similar incidence of submission as the other case management codes, D9991 through D9994. The beauty of the use of D9997 is that it allows potential identification of services provided to patients with special health care needs. Unfortunately, it is too early in the life of D9997 to have meaningful data which could help lead to improved access to dental care as well as help to identify those willing to treat patients with these special needs.

The definition of what would be considered a patient with special health care needs is in an earlier part of this chapter titled "Key Definitions and Concepts." This definition enables a provider to properly understand when this procedure would apply and be documented in the patient's record and on a claim. Historically, most commercial dental benefit plans do not provide coverage for the case management family of codes, however many of the government programs (Medicaid) can consider these encounters for potential reimbursement.

CDT 2019 had a unique code (D9613) added to help address the national opioid epidemic and crisis. The opioid epidemic resulted in new federal and state laws and regulations in 2018 and 2019. In response to the opioid crisis, the American Dental Association developed an opioids policy, which defines the role dentists play in the provision of opioids to patients as well as suggestions to reduce the number of prescriptions for opioids provided to dental patients. Reporting of the D9613 provides a means to document delivery of a non-opioid medication directly in the surgical site that aids in the management of post-surgical pain (for example, after third molar removal):

D9613 infiltration of sustained release therapeutic drug – single or multiple sites
Infiltration of a sustained release pharmacologic agent for long acting surgical site pain control. Not for local anesthesia purposes.

A review of claims data shows D9613 has been used more and more frequently and this code can offer a metric to track and trend the utilization and its relationship to the desired reduction in the use of prescriptions for opioids. Coupling provider education with utilization of this procedure and code, there has been a reduction in the number of prescriptions of opioid medications following oral surgical procedures. It may be some time before it will be possible to assess how the use of this type of medication impacts the opioid crisis. Most addictions to opioids are reflected years after first exposure, thus accounting for the time lag before accurate reporting of impact this procedure to the opioid epidemic is available. The current accurate data to report, is that the global number of prescriptions for an opioid pain medication has been reduced, thanks to education, counseling and development of medications such as the D9613. It is with optimism that the newly approved ibuprofen-acetaminophen combination oral analgesic will provide additional resources to continue reducing the number of opioid prescriptions given.

Chapter 12: D9000–D9999 Adjunctive General Services

Clinical Coding Scenario #1:

Dental Emergency during Mandatory Dental Office Closure

Note: This scenario describes a virtual encounter that occurs during a National Health Emergency. A virtual encounter with services rendered can occur at other times under various environmental (e.g., health and safety) circumstances. The procedures and coding described herein are not limited to the scenario's environmental (i.e., COVID-19) conditions.

The dental office was closed for compliance with federal, state, and local demands in response to the 2020 COVID-19 pandemic. A patient calls the office and states they are having a dental emergency. Office staff make arrangements for a virtual encounter where the dentist to meet with the patient via the Zoom™ conferencing application. During the virtual encounter the dentist has the patient explain their history, symptoms and issue of concern. The dentist asks the patient to hold the phone so they can visualize the area of the mouth and the condition that exists. The patient opens their mouth and shows the area, tissues and teeth. The dentist makes a diagnosis based on information gathered during this encounter, and then determines a course of treatment to palliate the patient's issues until the dental office can open again and definitively address the concerns presented. The dentist provided appropriate medications and advice based on the Zoom™ encounter.

How do you code this remote care?

D9995 teledentistry – synchronous; real-time encounter

Note: D9995 is used since the entire encounter, including the dentist's viewing of the patient's oral cavity, is live and completed without interruption.

D0140 limited oral evaluation – problem focused

or

D0170 re-evaluation – limited, problem focused (established patient; not post-operative visit)

or

D0171 re-evaluation – post-operative office visit

Note: Only one of these evaluation codes is reported. The appropriate code is selected based on the history of the condition being presented. If it is the first experience of this issue, the D0140 is the proper code. If the condition involves a previously known, addressed or treated condition, the re-evaluation code can be selected based on whether or not this is it is a post-operative encounter.

D9110 palliative (emergency) treatment of dental pain – minor procedure

Note: Reporting D9110 is appropriate as the provider gave the patient advice and medications based on the evaluation.

It is of vital importance that the D9995 be listed on the dental claim form to identify this as a teledentistry claim. Many individual states have mandated special handling of claims identified as "telehealth" and such identification is afforded solely by using the D9995 (as above) or the D9996 CDT codes. Many dental plans view these two codes as reporting a modality to deliver services, with the additional diagnostic and/or treatment codes being required for accurate reporting and reimbursement of services performed.

Clinical Coding Scenario #2:
Anesthesia

A patient, referred by a general dentist, is scheduled for surgical removal of third molars. An evaluation for the use of general anesthesia was conducted, resulting in the decision to proceed with the anesthetic and surgery upon obtaining the appropriate informed consents. After the initial administration of the anesthetic agent the surgery was completed. The anesthesia start time was 10:05 A.M. and anesthesia services were completed at 11:10 A.M. The oral surgeon extracting the third molars is wondering how many units of anesthesia can be billed, or is it just a single flat rate procedure?

How would you code this care?

> **D9219** **evaluation for moderate sedation, deep sedation or general anesthesia**
>
> **D9222** **deep sedation/general anesthesia – first 15 minutes**
>
> **D9223** **deep sedation/general anesthesia – each subsequent 15 minute increment**

(Report D9223 four times.)

A copy of the anesthesia record should be submitted with the claim to verify the anesthesia. According to the D9220 descriptor (which is also applicable to D9223) anesthesia time begins when the anesthesia agent delivery and monitoring protocol start, and the procedure is completed when the patient may be safely left under the observation of trained personnel.

In this scenario 65 minutes elapsed between the procedure's start and completion, so the appropriate coding is: 1) D9222 for the initial 15 minutes; and 2) D9223 with a quantity of "4" for the additional 50 minutes. As anesthesia is reported in 15 minute (or portions thereof) increments the D9223 claim documents delivery of three full 15 minute increments and one five minute increment (i.e., Quantity = "4").

Clinical Coding Scenario #3:
Occlusal Equilibration

The patient says her spouse hears loud grinding sounds at night. However, the patient says that she has no pain in her jaws or joint area, but adds that she does have difficulty chewing food. The patient also says that her teeth seem to be sensitive when biting down and at times seem to make noise or "chatter" when chewing.

Based on this information and oral evaluation, the dentist determined that the patient needed her bite adjusted.

How would you code the "bite adjustment" procedure?

Occlusal equilibration, also known as occlusal adjustment, refers to the reshaping of the occlusal surfaces of teeth to create a harmonious contact relationship between the upper and lower teeth. One of the following codes should be used, with selection based on the procedure's extent:

    D9951   occlusal adjustment – limited

or

    D9952   occlusal adjustment – complete

There is no formal definition of limited or complete occlusal adjustment. ADA claim completion instructions (Guide to Reporting Area of Oral Cavity and Tooth Number by CDT Code) the applicable arch(s) or quadrant(s) should be reported along with either of these codes. A dentist selects the appropriate occlusal adjustment code after considering this guidance, time required and clinical experience. The patient's record should include the reasons for selecting either code.

If the occlusal equilibration is associated with or to accommodate the placement of a restoration or prosthesis, the billing of the equilibration may be considered incidental to the restoration or prosthesis. Likewise, if the occlusal adjustment is associated with the final step of a comprehensive orthodontic treatment, it may be considered incidental to the orthodontic treatment.

Clinical Coding Scenario #4:
Occlusal Guard with both Hard and Soft Attributes

In addition to the occlusal adjustment performed in clinical coding scenario #3, the dentist feels that a full arch occlusal guard should be fabricated and placed in the patient's mouth to prevent future damage to the teeth and jaws. The documentation dilemma is that the desired occlusal guard has a hard occlusal surface as well as other component parts that would also be found on a soft appliance.

There are three available occlusal guard procedure codes to use for this scenario, differentiated by extent of protection and the appliance material. But none of the three clearly describe an appliance with both hard and soft attributes.

D9944 occlusal guard – hard appliance, full arch

D9945 occlusal guard – soft appliance, full arch

D9946 occlusal guard – hard appliance, partial arch

How would you code this care?

D9944 occlusal guard – hard appliance, full arch

A full arch code is appropriate as the dentist stated that a full arch guard should be fabricated to provide the necessary protection. The differentiation between hard and soft appliance is based on the knowledge that the operative part of an occlusal guard is the occlusal surface, and the key determinant of reporting the type of occlusal guard is what the material is on the occlusal surface. In this scenario the occlusal surface is hard.

To clarify further, occlusal guards that have any hard occlusal component, regardless of the presence of a soft component, should be coded as a hard guard.

Clinical Coding Scenario #5:
Dry Socket

A student came home from college to have his third molars removed. He returned to college, with complaints of worsening pain in the mandibular extraction sites. He did not understand this as at the time of surgery he had a new material injected in the extraction sites and had been experiencing minimal if any pain until now (eight to ten days post-surgery). He sought the care of a local dentist in the college town. The dentist examined the patient and diagnosed condensing osteitis, or dry socket, in the mandibular extraction sites.

How would you code this care?

A dry socket is localized inflammation of the tooth socket following extraction due to failure of the development of a blood clot or the loss of the blood clot with resultant osteitis. The condition is very painful and characterized by bad breath and an unpleasant smell and taste in the mouth. The procedure could be coded as either:

D9930 treatment of complications (post-surgical) – unusual circumstances, by report

or

D9110 palliative (emergency) treatment of dental pain – minor procedure

D0140 limited oral evaluation – problem focused

D0140 would be appropriate in addition to D9930 or D9110 as the dentist did perform a limited oral evaluation in determining the source of the chief complaint.

Clinical Coding Scenario #6:
Gingival Irritation around a Partially Erupted Third Molar

A patient reported to the dentist with a complaint of inflammation and pain from the gums around an unerupted third molar. The patient complained that food was getting stuck in the flap of tissue. The dentist evaluated the area and diagnosed pericoronitis. The dentist irrigated the area to remove and flush out the trapped food and to gain relief for the patient.

How would you code this care?

D0140 **limited oral evaluation – problem focused**

and

D9110 **palliative (emergency) treatment of dental pain – minor procedure**
This is typically reported on a "per visit" basis for emergency treatment of dental pain.

Using D9110 is appropriate as the patient did present at the dental office on an emergency basis with the complaint of pain around the third molar. The minor procedure was the irrigation of the food entrapment. D9110 does not define what procedure needs to be performed to qualify nor that the procedure be completed.

There are some that feel the irrigation could be coded using **D4921 gingival irrigation – per quadrant**. This code's descriptor notes that the procedure is for irrigation of gingival pockets, which is not the case in this scenario and the reason why D4291 is not applicable.

While on the subject of the D4921, this code is not intended to be used to report the irrigation of a socket following an extraction or for the irrigation of a tooth in the process of endodontic treatment.

Clinical Coding Scenario #7:
Assessments at a Title I School: A "Real-time" Teledentistry Encounter

This scenario assumes that the persons and services involved are performing services in accordance and compliance with all local, state, federal laws, rules, and regulations (e.g., dental practice acts or laws).

A hygienist is scheduled to meet with students of a local Title I school in order to assess their potential need for dental treatment. The school does not have dedicated space or equipment for dental assessments, so the hygienist brings a laptop computer and an intraoral camera, as well as a portable dental chair, light and unit. There is also portable radiographic equipment. This equipment is used to enable information capture and a real-time connection with the dentists via a HIPAA-compliant secure connection that uses certified encryption technology.

During the visit the hygienist records patient information that includes a clinical examination, a perio evaluation, a visual oral cancer examination, and the capture of high-quality intraoral diagnostic images (photographic and periapical radiographs). The dentist through this real-time connection sees ten patients exhibiting evidence of the need for immediate or further care (e.g., restorations, prophylaxis, extraction and fluoride application). Several of the students schedule their care at the affiliated brick and mortar dental practice following consultation with their parents.

What CDT codes would be used to document the services provided on the day of this real-time encounter?

In this scenario, patients present for diagnostic and evaluative procedures. The dentist is at a different physical location with complete and immediate access to patient information being captured and the ability to interact vocally and visually with the patient and the hygienist.

The following procedure codes are reported by the oral health or general health practitioner, as applicable, for each patient who received the services described.

D0191   **assessment of a patient**

D0220   **intraoral periapical first radiographic image**

D0230   **intraoral periapical each additional periapical image**

D0350   **2D oral/facial photographic image obtained intra-orally or extra-orally**

D0351   **3D photographic image**

Note: The types of diagnostic photographic images (2D or 3D) and the number captured, as well as the number of periapical images captured, to adequately document the clinical condition would be determined by the dentist/hygienist.

D01xx ("...oral evaluation...") CDT code – determined and reported by the dentist)

D9995   teledentistry – synchronous; real-time encounter

Note: D9995 is reported once for each patient, in the same manner as CDT code **D9410 house/extended care facility call** (once per date of service per patient) to document the type of teledentistry interaction in this setting on the date of service.

Clinical Coding Scenario #8:
Screening Services at an Off-site Setting:
A "Store and Forward" Teledentistry Encounter

(This scenario assumes that the persons and services involved are performing services in accordance and compliance with all local, state, federal laws, rules, and regulations (e.g., dental practice acts or laws)).

A dental auxiliary in an off-site setting collects a full set of electronic dental records as allowed in the state where the facility is located. These records include periapical radiographs, photographs, charting of dental conditions, health history, consent, and applicable progress notes. This stored information is forwarded to the dentist via a secure HIPAA-compliant connection that uses encryption technology. The dentist completes the oral evaluation, diagnosis, and treatment plan.

What CDT codes would be used to document the services provided at the off-site setting?

In this scenario the patient interacts only with the dental auxiliary. The information collected is conveyed to the dentist for diagnosis, evaluation and treatment planning at a different time and location. This dentist has no live vocal or visual interaction with the patient or dental auxiliary during information collection.

The following procedure codes can be reported, as applicable, for each individual who received the services described:

D0191 **assessment of a patient**

D0220 **intraoral – periapical first radiographic image**

D0230 **intraoral – periapical each additional periapical image**

D0350 **2D oral/facial photographic image obtained intra-orally or extra-orally**

D0351 **3D photographic image**

Note: The types of diagnostic photographic image (2D or 3D) and the number captured, as well as the number of separate periapical images captured, would be determined by the clinical condition being documented.

D01xx ("...oral evaluation..." CDT code – determined and reported by the dentist)

D9996 **teledentistry – asynchronous; information stored and forwarded to dentist for subsequent review**

Note: D9996 is reported once for each patient to document the type of teledentistry interaction in this setting on the date of service.

Coding Q&A

1. *Who could document and report a D9995 or D9996 CDT code?*

    A dentist who oversees or performs the teledentistry event, and who, via diagnosis and treatment planning, completes the oral evaluation, may report the appropriate teledentistry procedure code. Applicable state regulations may also determine the oral health or general health practitioner who is permitted to document and report these CDT codes.

2. *What documentation should I maintain in my patient records, and what will be needed on a claim submission when reporting teledentistry codes D9995 and D9996?*

    The patient record should include the CDT code that reflects the type of teledentistry encounter, and there may be additional state documentation requirements to satisfy. Treatment records should be very specific and document the scenario in which the encounter occurred. A claim submission must include all required information as described in the completion instructions for the ADA paper claim form and the HIPAA standard electronic dental claim. Some government programs (e.g., Medicaid) may have additional claim reporting and coding requirements.

3. *Are there any special teledentistry reporting rules when I am delivering care during a virtual encounter that occurs during a National Health Emergency or at other times under various environmental (e.g., health and safety) circumstances?*

    Some commercial health plans have established rules and CDT code relationship reporting for these codes to be considered. Some of these plans consider the D9995 or D9996 to be for reporting the modality of how services are delivered and not a separately reimbursable service. In these situations, it would be wise to report the appropriate diagnostic code (D0140, D0170 or D0171) in addition to the teledentistry code for clarity of the service performed. Most of the encounters in response to the COVID-19 crisis are D9995.

4. *How may I report **D9110 palliative (emergency) treatment of dental pain – minor procedure** delivered during a real-time virtual encounter?*

    There is no language in the descriptor of D9110 that defines the procedure having to be performed in the dental office. Emergency treatment of dental pain could be achieved in a teledentistry model, with guidance given to the patient on how to relieve the pain or infection, and may also involve prescribing medication.

When this palliative procedure is performed in a real-time virtual encounter D9995 should also be reported on the same claim for consideration. Diagnostic procedure codes may also be included if these procedures were also delivered during the encounter. Some dental benefit plan limitations may exclude or not recognize certain combinations of codes performed together on the same day. Some dental benefit plans may limit payment for the D9110 procedure to reflect an in-office encounter only.

5. *How may I report local anesthesia as a separate procedure?*

   D9215 local anesthesia in conjunction with operative or surgical procedures and **D9210 local anesthesia not in conjunction with operative or surgical procedures** are available CDT codes to report these local anesthesia services. Benefit plan limitations may exclude separate reimbursement benefits for local anesthesia.

6. *I have administered Pacira's Exparel, a sustained release pharmacologic agent, for pain control after third molar extractions, as well as in some periodontal and implant surgical procedures. How do I code for delivery of this non-opioid medicament for pain control?*

   D9613   infiltration of sustained release therapeutic drug – single or multiple sites

   The use of this code is not site specific but is designed in reporting for all applications occurring at the same appointment. It should be billed once per appointment regardless of whether it is a single site or multiple sites of injection.

7. *Should a specialist who sees a patient referred by a general dentist for an evaluation of a specific problem report the consultation code (D9310) or a problem focused evaluation code (D0140 or D0160)? Also, does it matter if the specialist initiates treatment for the patient on the same visit?*

   Typically, a consultation (D9310) is reported when one dentist refers a patient to another dentist for an opinion or advice on a problem encountered by the patient. According to this CDT code's descriptor, the dentist who is consulted may initiate additional diagnostic or therapeutic services for the patient. These services are reported separately by their own unique CDT codes.

   Both D0140 and D0160 are problem-focused evaluations and may be reported if the consulting specialist believes either of these codes better describe the services that were provided. Please note that neither of these evaluation procedures' nomenclatures or descriptors contain language that prohibits the consulting specialist from initiating and reporting additional services.

8. *If a practitioner treats more than one patient in one nursing home on one day, is D9410 house/extended care facility call reported per patient or per facility?*

The descriptor for code D9410 states that it may be reported in addition to separate reporting of services provided to a patient seen at the facility. D9410 may be reported for each patient receiving service at the facility on a given day. However, benefit plan limitations and exclusions may place limits on reimbursement, such as once per facility visit, not per patient. It is important to remember to report for what you do, not for what you intend to be paid or understand your contract to be.

9. *A patient who is a college student was complaining of grinding their teeth. The symptoms are worsening as final examinations approach. The dentist makes something that was called an anterior deprogrammer to provide relief and get this patient through finals. What CDT code should be used to report this?*

D9946 is appropriate for reporting the services performed.

D9946 occlusal guard – hard appliance, partial arch

This code properly represents the described service performed as it notes the device is a "removable dental appliance designed to minimize the effects of bruxism or other occlusal factors." The guard provides partial occlusal coverage as an anterior deprogrammer would fit on a partial arch.

10. *How do I report external bleaching?*

You may use one of the following codes as applicable based on the extent of the service provided to the patient:

D9972 external bleaching – per arch – performed in the office
or
D9973 external bleaching – per tooth

11. *How do I report the fabrication of trays and the provision of bleaching agent to my patients for their use at home?*

When trays and material are provided to a patient for application of bleach at home the following code is applicable:

D9975 external bleaching for home application, per arch; includes materials and fabrication of custom trays

12. *Teeth #23, #24, #25 and #26 are very divergent in shape and have limited interproximal contact except in the incisal 1/3. In conjunction with the orthodontic treatment I am performing, I would like to adjust the divergent points, and make the teeth appear less divergent to facilitate final alignment and to have broader contact points. What CDT code should I use to report this?*

Report this procedure with a CDT code **D9971 odontoplasty – per tooth**.

Starting with CDT 2021, this is documented and reported as a per tooth procedure, therefore it would be submitted on a claim in a manner that reports the procedure and tooth (or teeth) involved. In this scenario the claim could report the procedure four times, each on a separate service line, or once where the individual tooth numbers involved are documented in the applicable field along with a "4" in the service line's "Quantity" field.

13. *After placing an occlusal guard, the dentist asks patients to return for approximately three to four office visits, as needed, to adjust the guard. What procedure code would be used to report visits to adjust the guard?*

D9943   occlusal guard adjustment

This procedure code is reported for each adjustment visit.

14. *Is there a CDT code for air abrasion?*

There is no procedure code specifically for air abrasion.

If the procedure delivered is consistent with the nomenclature and descriptor of D9970, that code may be reported. The code and nomenclature are as follows:

D9970   enamel microabrasion
　　　　The removal of discolored surface enamel defects resulting from altered mineralization or decalcification of the superficial enamel layer. Submit per treatment visit.

Many experts in the dental field view air abrasion as a technique utilized to perform or enable a restorative procedure. If there is a restorative procedure delivered on the same tooth on the same date of service it is possible that D9970 may not be reimbursed separately as the dental benefit plan could consider it inclusive in the restorative procedure reimbursement.

15. *I place desensitizer on teeth before completing the restoration.*
    What code should I use to report the desensitizer?

There is no procedure code specifically for desensitizer used in conjunction with restorative procedures.

Reporting **D9910 application of desensitizing medicament** is not appropriate if application conflicts with the closing sentence of this code's descriptor "...not to be used for bases, liners or adhesives used under restorations." Please note that the header for amalgam restorations states "liners and bases are included as part of the restoration..." and the composite restorations header states "...liners and bases and curing are included as part of the restoration..."

The full CDT Code entry for the D9910 procedure follows:

D9910   application of desensitizing medicament
Includes in-office treatment for root sensitivity. Typically reported on a "per visit" basis for application of topical fluoride. This code is not to be used for bases, liners or adhesives used under restorations.

Summary

The CDT Code's Adjunctive General Services category continues to be an important part of a dental care treatment planning because these codes can clarify the nature, number and scope of procedures to be delivered, and their efficacy. In an ever-changing healthcare environment, dentistry will continue to evolve and develop more ways to measure and increase the efficacy of our treatments. The value of this category of CDT codes was demonstrated during the COVID-19 pandemic. While some of the codes in this category represent actual dental procedures, others can and were used to help clarify the setting that services were performed in. This adjunctive action can provide a defense for a dental provider, if they ever were accused of violating a stay at home, or safer at home orders by performing dental services.

For example, the teledentistry codes provide the opportunity and means for a patient to receive services when the patient is in one physical location and a dentist overseeing the delivery of those services is in another location. This is key to identify the compliance with federal, state and local regulations for stay at home or safer at home. The CDT codes for teledentistry, have proven that access to care has been influenced and the potential to bring dental care to patients in areas without access to a dentist or to their dentist is now a reality. Teledentistry is possible in many areas of dentistry, including diagnostic, preventive, restorative, prosthetics and orthodontics. During the COVID-19 pandemic, the majority of the teledentistry claims were diagnostic in nature, with palliative procedures being the next most frequently used codes.

Equally exciting to the utilization of the teledentistry codes is the increasing utilization of code D9613, added for reporting the infiltration of sustained release therapeutic drug – single or multiple sites. This code represents the use of medication that can impact and potentially eliminate the need for an opioid prescription usually associated with oral surgery procedures. With education of both patients and dental providers, the use of medication represented by this procedure code can influence or eliminate one of the first potential exposures to an opioid, eliminating that first opioid prescription. The trend shows we are starting to achieve the goal of helping to address the current opioid epidemic, ultimately leading to the prevention of further abuse.

The Adjunctive codes continue to be referenced regularly when other CDT codes do not seem to fit the procedure being performed. Many times, the use of an Adjunctive code can provide the clarity and granularity that makes the difference between a claim being paid or rejected, and between being able to defend the circumstances of treatment or not. With the recent COVID-19 pandemic, many emergency actions were taken by federal, state and local governments. Some of these changes may result in permanent regulatory and compliance rules which may necessitate future changes to this category. The beauty of the CDT is that this code set is a living document which reflects the current state of and situations that impact the practice of dentistry.

Chapter 12: D9000–D9999 Adjunctive General Services

Contributor Biography

Charles D. Stewart, D.M.D. is currently President, CEO and Chairman of the Board of Directors for Aetna Dental of California, Inc. He is also National Director, Dental Networks, for Aetna Inc. Dr. Stewart is Chairman of the National Association of Dental Plans (NADP) Codes Workgroup, a part of the NADP Standards and Transactions Initiative, a role he has held since 2013. In this role he represents NADP on the ADA Code Maintenance Committee. Dr. Stewart was recognized by NADP with the 2018 Don Mayes Leadership award for excellence in leadership. He is currently Chairman of California Association of Dental Plans (CADP) Quality Management Committee, member of the CADP Board of Directors, and the lead instructor for CADP's quality assurance consultant certification courses. Dr. Stewart also maintains a private practice on evenings and weekends. Dr Stewart is a graduate of Oral Roberts University School of Dentistry.

Chapter 13: Dental Benefits: What Every Dentist Should Know

By ADA Staff
Center for Dental Benefits, Coding and Quality, Practice Institute

This chapter addresses facets of a dental practice's business side, things a dentist should be aware of that will help anticipate or resolve problems. Topics covered include ascertaining a patient's benefits, becoming a participating dentist, claim processing problems and audits. The chapter concludes with links to additional related resources available from the American Dental Association.

Dental Benefit Coverage

The majority of patients with private dental benefits coverage have their plans provided by employers or unions. Employers offer dental plans to help attract and retain employees and to help employees maintain good oral health. However, most dental plans are not designed to cover all dental procedures and many procedures require the patient to meet a deductible or incur a high co-insurance payment. It is very important for dental offices to explain to their patients that a dental benefit plan is actually not insurance but simply a benefit. Thus, it is essential to educate your patients about costs and recommend they take their dental benefit grievances to their employer's human resources department when necessary.

Making the Decision to Participate with a Managed Care Plan

Making the decision to sign a managed care contract is one of the most important business decisions a dentist may make. When you sign a contract, you make promises that will be legally binding on you. Thus, it is extremely important that you carefully review any contract before you sign it.

It is highly recommended you consult your personal attorney before signing any contract. The ADA also offers an important resource for ADA members – the ADA Contract Analysis Service. Prior to signing a proposed contract, member dentists may submit a dental provider contract with a third-party payer or a dental management service organization to their state or local dental society who will forward it to the Service for a free analysis. The service provides a plain language explanation of proposed contract terms for each agreement analyzed. The service does not provide legal advice or recommend whether a contract should or should not be signed.

You have the right to negotiate the terms of a participating dentist agreement; however, the plan also has contractual rights that may affect your rights. It certainly doesn't hurt to ask if you have concerns with specific clauses in the participating dentist agreement.

Many times, if a dentist has contracted with a third-party payer, he or she may have agreed to abide by the carrier's processing policies, which may or may not appear in the contract itself. The processing policies of many carriers are published on their websites. Dentists should make it a point to understand the policies typically applied by payers.

And don't forget to ask for the plan's current dentist billing manual and be sure you understand how the plan processes the procedures that you most frequently perform.

Remember not to focus only on the contract itself – after all, you are making a business decision and data is very important. Your practice management software typically has reporting tools that many dentists may not be aware of and do not utilize to their own advantage. It may be a good time to call your software vendor to learn how to generate reports that will help you better understand your own practice metrics.

It is also important for dental offices to understand payer processing policies before treatment is started so that these policies can be adequately explained to patients. Patients often rely on their dentists and office staff to decode their dental benefits for them and the dentist-patient relationship can be affected by payer policies.

Treatment plans should cater to the needs of the patient rather than what is covered by the benefit plan. Always remember to "code for what you do and do what you coded for." Although the payer may bundle codes for the purpose of benefit determination, the patient record should always accurately describe the services that the patient received. You always have the right to appeal the claim decision, especially in instances where the payer has made a judgment regarding the medical necessity of a treatment you provided your patient.

Helping You After You Sign the Contract

Sometimes legislation may be the best approach to dealing with issues related to dental benefit plans. The ADA's Washington, DC office has many efforts underway to address dental benefit issues through legislative remedies.

Examples of current efforts include:

1. Non-Covered Services
2. Assignment of Benefits
3. Coordination of Benefits
4. Flexible Spending Accounts

Non-Covered Services
A key concern reported to ADA by dental offices has been carriers use of requiring dentists to charge patients the plan's maximum allowable fee for services not covered by the dental plan. The ADA is working closely with its state partners and has helped implement legislation in 39 states that prohibits dental plans from forcing dentists to accept the plan's maximum allowable fee for a non-covered procedure.

Bundling and Downcoding
Examples of provisions in the signed contract that limit reimbursement include bundling and downcoding, which has resulted in many dental offices calling the ADA asking for guidance. If the payer has applied some of these limitations and they are in accordance with the contract with which the dentist agreed, the dentist may be bound to the policies set forth by the payer.

The ADA defines bundling of procedures as the systematic combining of distinct dental procedure codes by third-party payers that results in a reduced benefit for the patient/beneficiary.

Downcoding is a practice of third-party payers in which the benefit code has been changed to a less complex or lower cost procedure than was reported, except where delineated in contract agreements.

Let's look at an example of downcoding. A 13-year-old patient with adult dentition is treated and the dentist has rendered a **D0120 periodic oral evaluation – established patient** and **D1110 prophylaxis – adult**.

The payer rejected the claim for D1110 and returned an explanation of benefits (EOB) statement indicating the correct code is **D1120 prophylaxis – child**, as this is the correct code because the dental benefit plan defines a patient under age 15 as a child, no matter what dentition is present. This is worth an appeal because the message implies that that the dentist miscoded the claim, which is not true.

An appeal could be avoided if the EOB acknowledged that the reimbursement was based on benefit plan design. It is important to note that appealing a claim may not always result in greater reimbursement but could simply help prevent misperceptions by the patient.

In this scenario, the claim was not adjudicated correctly as the payer ignored the D1110 descriptor and asked the dentist to report the wrong procedure code. The only proper action for the dentist is to code for what you do.

Now let's look at an example of bundling. The dentist provided a **D0120 periodic oral evaluation**, **D1120 prophylaxis – child** and **D1208 topical application of fluoride – excluding varnish** to a 6 year old patient. The payer rejected the claim and the EOB implied that all three procedures were part of the same CDT Code. Once again, this is a situation that should be appealed to correct the language within the EOB statement.

In this case, the payer ignored the nomenclatures and descriptors of these discrete codes and redefined procedure code D0120. A third-party payer is supposed to use the code number, its nomenclature and its descriptor as written.

It is not acceptable when a payer says the procedure reported with D0120 includes other procedures, in this instance – D1120 and D1208 – that are appropriately reported separately on the claim form. In this particular example the payer may even be in violation of its CDT Code license.

It is okay when a payer benefits procedures in combination with others as part of its payment policies, but the payer cannot claim that discrete procedures are actually part of other procedures.

Refund Requests and Overpayments

Some contracts may have clauses that contractually bind you to refund any overpayments. Many times when a third-party payer mistakenly pays a dentist, the payer will request a refund of the overpaid amount. In some cases, refund requests have been sent to dentists more than two years after the payment was made and the patient may no longer be a patient of record. In most instances, the overpaid amount is deducted from future benefits paid to the dentist. In some cases, overpayments made to other dentists for the same patient may be deducted from future benefit payments to the current treating dentist. Many members and the ADA question the fairness of this practice.

Several states have enacted legislation that restricts how far back a carrier can ask for a refund and a period of one year seems to be the most common. Ensuring you understand these clauses is of the utmost importance before signing a participating dentist agreement with a third-party payer.

Removal From Network Lists

If a dentist wants to terminate an agreement, there is usually a range of 30 to 90 days before a termination will take effect. Dental offices have reported that although a contract with a third-party payer was terminated previously, the carrier did not update its website with correct information. Patients were under the false impression that the dentist was still contracted with the plan and were expecting the carrier's discounted fees, not the dentist's full fees.

This can cause major problems for the patient and the dental office and may even interfere with the dentist–patient relationship. As a best practice, at the time of cancellation dentists should submit in writing, to the carrier (sent via certified mail) a request specifically to remove their names from any participating dentist list.

Dentists should follow up with carriers who fail to remove their name in a timely manner. Please call the ADA for assistance if your name has not been removed from the plan's website after the termination date.

What Fee Should I Submit?

A question frequently asked by dental offices is what fee to report on the claim form: the discounted fee or the dentist's full fee? Irrespective of whether you are contracted or not contracted, the ADA recommends that dentists should always submit their full fee to carriers. The carriers will be certain to only allow the agreed upon fees for payment.

Tips to Negotiate a Contract

If you are a participating provider with one or more dental benefit plans, you may need to negotiate your fee increases. This negotiation should be done individually, between only you and your plan, and not with or on behalf of other dentists. Before you enter negotiations with a payer, prepare your talking points and do your homework.

- Your strengths: Do you have advantages in terms of access?
    - Number of dentists in your locality
    - Wait times for available appointments, impacting the patients covered under the plan
    - Influx of new patients covered under the plan
- Your numbers: What data do you need to effectively negotiate?
    - Know which procedure codes generate the highest total revenue for your practice, including:
        - Frequency with which each procedure is reported

- Current allowed amount (i.e., your current discounted fee)
- Extent of these procedure codes' contribution to your overall practice revenue
- Your desired fee for each procedure code
  - Extent of preventive services that your office provides
  - Costs associated with operating your business
  - Patient satisfaction rates (most recent available)
  - Date when your fees were last revised
- Efficiencies you offer: Which of your business practices are favorable to the payer?
  - Electronic claims submission
  - Use of online portals to verify eligibility and benefits
  - EFT enabled for receipt of claim payments
- Review the *ADA Survey on Dental Fees*
- Use all of the above the information you have gathered to "tell your story".
- Identify the payer's provider representative assigned to your region who you can contact to begin to make your case. This may be someone known to your business staff, typically with the title of "provider relations manager".
- Begin with email introductions. If comfortable, request a phone call or continue making your case in writing.
- Always be respectful. Let the provider relations representative know that you value the patients garnered from being a network dentist.
- Be patient and don't give up! The first offer you receive may not be the best offer.
- Request information on whether the carrier leases their network and whether the revised fees will apply to any networks you have been leased into.
- After you succeed, make sure you have copies of all signed documents.
- Check the next Explanation of Benefits (EOB) documents to ensure the fee changes are appropriately reflected.
- Remember to renegotiate periodically.

It is good practice to always review your contracted fee schedules annually. Additionally, don't forget that it is very important to always report your full fee on the claim form. Several payers set fees based on market rates and the charges you submit will be used by payers to determine maximum allowable fees.

The fee schedules are typically part of the participating provider agreement – a legal contract between the dentist and the third-party payer. There are other clauses in the contract (along with documents referenced in the contract, i.e., the provider's office reference manual) that impact the final payment from the third-party payer. For example, a policy that bundles the fee for a core buildup with the fee for the crown is typically detailed in the provider's office reference manual along with other processing policies. It is important to review these documents carefully before trying to project revenues and negotiating fees with the payer.

Helping the Non-Contracted Dentist

Many dental carriers will not honor assignment of benefits to non-contracted dentists. These plans claim that assignment of benefits is a contracted dentist benefit. The good news is that 22 states have passed legislation requiring that assignment of benefits be honored. These laws generally apply only to fully insured plans which are governed by state insurance statutes and approximately 52% of patients with a dental benefit have a plan that is insured and subject to state laws. If your state has not passed assignment of benefits legislation, it is recommended you talk to your state dental society about doing so.

Helping All Dentists

Payment Delay and Lost Submissions

One of the biggest complaints concerning third-party claim payment is lost claim forms and radiographs. Many dentists report sending in claim forms or radiographs several times before the dental plan will acknowledge receipt. Often radiographs are submitted with the claim, but the dentist will receive an EOB requesting the radiographs.

In some instances, the method by which claims are submitted increases the possibility of loss. Attachments that are not firmly affixed to a claim form can get separated when the mail is opened; this is especially true when multiple claims are submitted in one envelope. If radiographs are not labeled and get detached from claim forms, they may not be able to be matched back to the appropriate claim form. Privacy and security standards require that personal medical information be protected so unmatched attachments would most likely be destroyed.

When a payer does not require a radiograph for a claim, the process established by that payer may require that the radiograph be removed and returned or destroyed. If a subsequent issue moves the claim from auto-adjudication to a manual review, a radiograph may be requested at that time.

Submitting electronic claims and the appropriate attachments to them is the best way to avoid the loss of claims, radiographs and other attachments.

There is no uniformity within the payer community regarding submission of radiographs, partly due to different business structures within the industry. Some companies would prefer that no radiographs be sent unless requested. Others want to see images at the time specific procedure codes are reported.

Top Procedure Denials

Periodontal scaling and root planing (D4341, D4342) and periodontal maintenance (D4910)

Scaling and root planing (SRP) denials are one of the most reported concerns to the ADA. Dentists believe that submitted radiographs show bone loss substantial enough to warrant coverage for SRP and have reported that dentist consultants working for payers deny these claims indicating there is no radiographic evidence of bone loss. Upon appeal some of these claims have been paid.

Dentists and their staff may not always understand what appears to be inconsistent SRP claim adjudication as payer adjudication policies vary substantially. One plan may require at least 4 mm pocket depth while another may have different depth criteria. Many plans will require radiographic evidence of bone loss before paying an SRP claim. Some payers may not benefit more than two quadrants of scaling and root planing performed on the same date of service.

It is very difficult for a small dental office to be familiar with the various payer requirements for payment of SRP claims as it is typical for a dental office to have patients present with well over 100 different dental plans.

A major concern of dental offices is that the denial language used on the EOB statement may lead the patient to think that the procedure was not necessary. Denial of benefits may not mean the SRP was unnecessary – it simply means the patient's clinical condition did not satisfy the benefit plan's threshold for reimbursement.

In addition to radiographic evidence of bone loss, it is not uncommon for payers to request periodontal charting and a narrative description for SRP coverage consideration.

Claim denials for **D4910 periodontal maintenance** occur because some carriers have limited benefits for D4910. Some plans reimburse only if periodontal maintenance was delivered within 2 to 12 months of scaling and root planing while others may require a 3-month wait after therapy. Some plans deny benefits unless 2 or more quadrants have received prior therapy; however, there are no such limitations in the CDT Code.

It is recommended that dental office staff determine how a patient's plan covers this procedure before delivery in order to better inform the patient of the coverage parameters so as to avoid any claim surprises. If known, tell patients in advance that plan provisions may not provide for reimbursement of D4910 for extended periods of time and that the patient may be responsible for the costs.

Crowns (D2710–D2799) and core buildups (D2950)

The ADA receives many calls on crown and core buildup denials and there are myriad reasons for these denials. Some carriers use a policy for crowns that is along the lines of requiring that at least 50% of the incisal angle must need replacement due to decay or fracture. In addition, many carriers will deny crowns for a tooth with a poor prognosis and due to abrasion and attrition. Core buildups are typically covered once every 5 years if there is less than 50% tooth structure due to disease or fracture. Many payers will require documentation, including radiographs and a narrative description, for coverage consideration.

The ADA has received calls from dental offices where carriers' EOBs have stated that only the crown should be reported as it includes the core buildup. In this example, the payer is incorrect per the CDT Code's perspective as the buildup procedure and crown procedure are separate and distinct from each other as not all crowns require a buildup.

It is understood that the payer can make single reimbursement based on benefit plan design, and this should be made clear on the EOB statement sent to the patient. The dentist should be able to balance bill the patient; however, the ability to balance bill is subject to the participating dentist agreement, if any.

To avoid post-treatment complaints, dental offices should help patients understand the clinical basis for treatment and should appeal the benefit decision if it is thought the claim has not been properly adjudicated.

Compliance Audits and Utilization Review

Many dental offices call the ADA when confronted with a compliance audit or with questions on utilization review. When a dentist is placed under utilization review, the office is often required to submit additional documentation for the procedures being questioned. These claims are then manually reviewed to determine the benefit.

Some carriers require that claims being reviewed be sent to a different address than where you would normally send claims. If you are being audited, please be sure to send audit documentation to the correct address provided by the dental plan. Otherwise it will slow down the processing of your claim submission.

When you are notified of being placed under review or are suddenly receiving requests for additional documentation, it is recommended you contact the dental plan's consultant or your provider relations manager to determine if a review is being undertaken and, if it is, why you were placed on utilization review and what it will take to get you off of the plan's utilization review.

The plan is obligated to disclose the results of your review. Please do not forget your right to appeal. You have the right to appeal the reasons why you have been placed on utilization review.

It is recommended you work with the plan to explain and justify potential differences in practice patterns, e.g., a dental office that caters to elderly patients may indeed have higher utilization patterns for bridges. This is something that could be explained and taken into consideration by the dental plan. Helping the dental plan understand the rationale for your recommended treatment plans can help significantly.

Remember to properly and accurately document your patient records to the very last detail, even if something appears obvious to you. It may be a good idea to submit pre-treatment estimates when you are under review, so as to minimize any surprises.

Over time if the payer is assured that treatment patterns are justified then the payer will remove the dentist from further review. However, in some instances the payer may choose to follow up with an in-office audit.

In the event of an in-office audit, plan representatives will personally visit your office to review patient files and records. The plan will request that a separate work area be set up for them to conduct the review and you will be asked in advance to have specific patient records available for review by plan representatives.

Auditors and plan representatives may look at claims as far back as state laws allow. Please note that in-office reviews can last one or more days depending on the number of records to be reviewed.

If you are contracted with the plan and have agreed to such audits, it is recommended that you read and familiarize yourself with your contract and the plan's policies before the audit begins.

We also encourage dentists to obtain a written description of the scope of the audit procedures. Consulting with your personal attorney so that you understand your rights and obligations in such a situation is also recommended.

It may be a good idea to talk with your plan representative about the following before the audit begins:

- Clinical review criteria
- Analytical methods
- Time periods for conducting reviews
- Qualifications of individuals conducting the review
- Confidentiality
- Disclosure of the process to insured's
- Access to review staff
- Appeals process for adverse determinations

A question we often receive is whether the dentist is allowed to disclose a patient's record to the plan in cases of an audit. The HIPAA Privacy Rule permits a dental practice to disclose such information in response to such a request if the dental plan has or had relationships with the individuals who are the subjects of the requested information. An important point to note is that for patients who have been beneficiaries of the plan in the past and are no longer deriving benefits from that plan, the payer's auditor can only look at the patient's records for the time the patient was part of the plan.

Individual patients have a right to request that disclosures not be made to a health or dental plan for services that the patient has paid for out of pocket and in full. A covered dental practice may not disclose information regarding patients who are not, and have never been beneficiaries of that plan, even if a participating dentist agreement requires it. Disclosing the information may be in violation of HIPAA.

When a patient has paid for a service in full and asks the practice not to disclose the service to the plan, the dental practice must comply with that request. As a best practice, a notice of privacy practices (NPP) should be given to individuals at their first visit. The NPP should contain information about the patient's rights with regards to HIPAA and how the patient may request restrictions on disclosures of information. Your practice must also have procedures for your staff to flag such requests in the event of such a request coming from a patient, written or otherwise.

Resources

- The Center for Professional Success website offers a plethora of information on dental benefits at *ADA.org/dentalbenefits*.

- Information on the Code on Dental Procedures and Nomenclature (CDT Code), as well as the review and revision process, is available at *ADA.org/cdt*.

- *Why Doesn't My Insurance Pay for This?* (W265) is a brochure designed to help patients understand dental benefit plans by explaining why some procedures are not covered and it describes annual maximums, least expensive alternative treatment clauses, pre-existing conditions, exclusions and more. Available at *ADAcatalog.org*.

- *What Every Dentist Should Know Before Signing a Dental Provider Contract* is a publication that answers common questions dentists may wish to consider before signing a dental contract with third-party payers. Available at *www.ADA.org/thirdpartycontract*.

- *CDT 2021: Current Dental Terminology* (J021) is the most up-to-date coding resource on the market and will help you document codes for dental procedures quickly and accurately. This book not only helps fill documentation gaps but can help reduce rejected dental claims. Available at *ADAcatalog.org*.

- *Third-Party Concerns* is a series of articles published in ADA News on third-party problems reported by dental offices. Available at *success.ADA.org/en/dental-benefits/member-support-on-third-party-issues*.

- *Decoding Dental Benefits* is a series of *ADA News* articles that seeks to educate dentists so informed decisions on dental plan participation can be made. Available at *success.ADA.org/en/dental-benefits/decoding-dental-benefits-series*.

- *Responding to Claim Rejections* is a publication that educates dentists and dental offices on the proper way to handle and respond to claim rejections from third-party payers. Available at *ADAcatalog.org/cpspdf.aspx?assets=2187&day=b1mygiq+JiA*.

- *Dental Benefit Series Videos* are short video tutorials, created by the ADA Center for Dental Benefits, Coding and Quality, are designed to help dental professionals understand a key issue in dentistry: how third-party programs interface with dental offices. Available at *success.ADA.org/en/dental-benefits/dental-benefit-videos?utm_source=promospots&utm_content=dentalbenefitslp&utm_medium=fb&utm_campaign=easy*.

- Dental Benefit Webinars are a series of recorded webinars on various dental benefit topics *success.ADA.org/en/dental-benefits/dental-benefit-webinars?utm_source=promospots&utm_content=dentalbenefitslp&utm_medium=fb&utm_campaign=easy*.

- *Dental Communications: Letters, Templates, and Forms (J05321)* contains sample letters addressing third-party issues, including UCR and EOB language which may be customized to send to patients' employers and third-party payers as appropriate. Available at *ADAcatalog.org*.

- ADA Contract Analysis Service (ADA members only) is available at *ADA.org/en/member-center/member-benefits/legal-resources/contract-analysis-service*.

Section 3

Appendices

Appendix 1: CDT Code to ICD (Diagnosis) Code Cross-Walk

CDT Code(s)	
D0120	periodic oral evaluation – established patient
D0140	limited oral evaluation – problem focused
D0150	comprehensive oral evaluation – new or established patient
D0210	intraoral – complete series of radiographic images
D0709	intraoral – complete series of radiographic images – image capture only
D0220	intraoral – periapical first radiographic image
D0707	intraoral – periapical radiographic image – image capture only
D0230	intraoral – periapical each additional radiographic image
D0251	extra-oral posterior dental radiographic image
D0272	bitewings – two radiographic images
D0274	bitewings – four radiographic images
D0708	intraoral – bitewing radiographic image – image capture only
D0330	panoramic radiographic image
D0701	panoramic radiographic image – image capture only
D0999	unspecified diagnostic procedure, by report
Suggested ICD-10-CM Diagnosis Code(s)	
Z01.20	Encounter for dental examination and cleaning without abnormal findings
Z01.21	Encounter for dental examination and cleaning with abnormal findings
Z13.84	encounter screening for dental disorders

CDT Code(s)	
D1110	prophylaxis – adult
D1120	prophylaxis – child
Suggested ICD-10-CM Diagnosis Code(s)	
E11.9	Type 2 diabetes mellitus without complications
K03.6	Deposits [accretions] on teeth
K05.1	Chronic gingivitis
K05.10	Chronic gingivitis, plaque induced
K05.30	Chronic periodontitis
Z33.1	Pregnant state, incidental
Z72.0	Tobacco Use

CDT Code(s)	
D1206	topical application of fluoride varnish
D1208	topical application of fluoride, excluding varnish
Suggested ICD-10-CM Diagnosis Code(s)	
K02.3	Arrested dental caries
K02.61	Dental caries on smooth surface limited to enamel
K02.7	Dental root caries
K03.1	Abrasion of teeth
K03.2	Erosion of teeth
M35.00	Sicca syndrome*, unspecified

* also known as Sjögren's Syndrome

CDT Code(s)	
D1330	oral hygiene instructions
Suggested ICD-10-CM Diagnosis Code(s)	
E11.9	Type 2 diabetes mellitus without complications
K02.3	Arrested dental caries
K02.52	Dental caries on pit and fissure surface penetrating into dentin
K02.61	Dental caries limited to enamel
K02.62	Dental caries on smooth surface penetrating into dentine
K02.7	Dental root caries
K02.9	Dental caries, unspecified
K03.2	Erosion of teeth
K03.6	Deposits [accretions] on teeth
K05.00	Acute gingivitis, plaque induced
K05.01	Acute gingivitis, non-plaque induced
K05.10	Chronic gingivitis, plaque induced
K05.30	Chronic periodontitis, unspecified
K05.5	Other periodontal diseases
M35.00	Sicca syndrome*, unspecified
Z33.1	Pregnant state, incidental
Z72.0	Tobacco use

* also known as Sjögren's Syndrome

CDT Code(s)	
D1351	sealant – per tooth
D1354	interim caries arresting medicament application – per tooth
D2990	resin infiltration of incipient smooth surface lesions
Suggested ICD-10-CM Diagnosis Code(s)	
K02.51	Dental caries on pit and fissure surface limited to enamel
K02.61	Dental caries on smooth surface limited to enamel
M35.00	Sicca syndrome*, unspecified

* also known as Sjögren's Syndrome

CDT Code(s)	
D1352	preventive resin restoration in a moderate to high caries risk patient – permanent tooth
Suggested ICD-10-CM Diagnosis Code(s)	
K02.51	Dental caries on pit and fissure surface limited to enamel

CDT Code(s)	
D2140	amalgam – one surface; primary or permanent
D2150	amalgam – two surfaces; primary or permanent
D2160	amalgam – three surfaces; primary or permanent
D2161	amalgam – four or more surfaces; primary or permanent
Suggested ICD-10-CM Diagnosis Code(s)	
K02.51	Dental caries on pit and fissure surface limited to enamel
K02.52	Dental caries on pit and fissure surface penetrating into dentin
K02.61	Dental caries on smooth surface limited to enamel
K02.62	Dental caries on smooth surface penetrating into dentin
K03.81	Cracked tooth
S02.5XXA	Fracture of tooth (traumatic), initial encounter for closed fracture

CDT Code(s)	
D2330	resin-based composite – one surface; anterior
D2331	resin-based composite – two surfaces; anterior
D2332	resin-based composite – three surfaces; anterior
D2335	resin-based composite – four or more surfaces or involving incisal angle (anterior)
Suggested ICD-10-CM Diagnosis Code(s)	
K00.2	Abnormalities of size and form of teeth
K02.51	Dental caries on pit and fissure surface limited to enamel
K02.52	Dental caries on pit and fissure surface penetrating into dentin
K02.61	Dental caries on smooth surface limited to enamel
K02.62	Dental caries on smooth surface penetrating into dentin
K03.1	Abrasion of teeth
K03.2	Erosion of teeth
K03.81	Cracked tooth
S02.5XXA	Fracture of tooth (traumatic), initial encounter for closed fracture

CDT Code(s)	
D2391	resin-based composite – one surface; posterior
D2392	resin-based composite – two surfaces; posterior
D2393	resin-based composite – three surfaces; posterior
D2394	resin-based composite – four or more surfaces; posterior
Suggested ICD-10-CM Diagnosis Code(s)	
K02.51	Dental caries on pit and fissure surface limited to enamel
K02.52	Dental caries on pit and fissure surface penetrating into dentin
K02.61	Dental caries on smooth surface limited to enamel
K02.62	Dental caries on smooth surface penetrating into dentin
K02.7	Dental root caries
K03.1	Abrasion of teeth
K03.2	Erosion of teeth
K03.81	Cracked tooth
S02.5XXA	Fracture of tooth (traumatic), initial encounter for closed fracture

CDT Code(s)	
D2740	crown – porcelain/ceramic
D2750	crown – porcelain fused to high noble metal
D2751	crown – porcelain fused to predominantly base metal
D2752	crown – porcelain fused to noble metal
D2753	crown – porcelain fused to titanium and titanium alloys
D2790	crown – full cast high noble metal
D2792	crown – full cast noble metal
D2794	crown – titanium and titanium alloys
D2950	core buildup, including any pins when required
D2951	pin retention – per tooth; in addition to restoration
D2952	post and core in addition to crown; indirectly fabricated
D2954	prefabricated post and core in addition to crown
Suggested ICD-10-CM Diagnosis Code(s)	
K00.2	Abnormalities of size and form of teeth
K02.52	Dental caries on pit and fissure surface penetrating into dentin
K02.53	Dental caries on pit and fissure surface penetrating into pulp
K02.62	Dental caries on smooth surface penetrating into dentin
K02.63	Dental caries on smooth surface penetrating into pulp
S02.5XXA	Fracture of tooth (traumatic), initial encounter for closed fracture

CDT Code(s)	
D2928	prefabricated porcelain/ceramic crown – permanent tooth
D2930	prefabricated stainless steel crown – primary tooth
Suggested ICD-10-CM Diagnosis Code(s)	
K00.2	Abnormalities of size and form of teeth
K02.52	Dental caries on pit and fissure surface penetrating into dentine
K02.53	Dental caries on pit and fissure surface penetrating into pulp
K02.62	Dental caries on smooth surface penetrating into dentine
K02.63	Dental caries on smooth surface penetrating into pulp
S02.5XXA	Fracture of tooth (traumatic), initial encounter for closed fracture

CDT Code(s)	
D2940	protective restoration
Suggested ICD-10-CM Diagnosis Code(s)	
K02.9	Dental caries, unspecified
S02.5XXA	Fracture of tooth (traumatic), initial encounter for closed fracture

CDT Code(s)	
D3110	pulp cap – direct (excluding final restoration)
D3120	pulp cap – indirect (excluding final restoration)
Suggested ICD-10-CM Diagnosis Code(s)	
K02.52	Dental caries on pit and fissure surface penetrating into dentin
K02.53	Dental caries on pit and fissure surface penetrating into pulp
K02.62	Dental caries on smooth surface penetrating into dentin
K02.63	Dental caries on smooth surface penetrating into pulp
K04.0	Pulpitis
S02.5XXA	Fracture of tooth (traumatic), initial encounter for closed fracture

CDT Code(s)	
D3220	therapeutic pulpotomy (excluding final restoration) – removal of pulp coronal to the dentinocemental junction and application of medicament
D3310	endodontic therapy; anterior tooth (excluding final restoration)
D3320	endodontic therapy; premolar tooth (excluding final restoration)
D3330	endodontic therapy; molar tooth (excluding final restoration)
Suggested ICD-10-CM Diagnosis Code(s)	
K02.53	Dental caries on pit and fissure surface penetrating into pulp
K02.63	Dental caries on smooth surface penetrating into pulp
K03.81	Cracked tooth
K03.89	Other specified diseases of hard tissues of teeth
K04.0	Pulpitis
K04.1	Necrosis of pulp
K04.5	Chronic apical periodontitis
K04.6	Periapical abscess with sinus
K04.7	Periapical abscess without sinus
K04.8	Radicular cyst
K04.90	Unspecified diseases of pulp and periapical tissues
K04.99	Other diseases of pulp and periapical tissues
K05.5	Other periodontal diseases
K08.8	Other specified disorders of teeth and supporting structures
S02.5XXA	Fracture of tooth (traumatic), initial encounter for closed fracture

CDT Code(s)	
D3346	retreatment of previous root canal therapy – anterior
D3347	retreatment of previous root canal therapy – premolar
D3348	retreatment of previous root canal therapy – molar
Suggested ICD-10-CM Diagnosis Code(s)	
K08.59	Other unsatisfactory restoration of tooth
M27.5	Periradicular pathology associated with previous endodontic treatment

CDT Code(s)	
D4210	gingivectomy or gingivoplasty – four or more contiguous teeth or tooth bounded spaces per quadrant
D4211	gingivectomy or gingivoplasty – one to three contiguous teeth or tooth bounded spaces per quadrant
Suggested ICD-10-CM Diagnosis Code(s)	
K05.30	Chronic periodontitis, unspecified
K05.31	Chronic periodontitis, localized
K05.32	Chronic periodontitis, generalized
K06.1	Gingival enlargement

CDT Code(s)	
D4249	clinical crown lengthening – hard tissue
Suggested ICD-10-CM Diagnosis Code(s)	
K02.9	Dental caries, unspecified
K03.81	Cracked tooth
K05.5	Other periodontal diseases
S02.5XXA	Fracture of tooth (traumatic), initial encounter for closed fracture

CDT Code(s)	
D4260	osseous surgery (including elevation of a full thickness flap and closure) – four or more contiguous teeth or tooth bounded spaces per quadrant
D4261	osseous surgery (including elevation of a full thickness flap and closure) – one to three contiguous teeth or tooth bounded spaces per quadrant
D4263	bone replacement graft – retained natural tooth – first site in quadrant
D4264	bone replacement graft – retained natural tooth – each additional site in quadrant
Suggested ICD-10-CM Diagnosis Code(s)	
K05.21	Aggressive periodontitis, localized
K05.22	Aggressive periodontitis, generalized
K05.30	Chronic periodontitis
K05.31	Chronic periodontitis, localized
K05.32	Chronic periodontitis, generalized
K05.6	Periodontal disease, unspecified
K08.20	Unspecified atrophy of edentulous alveolar ridge
K08.21	Minimal atrophy of the mandible
K08.22	Moderate atrophy of the mandible
K08.23	Severe atrophy of the mandible
K08.24	Minimal atrophy of the maxilla
K08.25	Moderate atrophy of the maxilla
K08.26	Severe atrophy of the maxilla

CDT Code(s)	
D4270	pedicle soft tissue graft procedure
D4273	autogenous connective tissue graft procedure (including donor and recipient surgical sites) first tooth, implant or edentulous tooth position in graft
D4275	non-autogenous connective tissue graft (including recipient site and donor material) first tooth, implant, or edentulous tooth position in graft
D4276	combined connective tissue and double pedicle graft, per tooth
D4277	free soft tissue graft procedure (including recipient and donor surgical sites) first tooth, implant or edentulous tooth position in graft
D4278	free soft tissue graft procedure (including recipient and donor surgical sites) each additional contiguous tooth, implant or edentulous tooth position in same graft site
D4283	autogenous connective tissue graft procedure (including donor and recipient surgical sites) – each additional contiguous tooth, implant or edentulous tooth position in same graft site
D4285	non- autogenous connective tissue graft procedure (including recipient surgical site and donor material) – each additional contiguous tooth, implant or edentulous tooth position in same graft site
Suggested ICD-10-CM Diagnosis Code(s)	
K06.0	Gingival recession

CDT Code(s)	
D4341	periodontal scaling and root planing – four or more teeth per quadrant
D4342	periodontal scaling and root planing – one to three teeth per quadrant
D4346	scaling in the presence of generalized moderate or severe gingival inflammation – full mouth after oral evaluation
D4910	periodontal maintenance
D6081	scaling and debridement in the presence of inflammation or mucositis of a single implant, including cleaning of the implant surfaces, without flap entry and closure
Suggested ICD-10-CM Diagnosis Code(s)	
A69.1	Other Vincent's infections
E11.9	Type 2 diabetes mellitus without complications
K03.6	Deposits [accretions] on teeth
K05.20	Aggressive periodontitis, unspecified
K05.21	Aggressive periodontitis, localized
K05.22	Aggressive periodontitis, generalized
K05.30	Chronic periodontitis, unspecified
K05.31	Chronic periodontitis, localized
K05.32	Chronic periodontitis, generalized
K05.5	Other periodontal diseases
K05.6	Periodontal disease, unspecified
K06.1	Gingival enlargement
Z33.1	Pregnant state, incidental
Z72.0	Tobacco Use
Z87.891	Personal history of nicotine dependence

CDT Code(s)	
D4355	full mouth debridement to enable a comprehensive oral evaluation and diagnosis on a subsequent visit
Suggested ICD-10-CM Diagnosis Code(s)	
K03.6	Deposits [accretions] on teeth
Z72.0	Tobacco Use
Z87.891	Personal history of nicotine dependence

CDT Code(s)	
D5110	complete denture – maxillary
D5120	complete denture – mandibular
Suggested ICD-10-CM Diagnosis Code(s)	
K08.1	Complete loss of teeth

CDT Code(s)	
D5211	maxillary partial denture – resin base (including any retentive/clasping materials, rests, and teeth)
D5212	mandibular partial denture – resin base (including retentive/clasping materials, rests, and teeth)
D5213	maxillary partial denture – cast metal framework with resin denture bases (including any retentive/clasping materials, rests and teeth)
D5214	mandibular partial denture – cast metal framework with resin denture bases (including any retentive/clasping materials, rests and teeth)
D6010	surgical placement of implant body: endosteal implant
D6056	prefabricated abutment – includes modification and placement
D6057	custom fabricated abutment – includes placement
D6059	abutment supported porcelain fused to metal crown (high noble metal)
D6240	pontic – porcelain fused to high noble metal
D6750	retainer crown – porcelain fused to high noble metal
D6752	retainer crown – porcelain fused to noble metal
Suggested ICD-10-CM Diagnosis Code(s)	
K00.00	Anodontia
K08.409	Partial loss of teeth, unspecified cause, unspecified class
K08.419	Partial loss of teeth due to trauma, unspecified class
K08.429	Partial loss of teeth due to periodontal diseases, unspecified class
K08.439	Partial loss of teeth due to caries, unspecified class

CDT Code(s)	
D7111	extraction, coronal remnants – primary tooth
D7250	removal of residual tooth roots (cutting procedure)
Suggested ICD-10-CM Diagnosis Code(s) – ICD-10-CM	
K03.9	Disease of hard tissues of teeth, unspecified

CDT Code(s)	
D7140	extraction, erupted tooth or exposed root (elevation and/or forceps removal)
D7210	extraction, erupted tooth requiring removal of bone and/or sectioning of tooth, and including elevation of mucoperiosteal flap if indicated
Suggested ICD-10-CM Diagnosis Code(s)	
K02.53	Dental caries on pit and fissure surface penetrating into pulp
K02.63	Dental caries on smooth surface penetrating into pulp
K04.0	Pulpitis
K04.1	Necrosis of the pulp
K04.5	Chronic apical periodontitis
K04.6	Periapical abscess with sinus
K04.7	Periapical abscess without sinus
K04.8	Radicular cyst
K05.21	Aggressive periodontitis, localized
K05.3	Chronic periodontitis
K08.439	Partial loss of teeth due to caries, unspecified class
K09.0	Developmental odontogenic cysts
L02.91	Cutaneous abscess, unspecified
L03.90	Cellulitis, unspecified
L03.91	Acute lymphangitis, unspecified
R44.8	Other symptoms and signs involving general sensations and perceptions
R44.9	Unspecified symptoms and signs involving general sensations and perceptions
R69	Illness, unspecified
S02.5XXA	Fracture of tooth (traumatic), initial encounter for closed fracture
S02.5XXB	Fracture of tooth (traumatic), initial encounter for open fracture
S03.2XXA	Dislocation of tooth, initial encounter

Appendix 1. CDT Code to ICD (Diagnosis) Code Cross-Walk

CDT Code(s)	
D7220	removal of impacted tooth – soft tissue
D7230	removal of impacted tooth – partially bony
D7240	removal of impacted tooth – completely bony
Suggested ICD-10-CM Diagnosis Code(s)	
K00.1	Supernumerary teeth
K00.6	Disturbances in tooth eruption
K01.0	Embedded teeth
K01.1	Impacted teeth
K09.0	Developmental odontogenic cysts

CDT Code(s)	
D7953	bone replacement graft for ridge preservation – per site
Suggested ICD-10-CM Diagnosis Code(s)	
K02.53	Dental caries on pit and fissure surface penetrating into pulp
K02.63	Dental caries on smooth surface penetrating into pulp
K04.0	Pulpitis
K04.1	Necrosis of pulp
K04.5	Chronic apical periodontitis
K04.6	Periapical abscess with sinus
K04.7	Periapical abscess without sinus
K04.8	Radicular cyst
K05.21	Aggressive periodontitis, localized
K05.30	Chronic periodontitis, unspecified
K05.31	Chronic periodontitis, localized
K05.32	Chronic periodontitis, generalized
K09.0	Developmental odontogenic cysts
S02.5XXA	Fracture of tooth (traumatic), initial encounter for closed fracture
S02.5XXB	Fracture of tooth (traumatic), initial encounter for open fracture
S03.2XXA	Dislocation of tooth, initial encounter

CDT Code(s)	
D8080	comprehensive orthodontic treatment of the adolescent dentition
Suggested ICD-10-CM Diagnosis Code(s)	
K00.0	Anodontia
K00.6	Disturbances in tooth eruption
K08.8	Other specified disorders of teeth and supporting structures
M26.212	Malocclusion, Angle's class II
M26.213	Malocclusion, Angle's class III
M26.24	Reverse articulation
M26.29	Other anomalies of dental arch relationship
M26.30	Unspecified anomaly of tooth position of fully erupted tooth or teeth
M26.31	Crowding of fully erupted teeth
M26.35	Rotation of fully erupted tooth or teeth
M26.39	Other anomalies of tooth position of fully erupted tooth or teeth
M26.4	Malocclusion, unspecified
M26.81	Anterior soft tissue impingement
M26.82	Posterior soft tissue impingement
M26.89	Other dentofacial anomalies
Q67.4	Other congenital deformities of skull, face, and jaw

CDT Code(s)	
D9110	palliative (emergency) treatment of dental pain – minor procedure
Suggested ICD-10-CM Diagnosis Code(s)	
K02.53	Dental caries on pit and fissure surface penetrating into pulp
K02.63	Dental caries on smooth surface penetrating into pulp
K04.0	Pulpitis
K04.6	Periapical abscess with sinus
K04.7	Periapical abscess without sinus
M26.60	Temporomandibular joint disorder, unspecified
M26.69	Other specified disorders of temporomandibular joint

CDT Code(s)	
D9230	inhalation of nitrous oxide/anxiolysis, analgesia
Suggested ICD-10-CM Diagnosis Code(s)	
F41.9	Anxiety disorder, unspecified

CDT Code(s)	
D9910	application of desensitizing medicament
Suggested ICD-10-CM Diagnosis Code(s)	
K03.0	Excessive attrition of teeth
K03.1	Abrasion of teeth
K03.2	Erosion of teeth

CDT Code(s)	
D9944	occlusal guard – hard appliance, full arch
D9945	occlusal guard – soft appliance, full arch
D9946	occlusal guard – hard appliance, partial arch
Suggested ICD-10-CM Diagnosis Code(s)	
F59	Unspecified behavioral syndromes associated with physiological disturbances and physical factors
K03.0	Excessive attrition of teeth
M26.60	Temporomandibular joint disorder, unspecified
M26.69	Other specified disorders of temporomandibular joint
M26.89	Other dentofacial anomalies

CDT Code(s)	
D9951	occlusal adjustment – limited
Suggested ICD-10-CM Diagnosis Code(s)	
K03.0	Excessive attrition of teeth
K03.81	Cracked Tooth
K04.0	Pulpitis
K06.0	Gingival recession
M26.60	Temporomandibular joint disorder, unspecified

Appendix 2: ADA Guide to Dental Procedures Reported with Area of the Oral Cavity or Tooth Anatomy (or Both)

This guide's focus is on claim submission completion – identifying by CDT code whether or not oral cavity area codes or tooth information should accompany the procedure code reported. It is also available online as a PDF at:

https://www.ADA.org/en/publications/cdt/ADA-dental-claim-form

ADA Dental Claim Data Content Recommendation
Reporting Area of the Oral Cavity and Tooth Anatomy by CDT Code – v4, Effective Jan 1, 2021

Dental procedure codes, listed in numeric order, are as published in **CDT 2021** (© American Dental Association)

This recommendation:

1. Complements the ADA's online comprehensive claim form completion instructions at: *http://www.ADA.org/en/publications/cdt/ADA-dental-claim-form*

2. Is applicable to both the ADA Dental Claim Form (© 2019) and the HIPAA standard electronic dental claim transaction (837D v5010)

Notes:

a. For reference the Area of the Oral Cavity and the Tooth Anatomy code sets used on 837D and ADA Claim Form follow

Area of the Oral Cavity	entire oral cavity	00	upper right quadrant	10				
	maxillary arch	01	upper left quadrant	20				
	mandibular arch	02	lower left quadrant	30				
			lower right quadrant	40				
Tooth Anatomy	**Number**					**Primary**	**Permanent**	
		Maxillary (Patient Right to Left)				A - J	1 - 16	
		Mandibular (Patient Left to Right)				K - T	17 - 32	
	Surface	Mesial	M	Incisal	I	Facial (or Labial)		F
		Occlusal	O	Lingual	L			
		Distal	D	Buccal	B			

b. "X" in columns titled "N/R" = ADA does not recommend reporting any Area of the Oral Cavity or Tooth Anatomy information for that row's CDT code

c. "Y" in other columns under "Area of the Oral Cavity" or "Tooth Anatomy" = ADA recommends reporting the indicated information for that row's CDT code

CDT Code	Area of the Oral Cavity				Tooth Anatomy			
	N/R	Entire	Arch	Quadrant	N/R	#	# Range	Surface
D0120	X				X			
D0140	X				X			
D0145	X				X			
D0150	X				X			
D0160	X				X			
D0170	X				X			
D0171	X				X			
D0180	X				X			
D0190	X				X			
D0191	X				X			
D0210	X				X			
D0220	X					Y	Y	
D0230	X					Y	Y	
D0240	X						Y	
D0250	X						Y	
D0251	X						Y	
D0270	X						Y	
D0272	X						Y	
D0273	X						Y	
D0274	X						Y	
D0277	X						Y	
D0310	X				X			
D0320	X				X			
D0321	X				X			
D0322	X				X			
D0330		Y			X			
D0340	X				X			
D0350	X				X			
D0351	X				X			
D0364			Y	Y		Y	Y	
D0365	X				X			
D0366	X				X			
D0367	X				X			
D0368	X				X			
D0369	X				X			
D0370	X				X			
D0371	X				X			
D0380	Y		Y	Y		Y	Y	

Appendix 2. ADA Guide to Dental Procedures Reported with Area of the Oral Cavity or Tooth Anatomy (or Both)

CDT Code	Area of the Oral Cavity				Tooth Anatomy			
	N/R	Entire	Arch	Quadrant	N/R	#	# Range	Surface
D0381	X				X			
D0382	X				X			
D0383	X				X			
D0384	X				X			
D0385	X				X			
D0386	X				X			
D0391	X				X			
D0393	X				X			
D0394	X				X			
D0395	X				X			
D0411	X				X			
D0412	X				X			
D0414	X				X			
D0415	X				X			
D0416	X				X			
D0417	X				X			
D0418	X				X			
D0419	X				X			
D0422	X				X			
D0423	X				X			
D0425	X				X			
D0431	X				X			
D0460	X					Y		
D0470	X				X			
D0472	X				X			
D0473	X				X			
D0474	X				X			
D0475	X				X			
D0476	X				X			
D0477	X				X			
D0478	X				X			
D0479	X				X			
D0480	X				X			
D0481	X				X			
D0482	X				X			
D0483	X				X			
D0484	X				X			
D0485	X				X			

CDT Code	Area of the Oral Cavity				Tooth Anatomy			
	N/R	Entire	Arch	Quadrant	N/R	#	# Range	Surface
D0486	X				X			
D0502	X				X			
D0600	X					Y	Y	
D0601	X				X			
D0602	X				X			
D0603	X				X			
D0604	X				X			
D0605	X				X			
D0701		Y			X			
D0702	X				X			
D0703	X				X			
D0704	X				X			
D0705	X						Y	
D0706	X						Y	
D0707	X					Y	Y	
D0708	X						Y	
D0709	X				X			
D0999	X				X			
D1110		Y			X			
D1120		Y			X			
D1206		Y			X			
D1208		Y			X			
D1310	X				X			
D1320	X				X			
D1321	X				X			
D1330	X				X			
D1351	X					Y		
D1352	X					Y		
D1353	X					Y		
D1354	X					Y		Y
D1355	X					Y		Y
D1510				Y		Y	Y	
D1516	X					Y	Y	
D1517	X					Y	Y	
D1520				Y		Y	Y	
D1526	X					Y	Y	
D1527	X					Y	Y	
D1551	X					Y	Y	

CDT Code	Area of the Oral Cavity				Tooth Anatomy			
	N/R	Entire	Arch	Quadrant	N/R	#	# Range	Surface
D1552	X					Y	Y	
D1553				Y		Y	Y	
D1556				Y		Y	Y	
D1557	X					Y	Y	
D1558	X					Y	Y	
D1575				Y		Y	Y	
D1999				Y		Y	Y	
D2140	X					Y		Y
D2150	X					Y		Y
D2160	X					Y		Y
D2161	X					Y		Y
D2330	X					Y		Y
D2331	X					Y		Y
D2332	X					Y		Y
D2335	X					Y		Y
D2390	X					Y		
D2391	X					Y		Y
D2392	X					Y		Y
D2393	X					Y		Y
D2394	X					Y		Y
D2410	X					Y		Y
D2420	X					Y		Y
D2430	X					Y		Y
D2510	X					Y		Y
D2520	X					Y		Y
D2530	X					Y		Y
D2542	X					Y		Y
D2543	X					Y		Y
D2544	X					Y		Y
D2610	X					Y		Y
D2620	X					Y		Y
D2630	X					Y		Y
D2642	X					Y		Y
D2643	X					Y		Y
D2644	X					Y		Y
D2650	X					Y		Y
D2651	X					Y		Y
D2652	X					Y		Y

CDT Code	Area of the Oral Cavity				Tooth Anatomy			
	N/R	Entire	Arch	Quadrant	N/R	#	# Range	Surface
D2662	X					Y		Y
D2663	X					Y		Y
D2664	X					Y		Y
D2710	X					Y		
D2712	X					Y		
D2720	X					Y		
D2721	X					Y		
D2722	X					Y		
D2740	X					Y		
D2750	X					Y		
D2751	X					Y		
D2752	X					Y		
D2753	X					Y		
D2780	X					Y		
D2781	X					Y		
D2782	X					Y		
D2783	X					Y		
D2790	X					Y		
D2791	X					Y		
D2792	X					Y		
D2794	X					Y		
D2799	X					Y		
D2910	X					Y		
D2915	X					Y		
D2920	X					Y		
D2921	X					Y		
D2928	X					Y		
D2929	X					Y		
D2930	X					Y		
D2931	X					Y		
D2932	X					Y		
D2933	X					Y		
D2934	X					Y		
D2940	X					Y		Y
D2941	X					Y		Y
D2949	X					Y		Y
D2950	X					Y		
D2951	X					Y		

CDT Code	Area of the Oral Cavity				Tooth Anatomy			
	N/R	Entire	Arch	Quadrant	N/R	#	# Range	Surface
D2952	X					Y		
D2953	X					Y		
D2954	X					Y		
D2955	X					Y		
D2957	X					Y		
D2960	X					Y		
D2961	X					Y		
D2962	X					Y		
D2971	X					Y		
D2975	X					Y		
D2980	X					Y		
D2981	X					Y		
D2982	X					Y		
D2983	X					Y		
D2990	X					Y		Y
D2999	X					Y	Y	Y
D3110	X					Y		
D3120	X					Y		
D3220	X					Y		
D3221	X					Y		
D3222	X					Y		
D3230	X					Y		
D3240	X					Y		
D3310	X					Y		
D3320	X					Y		
D3330	X					Y		
D3331	X					Y		
D3332	X					Y		
D3333	X					Y		
D3346	X					Y		
D3347	X					Y		
D3348	X					Y		
D3351	X					Y		
D3352	X					Y		
D3353	X					Y		
D3355	X					Y		
D3356	X					Y		
D3357	X					Y		

CDT Code	Area of the Oral Cavity				Tooth Anatomy			
	N/R	Entire	Arch	Quadrant	N/R	#	# Range	Surface
D3410	X					Y		
D3421	X					Y		
D3425	X					Y		
D3426	X					Y		
D3428	X					Y		
D3429	X					Y		
D3430	X					Y		
D3431	X					Y		
D3432	X					Y		
D3450	X					Y		
D3460	X					Y		
D3470	X					Y		
D3471	X					Y		
D3472	X					Y		
D3473	X					Y		
D3501	X					Y		
D3502	X					Y		
D3503	X					Y		
D3910	X					Y		
D3920	X					Y		
D3950	X					Y		
D3999	X					Y	Y	
D4210				Y			Y	
D4211				Y			Y	
D4212	X					Y		
D4230				Y			Y	
D4231				Y			Y	
D4240				Y			Y	
D4241				Y			Y	
D4245	X						Y	
D4249	X					Y		
D4260				Y			Y	
D4261				Y			Y	
D4263				Y		Y		
D4264				Y		Y		
D4265	X					Y		
D4266	X					Y	Y	
D4267	X					Y	Y	

CDT Code	Area of the Oral Cavity				Tooth Anatomy			
	N/R	Entire	Arch	Quadrant	N/R	#	# Range	Surface
D4268	X					Y		
D4270	X					Y	Y	
D4273	X					Y		
D4274	X					Y		
D4275	X					Y		
D4276	X					Y		
D4277	X					Y		
D4278	X					Y		
D4283	X					Y		
D4285	X					Y		
D4320	X					Y		
D4321	X					Y		
D4341				Y		Y	Y	
D4342				Y		Y	Y	
D4346	X				X			
D4355	X				X			
D4381	X					Y		
D4910	X				X			
D4920	X					Y	Y	
D4921				Y	X			
D4999	X					Y	Y	
D5110	X				X			
D5120	X				X			
D5130	X				X			
D5140	X				X			
D5211	X						Y	
D5212	X						Y	
D5213	X						Y	
D5214	X						Y	
D5221	X						Y	
D5222	X						Y	
D5223	X						Y	
D5224	X						Y	
D5225	X						Y	
D5226	X						Y	
D5282	X						Y	
D5283	X						Y	
D5284				Y			Y	

CDT Code	Area of the Oral Cavity				Tooth Anatomy			
	N/R	Entire	Arch	Quadrant	N/R	#	# Range	Surface
D5286				Y			Y	
D5410	X				X			
D5411	X				X			
D5421	X				X			
D5422	X				X			
D5511	X				X			
D5512	X				X			
D5520	X					Y		
D5611	X				X			
D5612	X				X			
D5621	X				X			
D5622	X				X			
D5630	X					Y		
D5640	X					Y		
D5650	X					Y		
D5660	X					Y		
D5670	X				X			
D5671	X				X			
D5710	X				X			
D5711	X				X			
D5720	X						Y	
D5721	X						Y	
D5730	X				X			
D5731	X				X			
D5740	X						Y	
D5741	X						Y	
D5750	X				X			
D5751	X				X			
D5760	X						Y	
D5761	X						Y	
D5810	X				X			
D5811	X				X			
D5820	X						Y	
D5821	X						Y	
D5850	X				X			
D5851	X				X			
D5862	X				X			
D5863	X				X			

CDT Code	Area of the Oral Cavity				Tooth Anatomy			
	N/R	Entire	Arch	Quadrant	N/R	#	# Range	Surface
D5864	X						Y	
D5865	X				X			
D5866	X						Y	
D5867				Y		Y	Y	
D5875			Y		X			
D5876			Y		X			
D5899	X					Y	Y	
D5911	X				X			
D5912	X				X			
D5913	X				X			
D5914	X				X			
D5915	X				X			
D5916	X				X			
D5919	X				X			
D5922	X				X			
D5923	X				X			
D5924	X				X			
D5925	X				X			
D5926	X				X			
D5927	X				X			
D5928	X				X			
D5929	X				X			
D5931			Y		X			
D5932			Y		X			
D5933			Y		X			
D5934	X				X			
D5935	X				X			
D5936			Y		X			
D5937			Y		X			
D5951	X				X			
D5952			Y		X			
D5953			Y		X			
D5954	X				X			
D5955	X				X			
D5958	X				X			
D5959	X				X			
D5960			Y		X			
D5982			Y		X			

CDT Code	Area of the Oral Cavity				Tooth Anatomy			
	N/R	Entire	Arch	Quadrant	N/R	#	# Range	Surface
D5983			Y		X			
D5984			Y		X			
D5985			Y		X			
D5986			Y		X			
D5987			Y		X			
D5988			Y			Y		
D5991			Y		X			
D5992			Y		X			
D5993			Y		X			
D5995			Y			Y		
D5996			Y			Y		
D5999	X				X			
D6010	X					Y		
D6011	X					Y		
D6012	X					Y		
D6013	X					Y		
D6040	X					Y		
D6050	X					Y		
D6051	X					Y		
D6055	X						Y	
D6056	X					Y		
D6057	X					Y		
D6058	X					Y		
D6059	X					Y		
D6060	X					Y		
D6061	X					Y		
D6062	X					Y		
D6063	X					Y		
D6064	X					Y		
D6065	X					Y		
D6066	X					Y		
D6067	X					Y		
D6068	X					Y		
D6069	X					Y		
D6070	X					Y		
D6071	X					Y		
D6072	X					Y		
D6073	X					Y		

CDT Code	Area of the Oral Cavity				Tooth Anatomy			
	N/R	Entire	Arch	Quadrant	N/R	#	# Range	Surface
D6074	X					Y		
D6075	X					Y		
D6076	X					Y		
D6077	X					Y		
D6080	X					Y		
D6081	X					Y		
D6082	X					Y		
D6083	X					Y		
D6084	X					Y		
D6085	X					Y		
D6086	X					Y		
D6087	X					Y		
D6088	X					Y		
D6090	X					Y		
D6091	X					Y		
D6092	X					Y		
D6093	X					Y		
D6094	X					Y		
D6095	X					Y		
D6096	X					Y		
D6097	X					Y		
D6098	X					Y		
D6099	X					Y		
D6100	X					Y		
D6101	X					Y		
D6102	X					Y		
D6103	X					Y	Y	
D6104	X					Y	Y	
D6110	X				X			
D6111	X				X			
D6112				Y	X			
D6113				Y	X			
D6114	X				X			
D6115	X				X			
D6116	X			Y	X			
D6117	X			Y	X			
D6118	X				X			
D6119	X				X			

CDT Code	Area of the Oral Cavity				Tooth Anatomy			
	N/R	Entire	Arch	Quadrant	N/R	#	# Range	Surface
D6190		Y		Y	X			
D6194	X					Y		
D6195	X					Y		
D6199	X					Y	Y	
D6205	X					Y	Y	
D6210	X					Y	Y	
D6211	X					Y	Y	
D6212	X					Y	Y	
D6214	X					Y	Y	
D6240	X					Y	Y	
D6121	X					Y		
D6122	X					Y		
D6123	X					Y		
D6124	X					Y		
D6191	X					Y		
D6192	X					Y		
D6241	X					Y	Y	
D6242	X					Y	Y	
D6243	X					Y	Y	
D6245	X					Y	Y	
D6250	X					Y	Y	
D6251	X					Y	Y	
D6252	X					Y	Y	
D6253	X					Y	Y	
D6545	X					Y		
D6548	X					Y		
D6549	X					Y		
D6600	X					Y		Y
D6601	X					Y		Y
D6602	X					Y		Y
D6603	X					Y		Y
D6604	X					Y		Y
D6605	X					Y		Y
D6606	X					Y		Y
D6607	X					Y		Y
D6608	X					Y		Y
D6609	X					Y		Y
D6610	X					Y		Y

CDT Code	Area of the Oral Cavity				Tooth Anatomy			
	N/R	Entire	Arch	Quadrant	N/R	#	# Range	Surface
D6611	X					Y		Y
D6612	X					Y		Y
D6613	X					Y		Y
D6614	X					Y		Y
D6615	X					Y		Y
D6624	X					Y		
D6634	X					Y		
D6710	X					Y		
D6720	X					Y		
D6721	X					Y		
D6722	X					Y		
D6740	X					Y		
D6750	X					Y		
D6751	X					Y		
D6752	X					Y		
D6753	X					Y		
D6780	X					Y		
D6781	X					Y		
D6782	X					Y		
D6783	X					Y		
D6784	X					Y		
D6790	X					Y		
D6791	X					Y		
D6792	X					Y		
D6793	X					Y		
D6794	X					Y		
D6920			Y				Y	
D6930	X				X			
D6940	X					Y		Y
D6950	X					Y		
D6980	X				X			
D6985			Y	Y	X			
D6999			Y	Y		Y	Y	Y
D7111	X					Y		
D7140	X					Y		
D7210	X					Y		
D7220	X					Y		
D7230	X					Y		

CDT Code	Area of the Oral Cavity				Tooth Anatomy			
	N/R	Entire	Arch	Quadrant	N/R	#	# Range	Surface
D7240	X					Y		
D7241	X					Y		
D7250	X					Y		
D7251	X					Y		
D7260				Y	X			
D7261				Y	X			
D7270	X				X			
D7272	X				X			
D7280	X					Y		
D7282	X					Y		
D7283	X					Y		
D7285		Y			X			
D7286		Y			X			
D7287		Y			X			
D7288		Y			X			
D7290	X				X			
D7291	X				X			
D7292				Y	X			/
D7293				Y	X			
D7294				Y	X			
D7295				Y	X			
D7296				Y		Y	Y	
D7297				Y		Y	Y	
D7310				Y		Y	Y	
D7311				Y		Y	Y	
D7320				Y		Y	Y	
D7321				Y		Y	Y	
D7340				Y	X			
D7350				Y	X			
D7410			Y		X			
D7411			Y		X			
D7412			Y		X			
D7413			Y		X			
D7414			Y		X			
D7415			Y		X			
D7440			Y		X			
D7441			Y		X			
D7450			Y		X			

CDT Code	Area of the Oral Cavity				Tooth Anatomy			
	N/R	Entire	Arch	Quadrant	N/R	#	# Range	Surface
D7451			Y		X			
D7460			Y		X			
D7461			Y		X			
D7465			Y		X			
D7471			Y		X			
D7472	X				X			
D7473				Y	X			
D7485				Y	X			
D7490			Y		X			
D7510				Y		Y		
D7511				Y		Y		
D7520			Y		X			
D7521			Y		X			
D7530	X				X			
D7540	X				X			
D7550				Y	X			
D7560	X				X			
D7610	X				X			
D7620	X				X			
D7630	X				X			
D7640	X				X			
D7650	X				X			
D7660	X				X			
D7670	X				X			
D7671	X				X			
D7680	X				X			
D7710	X				X			
D7720	X				X			
D7730	X				X			
D7740	X				X			
D7750	X				X			
D7760	X				X			
D7770	X				X			
D7771	X				X			
D7780	X				X			
D7810	X				X			
D7820	X				X			
D7830	X				X			

CDT Code	Area of the Oral Cavity				Tooth Anatomy			
	N/R	Entire	Arch	Quadrant	N/R	#	# Range	Surface
D7840	X				X			
D7850	X				X			
D7852	X				X			
D7854	X				X			
D7856	X				X			
D7858	X				X			
D7865	X				X			
D7870	X				X			
D7871	X				X			
D7872	X				X			
D7873	X				X			
D7874	X				X			
D7875	X				X			
D7876	X				X			
D7877	X				X			
D7880	X				X			
D7881	X				X			
D7899	X				X			
D7910	X				X			
D7911	X				X			
D7912	X				X			
D7920	X				X			
D7921	X				X			
D7922	X					Y		
D7940	X				X			
D7941	X				X			
D7943	X				X			
D7944	X				X			
D7945	X				X			
D7946	X				X			
D7947	X				X			
D7948	X				X			
D7949	X				X			
D7950	X				X			
D7951	X				X			
D7952	X				X			
D7953	X				X			

CDT Code	Area of the Oral Cavity				Tooth Anatomy			
	N/R	Entire	Arch	Quadrant	N/R	#	# Range	Surface
D7955	X				X			
D7961	X				X			
D7962	X				X			
D7963	X				X			
D7970			Y		X			
D7971	X				X			
D7972				Y	X			
D7979	X				X			
D7980	X				X			
D7981	X				X			
D7982	X				X			
D7983	X				X			
D7990	X				X			
D7991	X				X			
D7993	X				X			
D7994	X				X			
D7995	X				X			
D7996	X				X			
D7997			X		X			
D7998	X				X			
D7999	X				X			
D8010			Y	Y	X			
D8020			Y	Y	X			
D8030			Y	Y	X			
D8040			Y	Y	X			
D8050		Y	Y	Y	X			
D8060		Y	Y	Y	X			
D8070		Y			X			
D8080		Y			X			
D8090		Y			X			
D8210		Y	Y	Y	X			
D8220		Y	Y	Y	X			
D8660		Y			X			
D8670		Y			X			
D8680		Y	Y	Y	X			
D8681			Y		X			
D8690		Y	Y	Y	X			
D8695		Y	Y	Y	X			

CDT Code	Area of the Oral Cavity				Tooth Anatomy			
	N/R	Entire	Arch	Quadrant	N/R	#	# Range	Surface
D8696	X				X			
D8697	X				X			
D8698	X				X			
D8699	X				X			
D8701	X				X			
D8702	X				X			
D8703	X				X			
D8704	X				X			
D8999	X				X			
D9110	X				X			
D9120	X				X			
D9130	X				X			
D9210			Y	Y	X			
D9211			Y	Y	X			
D9212			Y	Y	X			
D9215			Y	Y	X			
D9219	X				X			
D9222	X				X			
D9223	X				X			
D9230	X				X			
D9239	X				X			
D9243	X				X			
D9248	X				X			
D9310	X				X			
D9311	X				X			
D9410	X				X			
D9420	X				X			
D9430	X				X			
D9440	X				X			
D9450	X				X			
D9610	X				X			
D9612	X				X			
D9613	X				X			
D9630	X				X			
D9910			Y	Y	X			
D9911	X					Y		
D9920	X				X			
D9930	X				X			

CDT Code	Area of the Oral Cavity				Tooth Anatomy			
	N/R	Entire	Arch	Quadrant	N/R	#	# Range	Surface
D9932	X				X			
D9933	X				X			
D9934	X				X			
D9935	X				X			
D9944			Y		X			
D9945			Y		X			
D9946			Y		X			
D9941			Y		X			
D9942			Y		X			
D9943			Y		X			
D9950			Y		X			
D9951			Y	Y	X			
D9952			Y	Y	X			
D9961	X				X			
D9970	X				X			
D9971	X					Y		
D9972			Y		X			
D9973	X					Y		
D9974	X					Y		
D9975			Y		X			
D9985	X				X			
D9986	X				X			
D9987	X				X			
D9990	X				X			
D9991	X				X			
D9992	X				X			
D9993	X				X			
D9994	X				X			
D9995	X				X			
D9996	X				X			
D9997	X				X			
D9999	X				X			

Appendix 3: CDT and ICD-10 Coding Recommendations for Smoking Cessation

By Jean L Stevens, RHIT, CCS-P

Tobacco use is the leading cause of preventable disease, disability, and death in the United States. An estimated 34 million adults in the United States smoke,[1] and 16 million individuals in the U.S. live with a tobacco-related disease.[2]

Providers are encouraged to submit claims for tobacco cessation counseling services. However, plan benefits are subject to specific policies. Patients and providers should always check with individual Medicaid, managed care organizations, and private dental benefit plans to determine what treatments are included and the extent to which this treatment is reimbursed.

Additionally, payers may mandate specific documentation requirements for smoking cessation treatment. It is important to follow payer-specific guidance for this service. The general information contained here should meet or exceed various payer requirements.

Counseling and the Patient Record

Successful intervention begins with identifying users and appropriate interventions based on the patient's willingness to quit. According to the Agency for Healthcare Research and Quality (AHRQ), there are five major steps to intervention (the "5 A's"): Ask, Advise, Assess, Assist, and Arrange.

1. **Ask**. Identify and document tobacco use status for every patient at every visit.

2. **Advise**. In a clear, strong, and personalized manner, urge every tobacco user to quit.

3. **Assess**. Is the tobacco user willing to make a quit attempt at this time?

4. **Assist**. For the patient willing to make a quit attempt, use counseling and pharmacotherapy to help him or her quit.

5. **Arrange**. Schedule follow-up contact, preferably within the first week after the quit date.

---

[1] Smoking Cessation. A Report of the Surgeon General. Atlanta, GA: U.S. Department of Health and Human Services, Centers for Disease Control and Prevention, National Center for Chronic Disease Prevention and Health Promotion, Office on Smoking and Health, 2020 [accessed 2020 July 13]. *https://www.cdc.gov/tobacco/data_statistics/sgr/2020-smoking-cessation/index.html.*

[2] "Fast Facts," Atlanta, GA: Centers for Disease Control and Prevention. 2020 [Accessed 2020 July 13] *https://www.cdc.gov/tobacco/data_statistics/fact_sheets/fast_facts/index.htm.*
Smoking Cessation. A Report of the Surgeon General. Atlanta, GA: U.S. Department of Health and Human Services, Centers for Disease Control and Prevention, National Center for Chronic Disease Prevention and Health Promotion, Office on Smoking and Health, 2020 [accessed 2020 July 13]. *https://www.cdc.gov/tobacco/data_statistics/sgr/2020-smoking-cessation/index.html.*

The following items should be documented for each counseling session:

- The patient's willingness to attempt to quit
- A detailed description of the discussion during counseling session
- The exact amount of time spent counseling
- The amount of tobacco use
- The provider's advice to quit and impact of smoking discussed with the patient
- The methods and skills suggested to support tobacco cessation
- Details of medication management, when provided
- Proposing a quit date with the patient
- Scheduling an appointment for follow-up counseling
- Note any resources that are made available to the patient

Additional Documentation Hints and Coding Tips

- The F17 Nicotine Dependence category codes are assigned when the record reflects the patient is currently dependent upon tobacco.
- Z72.0 Tobacco use (Tobacco use NOS, not otherwise specified) is to be assigned when the patient is not dependent upon tobacco.
- The Z and F17 codes cannot be combined.
- When the record states a patient has a "personal history of," it is interpreted to indicate the condition is part of the past history and it no longer exists, therefore, tobacco counseling would not be provided. (ICD-10 code Z87.891 Personal history of nicotine dependence.)
- Be sure to document "counseling" activities (advising about specific changes to routines, arranging for services or follow up) and not just "evaluation."

Clinical Coding Scenario

A 32-year-old female patient is currently nicotine dependent, smoking one pack of cigarettes per day. She has had multiple failed attempts at quitting using nicotine gum. Approximately 10 minutes were spent counseling the patient in cessation techniques. She understands continuing to smoke could lead to oral disease. The benefits of stopping were discussed. The patient has verbalized her desire to "give it another try." She will try a nicotine patch this time and has set her own goal of 30 days to be smoke-free. We will follow up in two weeks to check progress.

Diagnosis code:

F17.210 Nicotine dependence, cigarettes, uncomplicated

CDT code:

D1320 **tobacco counseling for the control and prevention of oral disease.**
Tobacco prevention and cessation service reduce patient risks of developing tobacco-related oral diseases and conditions and improves prognosis for certain dental therapies.

Resources

AHRQ Five Major Steps to Intervention (The "5 A's") provides a description of the five major steps to intervention; the "5 A's": Ask, Advise, Assess, Assist, and Arrange. More information is available at *www.ahrq.gov/prevention/guidelines/tobacco/5steps.html*.

You can find more information about smoking cessation at the Centers for Disease Control and Prevention (CDC): *www.cdc.gov/tobacco/data_statistics/fact_sheets/cessation/smoking-cessation-fast-facts/index.html*.

Appendix 4: Understanding and Procedure Coding for Patients with Special Health Care Needs

By Carol Roszel, R.D.H., B.S.D.H.

Introduction

This is a new topic for the *CDT 2021 Companion,* a high-level discussion of Special Health Care Needs (SHCN) patients who receive oral health care from a variety of dentists in diverse settings. What follows is a primer for those members of the dental community who may not have provided care to SHCN patients, as well as those who already do and seek additional insight on how necessary dental care is delivered and documented.

Comprehensive, preventive and therapeutic oral care for all individuals is the goal of the dental profession. Individuals with SHCN seek the same preventive and therapeutic oral care, often within unique circumstances. Appropriate treatment is attainable for these individuals with education and communication between dental and other healthcare providers, parents/guardians, and ancillary caregivers. Managing all these interactions might require mediation, communication and a little creativity to ensure optimal care.

SHCN Definition

The American Academy Pediatric Dentistry defines special healthcare needs as "any physical, developmental, mental, sensory, behavioral, cognitive, or emotional impairment or limiting condition that requires medical management, health care intervention, and/or use of specialized services or programs. The condition may be congenital, developmental, or acquired through disease, trauma, or environmental cause and may impose limitations in performing daily self-maintenance activities or substantial limitations in a major life activity."

According to the U.S. Census Bureau, special health care conditions affect approximately 18% of the population under 18 years old and an additional 37.9 million Americans.

Context for Dental Care Delivery

Patients with special healthcare needs are often accompanied by family members when seen for treatment in general dental practices. With better understanding of the challenges facing SCHN patients, more successful and complex treatments are now practiced.

People with SHCN receiving oral health treatment require special and unique considerations when compared with other patients. When treatment does not recognize the need for these special considerations, there can be a void in care for the individuals.

An example of an unrecognized need is when, after caring for a patient, a hygienist recommending that the patient is to use a mechanical toothbrush, fluoride toothpaste and floss twice a day. Such recommendations can, for a patient with SHCN, become daunting, overwhelming requests. The patient may be wondering: Who will get the mechanical toothbrush? The vibration of the toothbrush may be too intense to tolerate. How long do I have to brush? What is fluoride? Is the toothpaste okay to swallow because sometime spitting is hard to remember? I don't like the feeling of floss. I don't like different tastes of any kind. How will I remember to do this?

Understanding and addressing a SHCN patient is when the individual first becomes the dentist's patient of record. First contact at an "introductory appointment" is most helpful. This appointment can be done at the beginning or the end of the normal business day, allowing the individual to experience the sensations, such as the smells and noise, of the office, as well as to meet the dental team. This introductory session, which usually takes about 15 to 30 minutes, desensitizes the individual to the office, significantly reducing the anxiety of a new environment before the "real visit." Although there is no specific CDT code for such an "introductory appointment" the encounter can be documented with the case management code added in CDT 2021, **D9997 dental case management – patients with special health care needs**, as this encounter is ancillary to the first "real visit" for the patient's first examination – most likely documented as a **D0150 comprehensive oral evaluation – new or established patient**.

The narrative report that is required when a service is documented with a "999" code is where the dentist describes the nature and scope of services delivered during that encounter. This encounter would likely include review and completion of a "Get to Know Me" form. Information acquired from SHCN patients and their accompanying family members can help the dentist acquire necessary background and establish methods of communication, treatment and follow through of treatment instructions. Knowing where the individual lives allows insight into how their oral health is managed and addressed. Daily reminders of brushing, using oral health aids may fall to the responsibility of multiple people from different shifts or to different family members.

A sample "Get to Know Me" form is included in this appendix and can be modified as necessary by the dentist.

Understanding the life challenges of every patient is important for treatment success and their well-being. Extra time and effort is necessary for SCHN patients. There are existing CDT codes that enable accurate recording of SCHN patient care, as will be illustrated in the scenarios seen later in this part of the CDT Companion.

Living Arrangements and the Daily Dental Care for People with SCHN

People with SHCN have a variety of living arrangements. Sometimes people with SHCN live outside the family home because quality educational, training and employment opportunities are a distance from their families. Other times, parents who cared for people with SHCN from birth are no long able to assist with their daily care due to their own advancing age and health circumstances.

Government-funded Community Integrated Living Arrangements, or CILAs, or other independent living conditions offer independence, community and continuity of care for these individuals. Direct care assistance for their activities of daily life become an alternative option for these individuals, as well as their families. Supportive Living Arrangements (SLAs) are similar to CILAs, but are for individuals who need less direct support.

Federally-mandated SLAs and CILAs are required to provide individuals with a soft bristled toothbrush and fluoride toothpaste in a "hygiene box," per the ADA recommendation. Any prescription items, such as rinses and prescription toothpastes, are mandated to be kept with other medication and are dispensed by specifically-trained medical personnel.

Whether a person with SHCN is living at home with family or in a group home, a "care person" is needed to oversee the daily hygiene habits. The care person also can give verbal reminders or post visual cues for the individual to follow for daily oral hygiene, and personal care is often considered poor.

Individuals who assist with activities of daily living are either certified nursing assistants (CNAs) or have taken training classes in the facility to earn a Direct Care Worker Certificate. Their training for oral hygiene care and instruction is equivalent to a CNA's training.

Knowing the Players Within a SHCN Patient's Daily Life

Individuals with SHCN often have legal guardians who make all medical and financial decisions for the individual. Treatment of any kind must be approved through the legal guardian. The legal guardian may not live with or close to the SHCN individual, yet they remain the legal guardian.

If the individual participates in a school, day program, work training or any program outside the house will have a caseworker who is a social worker. The case worker is employed by a government agency, nonprofit organization, or another group to take on the cases of individuals and provide them with advocacy, information and solutions. This is the person to contact to assist in developing brushing habits, using oral aids products.

When an individual enters a group home, there is a nurse that will oversee the medical portion of their care. Any prescription item for the SHCN individuals, needs to be addressed with the registered nurse (RN) and introduced to the individual. Instructions on prescription items will be given by the RN to the direct care worker.

In federally-funded group homes the person assisting SHCN individuals with oral hygiene care are the direct care worker. These are the individuals that assist with holding the tooth brush, assist with applying the tooth paste if the individual cannot adequately brush by themselves. Additional training for the DCP is provided to allow them to dispense prescription medication on a daily basis earning them a "med passer" status.

Oral Health Intervention

Support and educational organizations provides services to assist individuals with developmental and intellectual disabilities along with their families. Many of these organizations provide education, training, skills and encouragement. Quality organizations recognizes the importance of oral health and its impact on physical health and well-being of Special Needs individuals. Dental personnel are in a position to be a liaison between the other oral health providers, nurses, case workers, families and most importantly, the individuals. The role is to assist in supporting and enhancing the oral health education, assistance, and support to the individuals and the direct care staff.

Often a lack of communication between dental providers, medical providers, parents and the direct care staff leads to mistakes or lack of treatment for the individual. Without intervention, oral care and the implementation of brushing, using oral health products, and following up with preventive care does not become interfaced into their daily routines.

Oral health interventions can occur in group homes (SLAs and CILAs) or where they attend life skills and job training classes and therapies. The meeting can be a one on one session of brushing, flossing, nutritional counseling. Or it can also consist of small group sessions on oral health education or nutritional counseling to supplement support between the traditional six-month preventive appointment done at their dental providers.

Bumpy, Outside, Inside, Tongue (BOIT) Brushing Method

One of the challenges for people with disabilities is the need for "muscle memory" to repeat an activity on a daily basis, as we ask in our patients with brushing their teeth. Research indicated that in group home situations the direct care staff had a 33% turnover rate. This means there was only a 1/3 chance that the person who assisted in brushing in the morning would be there in the evening. A standard method of brushing was necessary to bring consistency and muscle memory to the individuals. BOIT became the official method of brushing teeth for individuals: B=bumpy; O=outside; I=inside; T=tongue. This consistent acronym was adopted to bring uniformity in brushing to the care staff, individuals, and families. This consistent method allow the individuals to develop muscle memory, allowing it to become a long-term memory skill.

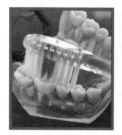 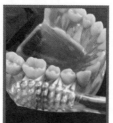 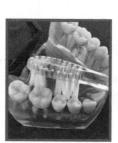 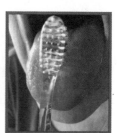

| **Bumpy** | **Outside** | **Inside** | **Tongue** |

Clinical Coding Scenarios

Clinical Coding Scenario #1

J.J. is a 25-year-old male with Down syndrome who lives with his elderly mother, his legal guardian. He attends classes five days a week in a job and life skills training center. J.J. was happy to join the oral care educator who addressed his dental condition during one of J.J.'s daily sessions at the life skill center. During this session the oral care educator captured intraoral photographic images that documented extensive decay in every tooth, with several teeth showing decay at the gum line. Significant food debris and plaque were present. Oral hygiene guidance was given along with a toothbrush and paste to take home.

Photos were shared with J.J. and a discussion on his teeth and their condition occurred. Photos were forwarded to local provider and to his case worker to share with his mother. J.J.'s mother was not aware of the severity of J.J.'s oral condition. Monitoring his oral hygiene habits was not something she is capable of doing on a daily basis. She is also unable to physically take him for dental treatment.

As J.J. has not seen a dentist routinely, the photos were sent to the local dental provider on campus via asynchronous teledentistry connection and appropriate preliminary services were arranged. J.J.'s case worker was able to arranged appropriate consent for treatment with J.J.'s mother. The dental provider's office is on the same campus as his training center. J.J. is escorted to the dental clinic and treatment commenced within 48 hours.

How would you code this encounter?

D0190 screening of a patient
A screening, including state and federally mandated screenings, to determine an individual's need to be seen by a dentist for diagnosis.

D1330 oral hygiene instructions
This may include instructions for home care. Examples include tooth brushing technique, flossing, and use of special oral hygiene aids.

D0350 2D oral/facial photographic image obtained intra-orally or extra-orally

Note: The number of photographic images captured is also documented.

D9996 teledentistry – asynchronous; information stored and forwarded to dentist for subsequent review

Reported in addition to other procedures (e.g., diagnostic) delivered to the patient on the date of service.

D9992 dental case management – care coordination

Assisting in a patient's decisions regarding the coordination of oral health care services across multiple providers, provider types, specialty areas of treatment, health care settings, health care organizations and payment systems. This is the additional time and resources expended to provide experience or expertise beyond that possessed by the patient.

D9997 dental case management – patients with special health care needs

Special treatment considerations for patients/individuals with physical, medical, developmental or cognitive conditions resulting in substantial functional limitations, which require that modifications be made to delivery of treatment to provide comprehensive oral health care services.

 © American Dental Association

Clinical Coding Scenario #2

During a visit to a CILA (Community Integrated Living Arrangements) home, a dental hygienist met Brad, a 29-year-old man on the autism spectrum disorder with limited verbal skills. Brad was asked if he would like to brush his teeth with the dental hygienist. While talking to Brad, the dental hygienist noticed his gingiva was bright red, with generalized food debris. The direct care staff person said, "Brad doesn't have a brush. He just rinses with this blue mouthwash," and handed the hygienist a bottle of chlorohexidine. After further questions it was noted that the bottle was brought back from a provider and the direct care staff was instructed to "have him rinse." Gentle brushing, with a soft bristle, hand brush and chlorohexidine was done for Brad. Gingival bleeding occurred and Brad's oral health was discussed with the direct care staff. While brushing his teeth, patches of decalcification on tooth surfaces were noted. Photos were taken for documentation and reference.

This void of oral care occurred for more than six months. Brad's dental care consisted of once a day rinsing and tooth brushing ceased. Miscommunication and an absence of information was preventing Brad from improving his oral health and risking further disease and inflammation. His case worker and RN were notified to follow up with the dental provider.

How would you code for this encounter?

Services documented by dental hygienist

> **D0191** **assessment of a patient**
> A limited clinical inspection that is performed to identify possible signs of oral or systemic disease, malformation, or injury, and the potential need for referral for diagnosis and treatment.

> **D1330** **oral hygiene instructions**
> This may include instructions for home care. Examples include tooth brushing technique, flossing, and use of special oral hygiene aids.

> **D9310** **consultation – diagnostic service provided by dentist or physician other than requesting dentist or physician**
> A patient encounter with a practitioner whose opinion or advice regarding evaluation and/or management of a specific problem; may be requested by another practitioner or appropriate source. The consultation includes an oral evaluation. The consulted practitioner may initiate diagnostic and/or therapeutic services.

D9996 **teledentistry – asynchronous; information stored and forwarded to dentist for subsequent review**
Reported in addition to other procedures (e.g., diagnostic) delivered to the patient on the date of service.

D9997 **dental case management – patients with special health care needs**
Special treatment considerations for patients/individuals with physical, medical, developmental or cognitive conditions resulting in substantial functional limitations, which require that modifications be made to delivery of treatment to provide comprehensive oral health care services.

Note: Knowing Brad's living situation, verbal skill levels, methods of communication and the players ahead of his appointment might have eliminated some of the information voids in this scenario. The dental provider might have contacted the RN and case worker directly to find out Brad's daily oral hygiene and sent a request for Brad to use the oral rinse in addition to his regular brushing routine. Once a case worker is clearly notified of treatment requests or changes to a routine, adjustments can be made in their system to track the continuity of care.

Summary

Knowing your patient's living situations and understanding their chain of communication can be the difference between treatment success and failure. This information can also open the door to inquiring about additional services that may be available for your SHCN patients. Certain states with more advanced practice acts may allow for caries risk assessments, saliva testing, application of fluoride varnish between their prophylactic appointments and radiographs. It's possible that there are other supportive procedures that may be performed at alternative locations.

Sample Get to Know Me Form

Name: _____ Birthdate: _____

Preferred Name: _____

Address: _____

Parents or Guardian: _____

Phone Number: _____

Email: _____

About Me

How I spend my days: ☐ School   ☐ Day Program   ☐ Home

My preferred method of communication: ☐ Verbal ☐ Pictures ☐ Sign Language

I need the following assistance with oral care: _____

My strengths: _____

My interests: _____

Physical limitations: _____

Behavioral information: _____

Words or things that make me happy: _____

Words or things that make me upset: _____

Words or things that calm me down: _____

I need the following assistance toileting: _____

My favorite snacks and drinks: _____

Any eating challenges or allergies to foods: _____

Any other information that would be helpful for us to know: _____

_____

Acknowledgement: Developed by Tina Marie Lowry, M.P.P.A., Little City Foundation, with a grant from Washington Square Health Fund and Autism Speaks created BOIT.

Numeric Index by CDT Code

Numeric Index by CDT Code

CDT Code	Page #(s)
D2950	93, 113, 114, 237, 320, 330
D2951	330
D2952	104, 242, 330
D2954	99, 104, 242, 330
D2955	105, 127–128
D2960	19, 24, 92, 95
D2961	19, 24, 92, 95
D2962	19, 24, 92, 94, 101
D2970	104
D2971	96, 102
D2980	105
D2990	328
D2999	103, 105, 106
D3110	331
D3120	331
D3220	331
D3221	98, 114, 117
D3230	97
D3310	117, 121, 331
D3320	98, 113, 331
D3330	114, 125, 126, 331
D3331	127
D3333	128
D3346	127, 332
D3347	99, 127, 332
D3348	127, 332
D3355	118
D3356	119
D3357	119
D3410	121
D3425	116
D3426	116
D3427	19, 24, 122, 124, 163, 270
D3428	116, 121
D3429	121
D3430	116

CDT Code	Page #(s)
D3431	116
D3471	19, 24, 112, 162, 163, 270
D3472	19, 24, 112, 162, 163, 270
D3473	19, 24, 112, 122, 162, 163, 270
D3501	19, 25, 112, 123, 124, 270
D3502	19, 25, 112, 270–271
D3503	19, 25, 112, 271
D3910	111
D3999	113, 125, 126
D4210	139, 332
D4211	332
D4212	237
D4230	150, 161, 164
D4231	161, 164
D4240	130
D4241	130, 155
D4249	157, 332
D4260	130, 136, 154, 163, 333
D4261	130, 157, 158, 163, 222, 333
D4263	137, 158, 159, 222, 255, 272, 333
D4264	137, 158, 159, 333
D4265	137, 154, 155, 255
D4266	137, 141, 155, 202, 205, 215, 250, 252, 255
D4267	205, 215, 250, 252, 255
D4270	334
D4273	156, 160, 225, 248, 334
D4274	158
D4275	147, 160, 216, 226, 248, 334
D4276	334
D4277	334
D4278	334
D4283	156, 248, 334
D4285	147, 160, 248, 334
D4321	154
D4341	51, 135, 153, 319, 335

CDT Code	Page #(s)		CDT Code	Page #(s)
D4342	84, 145, 161, 319, 335		**D5811**	176
D4346	83, 84, 142–143, 160, 225, 335		**D5820**	19, 26, 168, 202, 219
D4355	45, 60, 84, 133, 143, 161, 335		**D5821**	19, 26, 168
D4910	78, 140, 151, 159, 160, 161, 163, 225, 319, 320, 335		**D5851**	169
			D5862	8, 224
D4921	138, 141, 302		**D5867**	200
D5110	175, 336		**D5875**	169, 173, 208, 224
D5120	336		**D5876**	171, 175
D5130	175		**D5899**	219
D5140	170		**D5916**	185
D5211	336		**D5926**	190
D5212	336		**D5931**	181, 184, 187, 188
D5213	336		**D5932**	181, 184, 187, 188
D5214	336		**D5933**	181
D5221	172		**D5936**	180, 187, 188
D5225	19, 25, 167		**D5937**	183, 189
D5226	19, 25, 167		**D5951**	188
D5282	19, 25, 167, 176		**D5952**	190
D5283	19, 25, 168		**D5982**	180, 222
D5284	19, 25, 168		**D5984**	181, 184
D5286	19, 25, 168, 171		**D5986**	182, 188
D5421	175		**D5987**	189
D5512	171		**D5988**	186, 222
D5630	175		**D5991**	183, 189, 190
D5650	96, 175		**D5992**	184
D5660	96		**D5993**	184, 187, 190
D5720	175		**D5994**	19, 26, 179
D5721	175		**D5995**	19, 27, 179, 188, 190
D5730	19, 26, 168		**D5996**	19, 27, 179, 190
D5731	19, 26, 168, 170, 209		**D5999**	182, 188, 189
D5740	19, 26, 168		**D6010**	193, 203, 204, 206, 208, 212, 213, 226, 229, 230, 251, 252, 336
D5741	19, 168			
D5750	19, 26, 168			
D5751	19, 26, 168		**D6011**	19, 27, 173, 200, 203, 205, 207, 208, 218, 226, 229, 230
D5760	19, 26, 168			
D5761	19, 26, 168		**D6013**	193, 214, 221, 224, 230
D5810	176		**D6020**	223

CDT Code	Page #(s)
D6051	226
D6052	19, 27, 199, 230
D6055	195, 230
D6056	194, 208, 213, 221, 223, 225, 226, 228, 229, 230, 336
D6057	194, 203, 223, 226, 229, 230, 336
D6058	195, 203, 229
D6059	195, 221, 225, 229, 336
D6060	195, 229
D6061	195, 229
D6062	195, 229
D6063	195, 229
D6064	229
D6065	196, 221, 227, 229
D6066	196, 221, 229
D6067	196, 229
D6068	196, 229
D6069	196, 229
D6070	196, 229
D6071	196, 229
D6072	196, 229
D6073	196, 229
D6074	196, 229
D6075	196, 221, 229
D6076	196, 212, 229
D6077	196, 229
D6080	152, 217, 223–224
D6081	140, 152, 217, 225, 335
D6082	196, 229
D6083	196, 229
D6084	196, 229
D6085	196, 203, 224, 267
D6086	196, 229
D6087	196, 229
D6088	196, 229
D6090	220, 227

CDT Code	Page #(s)
D6091	19, 28, 174, 200, 205, 209, 220, 229
D6092	225
D6094	195
D6096	210, 273
D6097	195
D6098	19, 196, 200, 229
D6099	196, 229
D6100	8, 159, 215
D6101	141, 217
D6102	217, 222
D6103	141, 158, 222
D6104	159, 204, 252
D6110	197
D6111	169, 197, 205, 208, 214
D6112	197
D6113	197
D6114	207, 213, 228, 230
D6115	230
D6116	230
D6117	230
D6119	207, 213
D6120	196, 229
D6121	196, 229
D6122	196, 229
D6123	196, 229
D6190	180, 204, 206, 222, 265
D6191	19, 27, 173, 174, 176, 194, 199, 205, 208
D6192	19, 27, 169, 173, 194, 199, 205, 208, 214
D6194	196, 229
D6195	196, 229
D6199	214, 216, 226, 251
D6205	212, 222
D6240	212, 234, 336
D6242	235, 236, 237

CDT Code	Page #(s)
D6243	239, 243
D6245	238
D6253	238, 243
D6545	235
D6548	235
D6549	235
D6740	221, 238
D6750	212, 234, 336
D6752	236, 237, 336
D6753	239, 243
D6793	238, 243
D6930	240, 242
D6950	243
D6980	106
D6985	241
D6999	242, 244, 245
D7111	336
D7140	96, 155, 238, 268, 269, 337
D7210	202, 269, 337
D7220	338
D7230	261, 338
D7240	255, 338
D7241	270
D7250	268, 336
D7251	260
D7260	261
D7261	261
D7280	274
D7283	274
D7286	271
D7287	271
D7288	45, 64, 271
D7291	271
D7292	221
D7293	221, 258
D7294	221, 258

CDT Code	Page #(s)
D7295	249, 252
D7296	274
D7297	274
D7410	271
D7411	271
D7471	272
D7472	272
D7473	272
D7510	43, 125, 132, 144
D7550	256
D7880	262
D7899	262
D7910	259
D7921	158
D7922	266
D7950	250, 272
D7951	206, 272
D7952	206, 272
D7953	155, 159, 202, 215, 252, 272, 338
D7955	249
D7960	19, 28, 247
D7961	19, 28, 156, 247
D7962	19, 28, 247, 273
D7970	263
D7971	273
D7979	273
D7993	19, 28, 247, 273
D7994	19, 28, 247, 251
D7999	256, 259, 268
D8010	277, 287, 288
D8020	277, 280
D8030	277
D8040	277, 287, 288
D8050	278, 287
D8060	278, 287

CDT Code	Page #(s)
D8070	278, 287
D8080	279, 285, 286, 339
D8090	279
D8210	280, 289
D8220	280, 289
D8660	282, 285, 288
D8670	284, 286, 289
D8680	286
D8681	280, 286, 290
D8695	282, 283
D8696	283
D8697	289
D8699	283
D8702	289
D8703	288, 289
D8704	288
D8999	287, 289
D9110	43, 103, 132, 144, 297, 301, 302, 306–307, 339
D9130	262
D9210	307
D9215	101, 307
D9219	298
D9222	254, 261, 298
D9223	254, 261, 298
D9230	154, 340
D9239	137, 254
D9243	137, 254
D9248	141, 154, 254, 259
D9310	58, 260, 307, 373
D9311	134, 267
D9410	79, 304, 308
D9430	148, 150
D9440	93
D9450	281
D9610	259

CDT Code	Page #(s)
D9613	263, 295, 307
D9630	45, 120, 133, 137, 267
D9910	85, 310, 340
D9930	301
D9941	259
D9943	267, 309
D9944	300, 340
D9945	300, 340
D9946	300, 308, 340
D9951	146, 299, 340
D9952	299
D9970	309
D9971	19, 28, 288, 294, 309
D9972	308
D9973	308
D9975	40, 308
D9992	372
D9994	294
D9995	53, 296, 304, 306, 307
D9996	284, 305, 306, 372, 374
D9997	294–295, 367, 372, 374

Alphabetic Index by Topic

Alphabetic Index by Topic

R

radiation treatment, 181–184
radiographic imaging, 55–58
  2D/3D images, 57–58
  considerations, 30, 55–56, 244, 268
  full mouth series, 37–38
  off-site, 52–53
rapid palatal expander (RPE), 290
recession, 146–148, 156
referrals, 115–117
removable dentures, 230
resin laminate, 95
resin restoration, 46–47, 66, 75, 85
resin-based composite, 89–90
restorations
  considerations, 91
  crown, 90–91
  direct, 89–90
  final, 93–94
  indirect, 90–91, 94
  resin, 46–47, 66, 75, 85
  temporary, 104
  two-surface, 100, 101
  unspecified, 103
  using 3D printer, 264–265
Restorative category, 89–108
  changes, 92
  clinical coding scenarios, 93–100
  definitions/concepts, 89–91
  explanation of restorations, 91
  introduction, 89
  summary, 108
retainer crowns, 194, 196–197, 221, 243
retainers
  abutments, 201, 233
  adjusting/repairing, 283, 289, 290
  components, 233
  described, 233
  Essix, 219
  removable, 280
  replacing, 288
root canal therapy, 110
root canals
  considerations, 109, 126–128
  described, 110

emergency, 117
failed, 99
procedures, 109–110
pulpectomy, 110, 114, 117
retreating, 127–128
scenarios, 113, 117, 125
started in another state, 113
root caries, 73
root planing, 84, 145, 161, 165
root resorption, 270–271
root surface, 123–124
RPE (rapid palatal expander), 290

S

salivary flow, 63, 274
scaling, 140, 145, 161, 165, 319
Schweinebraten, Marie, D.M.D., 165
sealants, 66, 75, 76, 85, 86
sedation, 246
SHCN (Special Health Care Needs)
  patients, 293, 294, 366–375
sialolithotomy, 273
silver diamine fluoride therapy, 66,
  71–73, 85
sinus lift procedure, 272
site, 131
sleep apnea, 188–189
SNODENT, 11
snoring treatment appliances, 182, 188–189
soft tissue biopsies, 271
soft tissue impacted tooth, 247
space maintainers
  considerations, 87, 241, 288
  distal shoe, 67, 69
  re-cementing, 74
  removal of, 33, 86
Special Health Care Needs (SHCN)
  patients, 293, 294, 366–375
speech aid prosthesis, 190
splint, 178, 186
stent, 178
Stewart, Charles D., D.M.D., 311
strip crown, 106–107
subgingival decay, 157
supra-crestal fiberotomy, 271
surgery

flap surgery, 155, 162
implant, 173
orthognathic surgery, 41, 257–258
osseous, 158, 163
periodontal, 163
periradicular, 163
post-operative pain management, 263
root surface exposure, 123–124
surgical splint, 186
swelling, 43
synchronous teledentistry, 293

T

TAD (temporary anchorage device), 221
teeth
acute pulpitis, 98
bleaching, 308
brushing, 367, 369, 370, 373
cleaning. See prophylaxis
decay/damage. See caries
dry socket, 301
extracting. See extractions
foreign object stuck between, 144
fractured. See fractured teeth
full bone impacted, 247
grinding, 176, 299, 308
impacted, 247, 254–255, 270
missing, 227, 239, 243
pain, 43, 117, 263
partial bone impacted, 247
replacement of, 239
soft tissue impacted, 247
teledentistry, 52–53
asynchronous, 293
considerations, 291, 293, 306, 310
emergency treatment, 306–307
orthodontic exam, 284
resources, 53
scenarios, 303–305
synchronous, 293
temporary anchorage device (TAD), 221
temporomandibular disorder (TMD), 42,
262
temporomandibular joint (TMJ) disorder, 42
thumb sucking, 280

titanium/titanium alloys, 94, 100, 102, 239,
243
TMD (temporomandibular disorder), 42, 262
TMJ (temporomandibular joint) disorder, 42
tobacco cessation guidance, 77, 363–365
tobacco counseling, 21, 77, 87
tobacco use, 35, 77, 363–365
tongue presser appliance, 289
tooth. See teeth
Tooth Anatomy code, 341–362
tooth decay, 96, 157, 162, 371.
See also caries
tooth surfaces, 91
torus/exostosis, 272
traumatic wounds, 259
Trefoil bar, 227
trismus appliance, 189

U

utilization reviews, 321, 322

V

vaping, 21, 82, 267
veneers, 94, 95, 101
vesiculobullous diseases, 189, 190
Vidone, Linda, D.M.D., 231

X

xerostomia, 274

Z

zygomatic implants, 251

Notes:

_____

_____

_____

_____

_____

_____

_____

_____

_____

_____

_____

_____

Notes:

 © American Dental Association

Notes:

Notes

Notes:

© American Dental Association

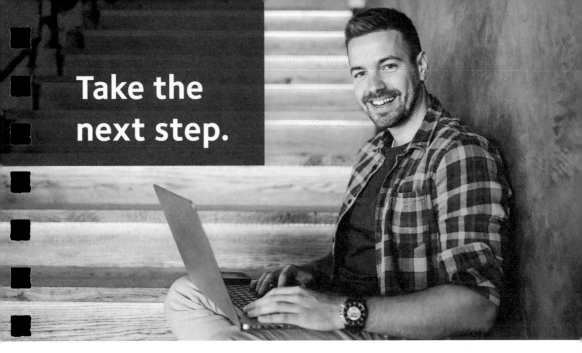

Take the next step.

You have the codes, now learn how to use them in practice.

Mastery of the CDT codes will make you a more valuable asset to the team and practice. Increase your coding skills and complete the **ADA Dental Coding Certificate: Assessment-Based CDT Course**. It helps new and experienced staff members achieve coding proficiency and help the dental office run more smoothly.

Participants will:

- Gain thorough knowledge of coding terms and tools
- Understand dental procedure codes and how to apply them
- Accurately complete the ADA Dental Claim Form
- Use the *CDT* and *CDT Companion* books correctly

As the official source for CDT® codes, the ADA has answered thousands of questions over the years. When dental teams have questions, we have the answers. Take advantage of our expertise and get up to code today!

After successfully passing the online assessment, **participants will earn 4 CE hours**. The course is available either with or without CDT books.

> **Save 20%** on this essential course and train your staff with promo scode **TRAIN2021** by 5.28.2021. Register today at **ADACEOnline.org**.

ADA American Dental Association®
America's leading advocate for oral health

This premier course is not included with CE Online Subscription and must be purchased separately.